Evolution of Machine Learning and Internet of Things Applications in Biomedical Engineering

This book provides a platform for presenting machine learning (ML)–enabled healthcare techniques and offers a mathematical and conceptual background of the latest technology. It describes ML techniques along with the emerging platform of the Internet of Medical Things used by practitioners and researchers around the world.

Evolution of Machine Learning and Internet of Things Applications in Biomedical Engineering discusses the Internet of Things (IoT) and ML devices that are deployed for enabling patient health tracking, various emergency issues, and the smart administration of patients. It looks at the problems of cardiac analysis in e-healthcare, explores the employment of smart devices aimed at different patient issues, and examines the usage of Arduino kits where the data can be transferred to the cloud for Internet-based uses. The book includes deep feedforward networks, regularization, optimization algorithms, convolutional networks, sequence modeling, and practical methodology. The authors also examine the role of IoT and ML in electroencephalography and magnetic resonance imaging, which play significant roles in biomedical applications. This book also incorporates the use of IoT and ML applications for smart wheelchairs, telemedicine, GPS positioning of heart patients, and smart administration with drug tracking. Finally, the book also presents the application of these technologies in the development of advanced healthcare frameworks.

This book will be beneficial for new researchers and practitioners working in the biomedical and healthcare fields. It will also be suitable for a wide range of readers who may not be scientists but who are also interested in the practices of medical image retrieval and brain image segmentation.

Emerging Trends in Biomedical Technologies and Health Informatics Series

Everyday Technologies in Healthcare
Chhabi Rani Panigrahi, Bibudhendu Pati, Mamata Rath, Rajkumar Buyya

Biomedical Signal Processing for Healthcare Applications
Varun Bajaj, G R Sinha, Chinmay Chakraborty

Deep Learning in Biomedical and Health Informatics
M. Jabbar, Ajith Abraham, Onur Dogan, Ana Madureira, Sanju Tiwar

Computational Approaches in Biotechnology and Bioinformatics
Pranav Deepak Pathak, Roshani Raut, Sebastian Jaramillo-Isaza, Padnya Borkar, and Rutvij H. Jhaveri

Computational Approaches in Biomaterials and Biomedical Engineering Applications
Pranav Deepak Pathak, Roshani Raut, Sebastian Jaramillo-Isaza, Padnya Borkar, and Rutvij H. Jhaveri

Healthcare Services in the Metaverse: Game Theory, AI, IOT, and Blockchain
Saurav Mallik, Anjan Bandyopadhyay, Ruifeng Hu, Pawan Kumar Singh, Soumadip Ghosh, and Sujata Swain

Evolution of Machine Learning and Internet of Things Applications in Biomedical Engineering
Arun Kumar Rana, Vishnu Sharma, Sanjeev Kumar Rana, and Vijay Shanker Chaudhary

For more information about this series, please visit: https://www.routledge.com/Emerging-Trends-in-Biomedical-Technologies-and-Health-informatics-series/book-series/ETBTHI

Evolution of Machine Learning and Internet of Things Applications in Biomedical Engineering

Edited by
Arun Kumar Rana, Vishnu Sharma,
Sanjeev Kumar Rana, and
Vijay Shanker Chaudhary

CRC Press
Taylor & Francis Group
Boca Raton London New York

CRC Press is an imprint of the
Taylor & Francis Group, an informa business

Designed cover image: © Shutterstock

First edition published 2025
by CRC Press
2385 NW Executive Center Drive, Suite 320, Boca Raton FL 33431

and by CRC Press
4 Park Square, Milton Park, Abingdon, Oxon, OX14 4RN

CRC Press is an imprint of Taylor & Francis Group, LLC

Library of Congress Cataloging-in-Publication Data
Names: Rana, Arun Kumar, editor. | Sharma, Vishnu, editor. | Rana, Sanjeev Kumar, editor. | Chaudhary, Vijay Shanker, editor.
Title: Evolution of machine learning and internet of things applications in biomedical engineering / edited by Arun Kumar Rana, Vishnu Sharma, Sanjeev Kumar Rana, and Vijay Shanker Chaudhary.
Description: First edition. | Boca Raton FL : CRC Press, 2025. | Includes bibliographical references and index.
Identifiers: LCCN 2024020363 (print) | LCCN 2024020364 (ebook) | ISBN 9781032759234 (hardback) | ISBN 9781032759258 (paperback) | ISBN 9781003476207 (ebook)
Subjects: MESH: Internet of Things | Machine Learning | Biomedical Technology | Medical Informatics Applications
Classification: LCC R855.3 (print) | LCC R855.3 (ebook) | NLM W 26.55.C7 | DDC 610.285—dc23/eng/20240806
LC record available at https://lccn.loc.gov/2024020363
LC ebook record available at https://lccn.loc.gov/2024020364

ISBN: 978-1-032-75923-4 (hbk)
ISBN: 978-1-032-75925-8 (pbk)
ISBN: 978-1-003-47620-7 (ebk)

DOI: 10.1201/9781003476207

Typeset in Times LT Std
by Apex CoVantage, LLC

Contents

Preface

The book includes deep feedforward networks, regularization, optimization algorithms, convolutional networks, sequence modeling, and practical methodology. It also presents the concepts of the Internet of Things and machine learning (ML), the set of technologies that develops traditional devices into smart devices. Finally, the book offers research perspectives, covering the convergence of ML and IoT. It also presents the application of these technologies in the development of healthcare frameworks.

ML and IoT is an emerging technology that integrates technologies and aspects coming from varied approaches. Pervasive computing, ubiquitous computing, communication technologies, sensing technologies, Internet protocol, and embedded devices are integrated to form a system where the digital and real worlds collaborate. A huge number of interconnected devices and enormous data open new opportunities to create services capable of bringing tangible benefits to the economy, environment, society, and individual citizens. In addition to connecting devices, ML and IoT connect people and other entities, thereby making every IoT component vulnerable to a huge range of attacks.

The book discusses IoT and ML devices that are deployed to enable patient health tracking, various emergency issues, smart administration of patients, and so on. It looks at the problems of cardiac analysis in e-healthcare, explores the employment of smart devices aimed at different patient issues, and examines the usage of Arduino kits where the data can be transferred to the cloud for Internet-based uses. The volume also considers the roles of IoT and ML in electroencephalography and magnetic resonance imaging, which play significant roles in biomedical applications. It also incorporates the use of IoT and ML applications for smart wheelchairs, telemedicine, GPS positioning of heart patients, smart administration with drug tracking, and more.

This book will be very beneficial for the new researchers and practitioners working in the biomedical and healthcare fields to quickly know the best-performing methods. It will also be suitable for a wide range of readers who may not be scientists but who are also interested in the practice of such areas as medical image retrieval and brain image segmentation.

About the Editors

Arun Kumar Rana is currently Assistant Professor-3 at Galgotias College of Engineering and Technology, Greater Noida, India, with more than 16 years of experience. His areas of interest include image processing, wireless sensor networks, Internet of Things, AI, and machine learning and embedded systems.

Vishnu Sharma is Professor and Dean of CSE at ITS College of Engineering, Greater Noida, India. Dr. Sharma completed his BTech, MTech, and PhD (CSE) in 2012 from the Government Autonomous Institute, Madhav Institute of Technology and Science (M.I.T.S.), Gwalior, MP, in Computer Science and Engineering, and was affiliated with the Rajiv Gandhi Technical University, Bhopal, India. His areas of interest are mobile computing, cybersecurity, and advanced mobile computing.

Sanjeev Kumar Rana is Professor of Computer Science and Engineering at Maharishi Markandeshwar (deemed to be a university), Mullana-Ambala, India. He earned his PhD from Maharishi Markandeshwar University, Mullana-Ambala, India, in 2012. He is also a CISCO-certified instructor. His research interests include distributed computing, network security, blockchain technology, and big data analytics.

Vijay Shanker Chaudhary is Assistant Professor (GCET, Greater Noida) and Researcher (photonic crystal fiber-based biosensors). He received his PhD from the Madan Mohan Malviya University of Technology, Gorakhpur, India. His research interests include photonic crystal fiber, optical fiber sensors, and terahertz sensing properties.

Contributors

Rahul Agrawal
GH Raisoni College of Engineering
Nagpur, India

Gaurav Kumar Ameta
Parul Institute of Technology
Parul University
Vadodara, Gujarat, India

Amit Arora
Galgotias University
Greater Noida, India

Anupam Bonkra
Department of Computer Science and Engineering Maharishi Markandeshwar (Deemed to be University)
Mullana 133207, India
anupam.bonkra@mmumullana.org

Joshua K Deepak
Department of Statistics and Data Science
CHRIST (Deemed to Be University)
Bengaluru, Karnataka, India

J. Deepika Roselind
Vellore Institute of Technology
Chennai Campus
Chennai, Tamilnadu, India

Priyanka Gauniya
HNB Garhwal University (A Central University)
Srinagar (Garhwal),
Uttarakhand, India

R. N. Muhammad Ilyas
The New College
Royapettah, Chennai, India

Sk Imran
Central University of South Bihar
Bihar, India

Poonam R. Inamdar
MIT World Peace University
Pune, India

Rishabh Jha
Lumbini Academic College
Kathmandu, Nepal

Atul Kabra
University Institute of Pharma Sciences
Chandigarh University
Mohali, India

Ruchin Kacker
Sagar Institute of Science and Technology
Bhopal, India

Divneet Kaur
Guru Nanak Dev Engineering College
Ludhiana, India

A. Ameer Rashed Khan
The New College
Chennai, India

Ganesh Khekare
Vellore Institute of Technology
Vellore, India

Urvashi Khekare
Vellore Institute of Technology
Vellore, India

Niharika Koch
Mahatma Gandhi Central University
Bihar, India

Mrunalini H. Kulkarni
Vishwakarma University
Pune, India

Aditya Kumar
Department of Computer Science
Central University of South Bihar
Bihar, India

G. Logeswari
Vellore Institute of Technology
Chennai, India

Jhansi Bharathi Madavarapu
University of the Cumberlands

M. Nagoor Meeral
Rose Mary College of Arts and Science
Tirunelveli, India

Anita Mohanty
Silicon University
Bhubaneswar, India

Subrat Kumar Mohanty
Electronics and Communication Engineering
Einstein Academy of Technology and Management
Odisha, India

Ambarish G. Mohapatra
Electronics Engineering
Silicon University
Bhubaneswar, Odisha, India

Kanchan Naithani
HNB Garhwal University
Srinagar Garhwal, India

Pallavi Pandey
Uttaranchal University, Prem Nagar
Dehradun, Uttarakhand, India

Subhendu Kumar Pani
Biju Patnaik University of Technology (BPUT)
Kausalya Ganga, Bhubaneswar
Odisha, India

Y. P. Raiwani
HNB Garhwal University
Srinagar Garhwal, India

Arun Kumar Rana
Galgotia College of Engineering, Knowledge Park I
Greater Noida, Uttar Pradesh, India

Sita Rani
Guru Nanak Dev Engineering College
Ludhiana, India

M. Umme Salma
Department of Statistics and Data Science
Christ (Deemed to be University)
Bengaluru, India

Pooja Sharma
School of Engineering and Technology
DY Patil University, Ambi, Pune, India

Rahul Sharma
Parul Institute of Technology
Parul University
Vadodara, Gujarat, India

Amrita Singh
Lumbini Academic College
Kathmandu, Nepal

Anish Singh
University Institute of Pharma Sciences
Chandigarh University
Mohali, India

Bharatdeep Singh
Guru Nanak Dev Engineering College
Ludhiana, India

Sanjay Kumar Singh
Sagar Institute of Science and Technology
Bhopal, India

G. Sudhakaran
Vellore Institute of Technology
Chennai, India

Shalu Surendran
Christ (Deemed to Be University)
Bengaluru, India

Ramya Thatikonda
University of the Cumberlands

Shrikant Tiwari
Galgotias University Greater Noida
India

Niva Tripathy
DRIEMS University
Cuttack, India

Subhranshu Sekhar Tripathy
KIIT Deemed to Be University
Bhubaneswar, India

Anil Turukmane
Department of Computer Science and Engineering
VIT-AP, University
Vijayawada, India

Jainath Yadav
Central University of South Bihar
Bihar, India

Nikhitha Yathiraju
University of the Cumberlands
Williamsburg, KY, USA

Pawan Whig
Vivekananda Institute of Professional Studies-TC
New Delhi, India

1 Applications of Artificial Intelligence and Internet of Things in Healthcare Industries

A. Ameer Rashed Khan, R. N. Muhammad Ilyas, and M. Nagoor Meeral

CONTENTS

1.1 INTRODUCTION

In recent years, the convergence of artificial intelligence (AI) and the Internet of Things (IoT) has significantly transformed various industries, with the healthcare sector experiencing revolutionary advancements. AI and IoT technologies have reshaped the landscape of healthcare by introducing innovative solutions, optimizing patient care, enhancing operational efficiency, and facilitating predictive analytics. This convergence has paved the way for personalized, efficient, and proactive healthcare systems that cater to individual patient needs while streamlining medical processes.

AI, with its ability to process large datasets and derive meaningful insights, when combined with IoT's network of interconnected devices and sensors, has opened up a plethora of possibilities in healthcare. This integration has led to the development

DOI: 10.1201/9781003476207-1

of smart medical devices, remote patient monitoring (RPM) systems, predictive analytics tools, and improved diagnostic capabilities, ultimately leading to better patient outcomes and operational excellence within healthcare organizations. The main contributions of the chapter are as follows.

1. It outlines different real-world applications of AI and the IoT in healthcare, ranging from RPM to personalized medicine.
2. It outlines several critical challenges associated with implementing AI and IoT applications in healthcare. These challenges encompass data security and privacy concerns, interoperability issues, regulatory compliance, clinical validation and reliability, health inequality and accessibility, ethical concerns, and bias. Each of these challenges represents significant hurdles that must be overcome to ensure the successful integration and responsible use of AI and IoT technologies in healthcare.

The chapter is organized as follows: Section 1.1 comprises an introduction, Section 1.2 includes a review of literature, and Section 1.3 describes real-world AI and IoT applications in healthcare. Section 1.4 discusses the challenges involved in AI and IoT applications in healthcare, and Section V incorporates a conclusion.

1.2 REVIEW OF LITERATURE

The diverse applications of AI in healthcare focus on machine learning, natural language processing, and computer vision. It discusses how AI aids in disease prediction, medical imaging analysis, drug discovery, and personalized medicine. Furthermore, it highlights the integration of AI with IoT for improved patient monitoring and clinical decision-making [1]. This structured literature review extracted 288 peer-reviewed papers from Scopus, indicating an emerging focus on AI in healthcare across disciplines like health services management, predictive medicine, patient data analytics, and clinical decision-making. The United States, China, and the UK led in research contributions. Keyword analysis highlighted AI's role in aiding diagnoses, disease prediction, and treatment customization. The study emphasized the need for data-intensive analysis skills and quality awareness in AI projects, offering valuable insights for future research in healthcare AI [2]. A comprehensive overview of IoT technologies in healthcare discusses the potential benefits, including remote monitoring, patient-centric care, and efficient data collection. It delves into the challenges and issues related to security, interoperability, and scalability when implementing IoT in healthcare settings [3].

The combined role of AI and IoT in healthcare, discussing wearable devices, sensors, and data analytics. The review highlights how these technologies support RPM, predictive analytics, and personalized healthcare interventions [4]. The current state of AI and IoT applications in healthcare emphasizes their impact on diagnostics, treatment planning, and healthcare management. It discusses challenges such as data privacy, regulatory hurdles, and the need for standardized protocols [5]. The convergence of AI and IoT emphasizes the opportunities it presents in enhancing patient care, optimizing healthcare processes, and improving decision-making. It also highlights challenges related to data security, ethical considerations, and interoperability among IoT devices [6].

The potential of IoT in healthcare focuses on RPM, smart medical devices, and real-time data analysis. It explores how AI algorithms leverage data collected from IoT devices to provide actionable insights for healthcare professionals [7]. It addresses the challenges and opportunities associated with the integration of AI and IoT in healthcare. It examines issues such as data security, interoperability, and ethical concerns while discussing the potential benefits of improving healthcare delivery [8]. Amid growing healthcare challenges, the synergy between the IoT and AI presents a promising avenue. Explored in this comprehensive survey is the realm of Artificial Intelligence of Things (AIoT) in healthcare. It outlines an integrated AIoT architecture, encompassing sensors, communication tech, and cross-layer AI. Through a multifaceted examination, it identifies technology potentials, healthcare-specific challenges, and opportunities. Real-world AIoT healthcare use cases underscore the transformative capabilities of these technologies, culminating in proposed future research directions for AIoT in healthcare [9].

This study examines the impact of IoT and AI in healthcare via a systematic review of 75 peer-reviewed journal articles, indicating a remarkable surge in publications over the past decade across diverse outlets. It highlights a global interest in these technologies, not solely in the United States but also in Europe and Asia. Key application categories such as wearables, disease detection, patient care, and sensor networks are identified, underscoring emerging trends. Moreover, the chapter identifies crucial research gaps concerning technology design, data security regulations, and system efficacy, emphasizing future research directions for these transformative healthcare technologies [10].

1.3 REAL-WORLD AI AND IoT APPLICATIONS IN HEALTHCARE

1.3.1 RPM

RPM is a transformative healthcare approach that utilizes advanced technologies to monitor patients' health outside of traditional healthcare settings, providing real-time data and improving the overall quality of care. With the advent of IoT devices and connected health technologies, RPM enables healthcare professionals to remotely track and analyze patients' vital signs, symptoms, and other health indicators.

In RPM, patients use wearable devices, such as smartwatches or medical-grade sensors, to continuously collect and transmit health-related data. These devices monitor metrics like heart rate, blood pressure, glucose levels, and activity levels. The collected data is then transmitted securely to healthcare providers, allowing them to assess patients' conditions without the need for frequent in-person visits.

This continuous stream of real-time data empowers healthcare professionals to detect potential health issues early, customize treatment plans, and intervene promptly when necessary. RPM is particularly beneficial for managing chronic conditions, post-surgery recovery, and keeping tabs on the health of aging populations. It enhances patient engagement by involving individuals in their own care and promoting a proactive approach to health management.

By reducing the need for hospital visits and enabling timely interventions, RPM not only improves patient outcomes but also contributes to the overall efficiency of healthcare systems. It represents a significant advancement in patient-centered care, offering a more personalized and data-driven approach to healthcare delivery.

1.3.2 Predictive Analytics

Predictive analytics is a data-driven approach that leverages statistical algorithms and machine learning techniques to analyze historical data and make predictions about future events or trends. By identifying patterns and relationships within large datasets, organizations can gain valuable insights to inform decision-making and anticipate outcomes.

The process begins with the collection and preparation of relevant data, followed by exploratory data analysis to understand patterns and select crucial features. Machine learning models are then trained on this data to recognize underlying relationships. Predictive analytics is versatile and finds applications across various industries, such as finance, marketing, and healthcare.

In healthcare, for instance, predictive analytics can forecast disease risks, anticipate patient readmission rates, and aid in personalized treatment planning. It enables proactive interventions, optimizing resource allocation and improving patient outcomes. In business, organizations use predictive analytics to optimize marketing strategies, enhance customer experiences, and streamline operations.

The power of predictive analytics lies in its ability to transform historical data into actionable insights, empowering decision-makers to anticipate trends and make informed choices, ultimately contributing to more efficient and effective processes in diverse fields. As technology continues to advance, predictive analytics will likely play an increasingly pivotal role in shaping the way organizations plan for the future.

1.3.3 Telemedicine

Telemedicine is a healthcare delivery model that utilizes technology to provide medical services remotely, allowing patients to consult with healthcare professionals without the need for in-person visits. This transformative approach leverages telecommunications tools, such as video conferencing, phone calls, and secure messaging, to facilitate virtual consultations and deliver a wide range of healthcare services.

In telemedicine, patients can connect with healthcare providers from the comfort of their homes or other remote locations, overcoming geographical barriers and increasing access to medical care. It encompasses various medical specialties, including primary care, mental health, dermatology, and chronic disease management.

Increased Accessibility: Especially beneficial for individuals in rural or underserved areas, telemedicine improves access to healthcare services, reducing the need for extensive travel.

Convenience: Patients can schedule virtual appointments at times that suit their schedules, promoting flexibility and reducing the time and effort associated with traditional clinic visits.

Cost-Effectiveness: Telemedicine can lower healthcare costs by minimizing travel expenses and time away from work for both patients and healthcare providers.

Remote Monitoring: In addition to consultations, telemedicine supports RPM using wearable devices and sensors, allowing healthcare professionals to track vital signs and manage chronic conditions.

Continuity of Care: Telemedicine enables ongoing care and follow-up appointments, contributing to better continuity of care for patients with chronic conditions or those in need of regular monitoring.

Especially notable in times of public health crises, such as the COVID-19 pandemic, telemedicine has become a critical tool for maintaining healthcare services while minimizing the risk of virus transmission.

Despite its advantages, challenges such as technology access and privacy concerns must be addressed to ensure equitable and secure telemedicine services for all. As technology continues to advance, telemedicine is expected to play an increasingly integral role in modern healthcare delivery, providing accessible and convenient medical care to a diverse range of patients.

1.3.4 Drug Discovery and Development

Drug discovery and development is a complex and multifaceted process that involves the identification, design, testing, and refinement of potential therapeutic compounds to address various diseases. This intricate journey typically spans many years and requires collaboration among scientists, researchers, and pharmaceutical professionals. The process can be broadly divided into several key stages.

Target Identification and Validation: Researchers identify specific molecular targets, such as proteins or genes, associated with a disease. Validation involves confirming that these targets play a crucial role in the disease's development.

Hit Discovery and Lead Optimization: Screening processes identify potential compounds (hits) that interact with the chosen targets. Lead optimization involves refining these hits to enhance their efficacy, selectivity, and safety.

Preclinical Testing: Promising leads undergo extensive testing in vitro (in the laboratory) and in vivo (in animals) to evaluate safety, efficacy, and potential side effects.

Investigational New Drug (IND) Application: Successful leads progress to the IND stage, where researchers submit an application to regulatory authorities, detailing the proposed clinical trials.

Clinical Trials (Phases I–III): Phase I assesses safety and dosage in a small group of healthy volunteers. Phase II evaluates efficacy and side effects in a larger group of patients. Phase III involves a more extensive patient population to confirm efficacy and monitor long-term side effects.

New Drug Application (NDA): If clinical trials are successful, researchers submit an NDA to regulatory agencies for approval to market the drug.

Post-Market Surveillance (Phase IV): Continuous monitoring of the drug's safety and effectiveness after it reaches the market. Throughout this process, advancements in technology, computational modeling, and data analytics play a crucial role. AI and machine learning algorithms assist in virtual screening, predicting potential drug interactions, and analyzing large datasets. These technologies accelerate the identification of promising candidates and enhance the efficiency of the drug development pipeline.

The drug discovery and development process is resource-intensive and involves significant risks, but successful outcomes contribute to the advancement of medicine, addressing unmet medical needs and improving patient outcomes. The integration of cutting-edge technologies continues to revolutionize this field, making the journey from laboratory discovery to effective therapies more efficient and targeted.

1.3.5 Personalized Medicine

Personalized medicine, also known as precision medicine, is a transformative approach to healthcare that tailors medical treatment and interventions to the individual characteristics of each patient. It recognizes that individuals differ in their genetic makeup, lifestyle, and environmental exposures, influencing their response to diseases and treatments. The goal of personalized medicine is to optimize therapeutic outcomes while minimizing side effects.

Genomic Information: Analysis of an individual's genetic makeup to identify specific genetic variations that may influence disease susceptibility and treatment response.

Biomarker Identification: Identification of biomarkers, which are measurable indicators of biological processes or responses, to guide treatment decisions.

Targeted Therapies: Development of treatments that target specific molecular pathways or genetic mutations associated with a particular disease, increasing treatment efficacy.

Companion Diagnostics: Use of diagnostic tests to identify patients who are most likely to benefit from a particular treatment, avoiding unnecessary exposure to ineffective therapies.

Tailored Treatment Plans: Customization of treatment plans based on individual patient characteristics, including genetic information, to maximize therapeutic benefits. Personalized medicine has made significant strides in oncology, where genetic profiling of tumors helps identify targeted therapies. It is also gaining prominence in other areas, such as cardiovascular diseases, neurology, and infectious diseases.

Advancements in technology, particularly in genomics and data analytics, have accelerated the adoption of personalized medicine. The integration of AI and machine learning enables the analysis of vast datasets, uncovering complex relationships between genetic variations and treatment responses.

While personalized medicine holds great promise for more effective and precise healthcare, challenges include the need for large-scale data sharing, ethical considerations, and addressing healthcare disparities. As technology continues to advance and our understanding of individual variability deepens, personalized medicine is expected to play an increasingly pivotal role in optimizing patient care and outcomes.

1.3.6 Operational Efficiency

Operational efficiency is a key business concept that refers to the optimization of processes and resources to achieve the highest level of productivity and performance within an organization. It involves streamlining workflows, minimizing waste, and maximizing output without compromising quality. The goal of operational efficiency is to enhance overall effectiveness, reduce costs, and improve the organization's ability to meet its objectives.

Process Optimization: Analyzing and redesigning workflows to eliminate bottlenecks, redundancies, and unnecessary steps. Implementing best practices to enhance the efficiency of routine tasks.

Resource Allocation: Efficiently assigning and managing resources, including human capital, technology, and financial assets, to ensure optimal utilization.

Technology Integration: Implementing and leveraging technology solutions to automate tasks, enhance communication, and improve decision-making processes.

Continuous Improvement: Adopting a culture of continuous improvement by regularly assessing and refining processes based on performance metrics and feedback.

Supply Chain Management: Optimizing the supply chain to reduce lead times, minimize excess inventory, and enhance coordination with suppliers.

Data-driven Decision-Making: Utilizing data analytics and business intelligence tools to make informed decisions, identify trends, and uncover areas for improvement.

Employee Training and Engagement: Providing employees with the necessary training and tools to perform their roles efficiently. Fostering a positive work environment to enhance employee engagement and productivity. Operational efficiency is crucial for businesses seeking to remain competitive in today's dynamic marketplaces. It allows organizations to respond more effectively to changing customer demands, market conditions, and technological advancements. By optimizing processes and resource utilization, businesses can achieve cost savings, improve customer satisfaction, and position themselves for sustainable growth.

Efforts to enhance operational efficiency often involve a combination of strategic planning, process reengineering, and the implementation of advanced technologies. Regular assessments and adjustments ensure that the organization remains agile and adaptable to evolving business landscapes. Ultimately, operational efficiency is a cornerstone of organizational success, enabling businesses to deliver value to customers and stakeholders in an effective and sustainable manner.

1.3.7 Patient Engagement

Patient engagement is a critical concept in healthcare that refers to the active involvement of patients in their own healthcare journey. It encompasses a range of activities and interactions between healthcare providers and patients, aiming to empower individuals to take an active role in managing their health and well-being. Effective patient engagement contributes to improved health outcomes, increased patient satisfaction, and more efficient healthcare delivery.

Health Education: Providing patients with information about their medical conditions, treatment options, and preventive measures to enhance their understanding.

Shared Decision-Making: Involving patients in the decision-making process regarding their treatment plans, considering their preferences, values, and goals.

Communication: Facilitating open and transparent communication between healthcare providers and patients to ensure a mutual understanding of health-related information.

Access to Health Information: Empowering patients with access to their health records, test results, and relevant educational resources, fostering informed decision-making.

Digital Health Tools: Leveraging technology, such as patient portals and mobile health apps, to facilitate communication, appointment scheduling, and remote monitoring.

Behavioral Support: Providing support for lifestyle changes and adherence to treatment plans through counseling, coaching, and resources.

Feedback and Input: Seeking and incorporating patient feedback to improve the quality of care and enhance patient experiences. Effective patient engagement is associated with several benefits, including increased medication adherence, better chronic disease management, and reduced healthcare costs. It also contributes to a more patient-centered healthcare approach.

Healthcare providers are increasingly recognizing the importance of patient engagement as a strategy to improve overall healthcare outcomes and enhance patient satisfaction. As technology continues to advance, digital tools and platforms play a crucial role in facilitating patient engagement, allowing for more seamless communication and interaction between patients and their healthcare providers. In essence, patient engagement is a collaborative effort that recognizes the patient as an active participant in their own healthcare journey.

1.3.8 Fraud Detection and Security

Fraud detection and security are critical components in various industries, particularly in finance, healthcare, and online transactions. These processes involve the use of advanced technologies and methodologies to identify and prevent fraudulent activities, safeguarding assets and sensitive information and maintaining the integrity of systems.

Data Analytics: Utilizing data analytics and machine learning algorithms to analyze patterns and anomalies in large datasets, identifying potentially fraudulent behavior.

Biometric Authentication: Implementing biometric measures such as fingerprints, facial recognition, or voice recognition to enhance user authentication and prevent identity theft.

Behavioral Analysis: Monitoring and analyzing user behavior, transactions, or system interactions to detect deviations from normal patterns that may indicate fraudulent activity.

Encryption and Secure Communication: Implementing robust encryption techniques to protect sensitive data during transmission and storage, preventing unauthorized access.

Access Controls and Authorization: Establishing strict access controls and authorization mechanisms to ensure that only authorized individuals have access to sensitive information or critical systems.

Real-time Monitoring: Employing real-time monitoring systems to promptly detect and respond to potential security threats or fraudulent activities as they occur.

Fraud Prevention Education: Providing education and awareness programs to employees and users to recognize and avoid potential fraudulent schemes and activities.

Regulatory Compliance: Adhering to industry-specific regulations and standards to ensure that security measures meet required standards and mitigate risks. In the financial sector, fraud detection systems analyze transaction patterns, detect unusual activities, and trigger alerts for further investigation. In healthcare, fraud detection involves monitoring billing practices, insurance claims, and patient records to identify potential fraudulent schemes.

As technology evolves, so do the methods employed by fraudsters. Consequently, organizations continuously update and enhance their fraud detection and security measures to stay ahead of emerging threats. Proactive and multi-layered security strategies are essential to protect against the ever-changing landscape of fraud and cybersecurity risks.

1.4 CHALLENGES INVOLVED IN AI AND IoT APPLICATIONS IN HEALTHCARE

Implementing AI and IoT applications in healthcare offers tremendous potential to enhance patient care, streamline operations, and revolutionize the industry. However, alongside these opportunities, numerous challenges must be addressed to ensure the successful integration of these technologies into the healthcare ecosystem.

1. **Data Security and Privacy Concerns:**

   Data security and privacy concerns in the context of AI and IoT applications in healthcare are paramount, given the sensitive nature of patient information.

   Sensitive Health Information: Healthcare data, including personal identifiers, medical records, and potentially genetic details, is highly sensitive. Unauthorized access to this information can lead to identity theft, fraud, and compromise patient privacy.

   Consent and Ownership: Obtaining informed consent for data collection and ensuring patients have control over their information is critical. Determining ownership of healthcare data, especially with the involvement of AI and IoT devices, poses ethical challenges.

   Cybersecurity Threats: Data breaches and cyberattacks are constant threats, exposing healthcare organizations to financial and reputational damage. Vulnerabilities in IoT devices can serve as entry points for hackers, necessitating robust security measures.

   Regulatory Compliance: Adherence to regulations such as the Health Insurance Portability and Accountability Act (HIPAA) and General Data Protection Regulation (GDPR) is mandatory to safeguard patient data. Regulatory frameworks need to evolve to address emerging challenges in AI and IoT-driven healthcare.

   Ethical Considerations: Continuous monitoring through IoT devices raises ethical questions about invasion of privacy.

   Ethical concerns also surround AI-driven decision-making, demanding transparency and accountability.

   Patient Trust and Perception: Data breaches can erode patient trust, necessitating transparent communication and robust security measures. Managing patient perception of the risks associated with data sharing and AI interventions is crucial for widespread acceptance.

   Addressing these concerns requires a holistic approach, involving technological solutions, regulatory frameworks, and ongoing education for healthcare stakeholders to ensure the responsible and secure integration of AI and IoT in healthcare.

2. **Interoperability Issues:**

   Interoperability issues are significant challenges in the integration of AI and IoT applications in healthcare. Interoperability refers to the seamless exchange and use of information among different systems, and, in healthcare, it is crucial for facilitating effective communication and collaboration. Here's a concise overview of interoperability issues:

   Integration of Systems: Healthcare organizations often use diverse systems for electronic health records, medical devices, and other applications. Ensuring smooth integration among these systems is challenging and crucial for the effective exchange of patient data.

   Data Exchange Protocols: Lack of standardized protocols for data exchange hampers interoperability. Establishing common standards is essential to enable different AI and IoT devices to communicate and share information seamlessly.

Heterogeneity of Devices: IoT devices come from various manufacturers, each with its own specifications and communication protocols. Achieving interoperability requires addressing the heterogeneity of these devices to ensure they can work cohesively within a healthcare environment.

Patient Data Portability: Patients may seek care from multiple providers, and ensuring the portability of their data across different healthcare systems is a challenge. A lack of interoperability can hinder the sharing of patient information, affecting the continuity and quality of care.

Standardization Challenges: Standardizing data formats, terminology, and communication methods is complex due to the diversity of healthcare practices and technologies. The absence of widely adopted standards impedes the seamless flow of information across different platforms.

Legacy Systems: Many healthcare organizations still rely on legacy systems that may not be designed for modern interoperability requirements. Integrating these older systems with new AI and IoT technologies poses compatibility challenges.

Regulatory Mandates: While regulations may mandate interoperability, achieving compliance can be challenging due to the diversity of systems and technologies in use. Meeting regulatory standards requires significant coordination and investment.

User Training and Adoption: Healthcare professionals may face challenges in adapting to new interoperable systems.

Adequate training and support are essential to ensure that users can effectively utilize and benefit from integrated AI and IoT solutions.

Addressing interoperability issues requires collaboration among healthcare stakeholders, standardization bodies, and technology developers. Establishing and adhering to interoperability standards, investing in modernizing infrastructure, and promoting a culture of collaboration can contribute to overcoming these challenges and unlocking the full potential of AI and IoT in healthcare.

3. Regulatory Compliance and Ethical Considerations:

Regulatory compliance and ethical considerations play a crucial role in shaping the responsible deployment of AI and IoT applications in healthcare. Ensuring adherence to existing regulations and addressing ethical concerns are vital for protecting patient rights, maintaining trust, and fostering innovation in the healthcare sector. Here's a concise overview of regulatory compliance and ethical considerations:

HIPAA and GDPR Compliance: Adhering to regulatory frameworks such as the HIPAA in the United States and the GDPR in the European Union is mandatory. Compliance involves safeguarding patient privacy, securing sensitive health information, and obtaining explicit consent for data use.

Evolution of Regulations: As technology advances, regulatory frameworks must evolve to address new challenges arising from AI and IoT applications in healthcare. Continuous efforts are required to update existing regulations and enact new ones that strike a balance between innovation and patient protection.

Informed Consent and Patient Rights: Ethical considerations include obtaining informed consent from patients before deploying AI and IoT technologies in their care. Respecting patient autonomy, ensuring transparency, and providing clear information about the purpose and implications of data usage are ethical imperatives.

Algorithmic Transparency and Accountability: Ethical concerns arise from the opacity of AI algorithms, especially when they contribute to critical healthcare decisions. Ensuring transparency in algorithmic decision-making and establishing accountability frameworks are essential to building trust among healthcare professionals and patients.

Equity and Fairness: Ethical considerations include addressing biases in AI algorithms that may disproportionately affect certain demographics. Striving for equity in healthcare delivery and ensuring that AI applications do not contribute to existing disparities are ethical imperatives.

Responsible Data Use: Ethical deployment of AI and IoT in healthcare involves responsible data stewardship. Healthcare organizations must establish clear policies on data collection, usage, and sharing, prioritizing patient well-being and privacy.

Human Oversight and Intervention: Maintaining a balance between automated decision-making and human intervention is crucial. Ethical considerations include ensuring that healthcare professionals retain the ability to override or intervene in AI-driven decisions when necessary.

Public Trust: Building and maintaining public trust is essential for the widespread acceptance of AI and IoT applications in healthcare. Demonstrating a commitment to ethical practices, regulatory compliance, and patient well-being contributes to a positive perception of these technologies. Addressing regulatory compliance and ethical considerations requires collaboration among healthcare organizations, regulatory bodies, technology developers, and other stakeholders. A shared commitment to upholding the highest ethical standards while navigating the evolving regulatory landscape is crucial for the responsible integration of AI and IoT in healthcare.

4. **Clinical Validation and Reliability:**

Clinical validation and reliability are critical aspects of integrating AI and IoT applications into healthcare. These factors ensure that the technologies can be trusted to provide accurate, clinically meaningful insights and recommendations. Here's a concise overview:

Algorithmic Accuracy: Clinical validation involves establishing the accuracy of AI algorithms in interpreting and analyzing healthcare data. Rigorous testing against real-world clinical scenarios is essential to verify the algorithm's ability to deliver reliable results.

Validation Studies: Conducting comprehensive validation studies is a crucial step in assessing the performance of AI and IoT applications. These studies involve comparing the technology's outputs to established clinical standards, ensuring its reliability in diverse patient populations and conditions.

Real-World Clinical Settings: Clinical validation must extend beyond controlled environments to real-world clinical settings. The technology's performance in everyday healthcare scenarios ensures that it can effectively integrate into existing workflows and contribute meaningfully to patient care.

Patient Safety: Reliability is paramount in healthcare, where decisions based on AI insights can directly impact patient safety. Thorough validation helps identify and mitigate potential errors, ensuring that AI and IoT applications contribute positively to patient outcomes.

Continuous Monitoring and Improvement: Reliability is an ongoing commitment that extends beyond initial validation. Implementing mechanisms for continuous monitoring, feedback, and improvement is crucial to address emerging issues and enhance the reliability of AI and IoT applications over time.

Standardization in Validation Protocols: Establishing standardized protocols for the validation of AI and IoT applications promotes consistency across the industry. Standardization allows for comparability between different technologies and ensures that all adhere to a common set of rigorous validation practices.

Incorporating Clinician Feedback: Involving healthcare professionals in the validation process is essential to gaining insights into the technology's usability and clinical relevance. Clinician feedback helps refine algorithms, making them more aligned with the practical needs of healthcare providers.

Ethical Considerations in Validation: Ethical considerations extend to the validation process, ensuring that patient data is handled responsibly and that the validation studies prioritize patient welfare. Transparency in the validation process helps build trust among healthcare professionals and patients.

In summary, clinical validation and reliability are pivotal in ensuring that AI and IoT applications in healthcare meet high standards of accuracy, safety, and effectiveness. By investing in rigorous validation processes, involving healthcare professionals, and adhering to ethical considerations, stakeholders can enhance the credibility of these technologies, fostering their acceptance and integration into routine clinical practice. Continuous improvement and a commitment to patient-centered outcomes are essential for the sustained success of AI and IoT applications in healthcare.

5. **Health Inequality and Accessibility:**

Health inequality and accessibility are critical considerations in the deployment of AI and IoT applications in healthcare. Addressing these issues is crucial to ensure that technological advancements benefit all individuals, regardless of socioeconomic status or geographic location.

Digital Divide: Health inequality can be exacerbated by a digital divide, where certain populations lack access to the necessary technologies. Disparities in Internet connectivity, smartphone ownership, and digital literacy can limit individuals' ability to benefit from AI and IoT healthcare solutions.

Access to Technology: Not all communities have equal access to advanced healthcare technologies, including AI-powered diagnostics and IoT devices. This lack of access can result in unequal distribution of healthcare benefits, disadvantaging individuals who may already face health disparities.

Remote and Underserved Areas: Rural or underserved areas may experience challenges in accessing high-speed Internet, hindering the implementation of telehealth solutions and RPM through IoT devices. AI applications may also face challenges in reaching these areas, limiting the potential impact on healthcare outcomes.

Affordability: The cost of AI and IoT technologies can be a barrier to accessibility for individuals with limited financial resources. Ensuring that these technologies are affordable and accessible to a broad spectrum of the population is essential to avoid perpetuating health disparities.

Cultural and Linguistic Diversity: AI and IoT applications need to be sensitive to cultural and linguistic diversity to ensure that they are accessible and relevant to diverse patient populations. Failure to consider cultural factors can contribute to health inequalities by excluding certain groups from the benefits of these technologies.

Digital Literacy: Limited digital literacy, particularly among older adults and disadvantaged populations, can impede the adoption and effective use of AI and IoT technologies. Education and support programs are necessary to enhance digital literacy and ensure that individuals can navigate and utilize these technologies for their health.

Inclusive Design: AI and IoT solutions must be designed with inclusivity in mind, considering the diverse needs and capabilities of users. Inclusive design helps ensure that these technologies are accessible to a wide range of individuals, minimizing health disparities.

Policy Interventions: Policymakers play a crucial role in addressing health inequality and accessibility issues by implementing policies that promote equal access to healthcare technologies. Initiatives to bridge the digital divide and ensure equitable distribution of resources can contribute to reducing health disparities.

By proactively addressing health inequality and accessibility challenges, stakeholders can work toward ensuring that the benefits of AI and IoT applications in healthcare are accessible to all, promoting health equity and improving outcomes for diverse populations. This requires a collaborative effort involving healthcare providers, technology developers, policymakers, and communities to create solutions that bridge gaps and promote inclusivity.

6. Ethical Concerns and Bias:

Ethical concerns and bias are significant considerations in the development and deployment of AI and IoT applications in healthcare. Ensuring fairness, transparency, and accountability is essential to avoid unintended consequences and uphold ethical standards. Here's a concise overview:

Algorithmic Bias: AI algorithms can inadvertently perpetuate and amplify biases present in the training data. This bias can lead to unfair and discriminatory outcomes, particularly affecting marginalized or underrepresented groups. Addressing algorithmic bias requires ongoing efforts to identify, understand, and mitigate biases in AI models.

Transparency in Decision-Making: Lack of transparency in how AI algorithms make decisions can raise ethical concerns. Understanding the rationale behind algorithmic decisions is crucial for healthcare professionals and patients. Transparent algorithms enable scrutiny, accountability, and trust-building in the use of AI applications in healthcare.

Impact on Vulnerable Populations: Vulnerable populations, such as those with limited access to healthcare or socioeconomically disadvantaged groups, may be disproportionately affected by biased algorithms. Ensuring that AI and IoT applications do not exacerbate existing health disparities is an ethical imperative.

Informed Consent and Autonomy: Obtaining informed consent becomes more complex with AI applications, especially when patients may not fully understand the implications of algorithmic decision-making. Respecting patient autonomy involves providing clear information about the role of AI in their care and obtaining informed consent for its use.

Privacy Concerns: AI and IoT applications often involve the processing of sensitive health data. Ensuring robust data privacy measures is an ethical obligation to protect patient confidentiality. Clear communication regarding data usage, storage, and sharing is necessary to maintain patient trust.

Explainability of AI Decisions: The lack of explainability in AI decision-making, often associated with complex neural networks, poses ethical challenges. Patients and healthcare professionals should have the ability to understand and question the rationale behind AI-driven recommendations or decisions.

Human Oversight and Intervention: Striking the right balance between automated decision-making and human oversight is an ethical consideration. Ensuring that healthcare professionals retain the ability to intervene in algorithmic decisions when necessary is crucial for maintaining ethical standards.

Diversity in Data and Development Teams: Lack of diversity in the data used to train algorithms and, in the teams, developing AI applications can contribute to biases. Promoting diversity ensures a more comprehensive understanding of healthcare needs and helps mitigate biases in the design and deployment of these technologies.

Addressing ethical concerns and biases requires a commitment to fairness, transparency, and inclusivity throughout the development and implementation of AI and IoT applications in healthcare. Ethical frameworks, guidelines, and ongoing monitoring are essential to ensure that these technologies contribute positively to healthcare outcomes while respecting the rights and dignity of individuals. Continuous efforts to identify and rectify biases and to involve diverse perspectives are critical for building trustworthy and ethically sound healthcare AI and IoT systems [11–14].

1.5 CONCLUSION

In conclusion, the integration of AI and IoT applications in healthcare presents a myriad of opportunities and challenges. The potential benefits are vast, promising improved patient care, enhanced diagnostics, efficient healthcare operations, personalized medicine, and cost reduction. These advancements have the power to transform the healthcare landscape, providing innovative solutions to longstanding issues and positively impacting patient outcomes.

However, the realization of these opportunities is accompanied by a set of formidable challenges. Data security and privacy concerns loom large, requiring robust measures to protect sensitive health information. Interoperability issues demand coordinated efforts to ensure seamless communication among diverse healthcare systems and devices. Regulatory compliance and ethical considerations must be navigated carefully to uphold patient rights, maintain trust, and foster responsible innovation.

Overcoming these challenges necessitates collaborative efforts from healthcare providers, technology developers, policymakers, and the broader community. Striking a balance between innovation and safeguarding patient welfare is crucial. As technologies continue to evolve, there is an ongoing need for a dynamic regulatory framework that keeps pace with advancements while upholding ethical standards.

In navigating this complex landscape, it is essential to prioritize patient-centric approaches, ensuring that the benefits of AI and IoT applications are accessible to all, while actively mitigating risks and addressing disparities. By fostering a culture of responsible innovation, healthcare stakeholders can harness the full potential of AI and IoT, ultimately leading to a more efficient, effective, and patient-centered healthcare ecosystem.

REFERENCES

1. Shaheen, M. Y. (2021). Applications of Artificial Intelligence (AI) in healthcare: A review. *ScienceOpen Preprints*, *20*, 300–309.
2. Secinaro, S., Calandra, D., Secinaro, A., Muthurangu, V., & Biancone, P. (2021). The role of artificial intelligence in healthcare: A structured literature review. *BMC Medical Informatics and Decision Making*, *21*, 1–23.
3. Shah, S. T. U., Yar, H., Khan, I., Ikram, M., & Khan, H. (2019). Internet of things-based healthcare: Recent advances and challenges. *Applications of Intelligent Technologies in Healthcare*, 153–162.
4. Yang, Y., Wang, H., Jiang, R., Guo, X., Cheng, J., & Chen, Y. (2022). A review of IoT-enabled mobile healthcare: Technologies, challenges, and future trends. *IEEE Internet of Things Journal*, 9(12), 9478–9502.
5. Shah, R., & Chircu, A. (2018). IoT and AI in healthcare: A systematic literature review. *Issues in Information Systems*, 19(3).
6. Shi, F., Ning, H., Huangfu, W., Zhang, F., Wei, D., Hong, T., & Daneshmand, M. (2020). Recent progress on the convergence of the Internet of Things and artificial intelligence. *IEEE Network*, 34(5), 8–15.
7. Kakhi, K., Alizadehsani, R., Kabir, H. D., Khosravi, A., Nahavandi, S., & Acharya, U. R. (2022). The internet of medical things and artificial intelligence: Trends, challenges, and opportunities. *Biocybernetics and Biomedical Engineering*, 42(3), 749–771.
8. Selvaraj, S., & Sundaravaradhan, S. (2020). Challenges and opportunities in IoT healthcare systems: A systematic review. *SN Applied Sciences*, 2(1), 139.
9. Baker, S., & Xiang, W. (2023). Artificial intelligence of things for smarter healthcare: A survey of advancements, challenges, and opportunities. *IEEE Communications Surveys & Tutorials, 70*, 803–813.
10. Shah, R., & Chircu, A. (2018). IoT and AI in healthcare: A systematic literature review. *Issues in Information Systems*, 19(3).
11. Davenport, T. H., & Kalakota, R. (2019). The potential for artificial intelligence in healthcare. *Future Healthcare Journal*, 6(2), 94–98.
12. Hassan, R., Qamar, F., Hasan, M. K., Aman, A. H. M., & Ahmed, A. S. (2020). Internet of Things and its applications: A comprehensive survey. *Symmetry*, 12(10), 1674.
13. Rajkomar, A., & Dean, J. (2019). *The evolution of machine learning in healthcare.* MIT Review.
14. Denecke, K., & Xing, W. (2020). Leveraging the internet of things for healthcare. *Studies in Health Technology and Informatics*, 270, 960–961.

2 Machine Learning for Internet of Medical Things Applications

Framework, Developments, and Challenges

Divneet Kaur, Bharatdeep Singh, and Sita Rani

CONTENTS

DOI: 10.1201/9781003476207-2

2.1 INTRODUCTION

Rapid advancements in information technology are impacting MedTech innovation and leading to the creation of more interconnected medical devices, which produce, gather, transmit, and analyze massive amounts of healthcare data. The integration of the Internet of Things (IoT) with machine learning (ML) has led to revolutionary advancements across a range of industries, including healthcare (Rani, Kataria, Kumar, & Tiwari, 2023; Rani, Kumar, Kataria, & Min, 2023). In a broader sense, the IoT is the network that connects common things so they can communicate and gather data. A component of the IoT, sometimes known as the healthcare IoT, is the Internet of Medical Things (IoMT) (shown in Figure 2.1). It is an integrated network of software programs, hardware, and healthcare systems and services that uses networking technologies to send real-time data. Thus, the integration of the IoT in medical equipment is known as the IoMT. An excellent example of a "thing" in the context of IoMT is a wearable fitness tracker, which is a wrist-worn device. This wearable, which has a wide range of sensors, records and keeps track of several health-related variables, such as steps done, heart rate, sleep patterns, and calories burned. This abundance of data is seamlessly transferred via the fitness tracker to the hospital's cloud-based software platform, creating a strong link between the patient's wearable gadget and the digital infrastructure of the healthcare provider. Particularly, ML is essential to the IoMT because it improves the functionality of medical equipment that is connected, makes intelligent decisions easier, and allows for customized healthcare solutions (Dutta, Neog, & Medhi, 2021; Qureshi et al., 2022). The IoMT connects and monitors every medical equipment through the Internet, allowing healthcare practitioners to monitor it all. Wearable sensors, remote monitoring devices, and smart medical implants are just a few examples of the interconnected gadgets that provide large amounts of medical data that are analyzed by IoMT apps using ML techniques. By providing real-time insights, predictive analytics, and early detection capabilities, this integration enables healthcare practitioners to provide patient

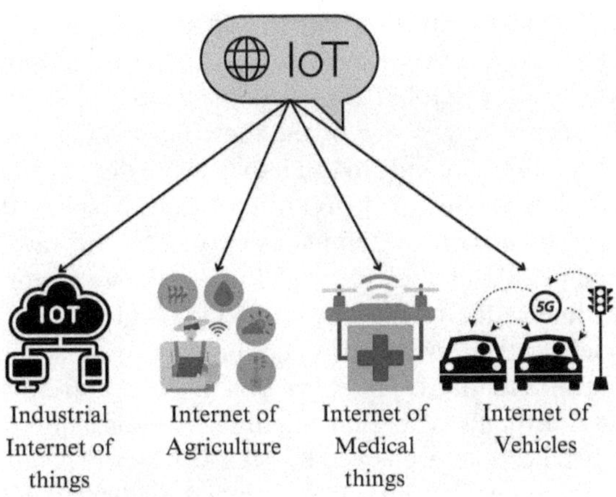

FIGURE 2.1 IoMT as a subset of IoT.

care, treatment plans, and diagnoses more effectively. A crucial part of developing healthcare technologies is creating ML frameworks specifically designed for IoMT applications. More people are becoming more conscious of their health as a result of the COVID-19 pandemic, which has raised the need for efficient eHealth initiatives and health monitoring tools that can measure vital signs like body temperature, heart rate, cholesterol, and sleep patterns. But there are drawbacks to this junction as well, such as issues with data privacy, interoperability, and the requirement for strong security measures to protect private medical data. Unlocking the full potential of ML in IoMT and assuring the provision of creative, patient-centered healthcare solutions depend on addressing these issues (Razdan & Sharma, 2022).

The healthcare industry has continuously adopted cutting-edge technologies, and artificial intelligence (AI) and ML are finding a wide range of uses that are comparable to their functions in business and e-commerce. With this technology, the possibilities are practically endless. Through innovative applications, ML significantly contributes to the advancement of the healthcare sector. Healthcare systems have already included big data tools for advanced data analytics due to the need for electronic medical records. ML techniques have the potential to improve this process even further, improving the level of automation and intelligent decision-making in public healthcare systems as well as primary and tertiary patient care. The prospective application of ML techniques could greatly raise billions of people's standards of living worldwide (Manickam et al., 2022). ML has several potential applications in research and clinical trials. Using ML-based predictive research, researchers may potentially recruit clinical trial participants by using a range of data sources, including past medical visits and social media activity. Instantaneous access to data is ensured by this technique, which also efficiently monitors trial participants. This allows for the discovery of the ideal sample size and the utilization of electronic procedures to minimize data inaccuracies. Finding patterns and abnormalities in the vast amount of electronically recorded medical imaging data may be accomplished through the use of various algorithms. Similar to an expert radiologist, ML algorithms are capable of analyzing imaging data and identifying abnormalities such as tumors, lesions, skin patches, and brain hemorrhages. Consequently, the extensive adoption of these platforms to assist radiologists is anticipated to experience a significant surge (Alsubaei, Abuhussein, Shandilya, & Shiva, 2019). The IoMT framework is described in Figure 2.2.

Among AI, ML technology is one of the most fascinating areas, attracting the attention of many businesses looking to use it to achieve their particular goals (Rani, Mishra, Kataria, Mallik, & Qin, 2023). With algorithms enabling data-driven learning across a variety of industries, including business and healthcare, ML is becoming more and more popular. Within the ever-evolving healthcare sector, ML has become an invaluable instrument due to the ongoing technological progress and creative thinking that define the field. Medical practitioners may find it useful in managing novel and changing situations. The extraction of insights from unstructured text, which was previously difficult to develop and implement on a big scale, is now possible, thanks to modern technology enabled by ML. This newly acquired abundance of ML-derived intelligence enables administrators and medical professionals to make timely, well-informed decisions regarding patient care and operational programs, impacting millions of lives.

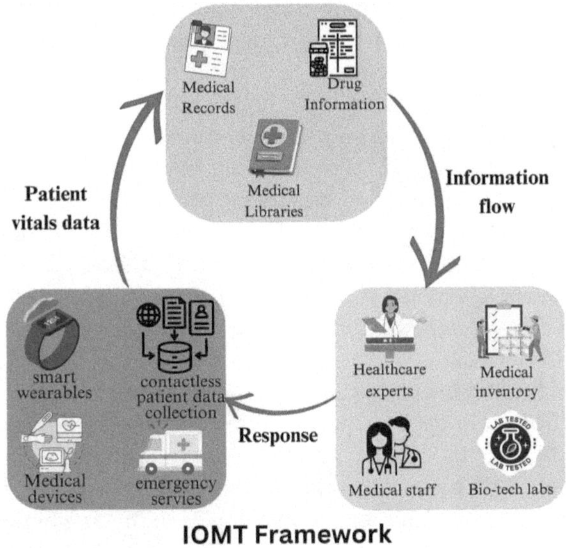

FIGURE 2.2 IoMT framework.

2.1.1 Objectives of the Chapter

The key objectives of this chapter are:

- To present the basic concepts of IoMT in diversified healthcare applications.
- To comprehensively explore the integration of ML in the context of IoMT.
- To elaborate on the ML–IoMT conflux in healthcare applications and associated challenges.
- To present possible future research directions.

The chapter is organized as follows: Section 2.1 consists of the introduction of the chapter. Section 2.2 describes the foundations of IoMT. The various framework of ML is described in Section 2.3. Further the applications and recent development in IoMT are described in Sections 2.4 and 2.5, respectively. Challenges and ethical considerations are described in Section 2.6. Later Sections 2.8 and Section 2.9 describe the future directions and conclusions.

2.2 FOUNDATIONS OF IOMT

Health stands as a universal aspiration for all individuals, and the safeguarding of people's well-being constitutes the fundamental responsibility of the healthcare system. On the one hand, medical methods and ideologies have advanced significantly due to the advances in contemporary technology. With the availability of more advanced diagnostic equipment and effective treatment options, modern doctors are better equipped to prevent illness and maintain patient health. However, there are significant obstacles facing the healthcare system. Chronic illnesses including heart disease and cancer still represent serious risks to people's health. Furthermore, infectious diseases like AIDS continue to be powerful enemies that are difficult to combat completely. The current coronavirus pandemic epidemic has highlighted how susceptible contemporary healthcare systems are to serious infectious diseases, underscoring the urgent need for novel solutions. Technological innovations are desperately needed to develop new approaches to illness prevention and treatment, which will ultimately make healthcare systems more resilient to public health emergencies. Researchers believe that in addition to increasing the effectiveness and capacity of medical systems, these new technologies will help them better meet the population's health demands. A new era of innovation and efficiency in healthcare is being ushered in by the innovative concept known as the IoMT, which connects Internet technology with a variety of medical devices. Compared to the Internet, which was often mentioned in the past, the IoT is fundamentally different. In the past, people were connected by the Internet. Individual people made up the Internet's nodes, and the connections between people on the network were what gave it its value. All entities in this physical world—people and objects alike—are connected by the IoT, not just individuals. In theory, a node in the IoT can be any entity that can be addressed independently. The interoperability of items is what gives the IoT its greater value (Noura, Atiquzzaman, & Gaedke, 2019). Smart homes, smart factories, smart cities, smart transportation, and other areas have all seen significant advancements with the IoT. The idea of the IoT permeates the medical field extensively, inspiring the creation of the novel idea of the IoMT. An intelligent healthcare system built on the IoMT consists of a collection of various smart medical devices that are networked together over the Internet. An IoMT-based smart healthcare system's architecture is divided into different stages. Initially, implantable devices or smart wearables with intelligent sensors integrated into them are used to collect medical data from the patient's body. Through a wireless sensor network or a body sensor network, these devices establish a network. The gathered data is then sent via the Internet to the following stage, which entails analysis and prediction. After the medical data is received, advanced analysis is performed using AI-based methods for data transformation and interpretation. This stage is essential for obtaining insightful conclusions and spotting possible health problems. When there are serious health issues, sophisticated AI-based applications built into smartphones can help swiftly notify medical specialists or other resources. This guarantees quick action in urgent circumstances, enabling prompt medical interventions. Based on the examination of the collected data, people can use self-preventive methods for less serious health concerns. Through early detection of possible health problems, this proactive method enables people to take preventive measures and preserve their well-being (Ramson, Vishnu, & Shanmugam, 2020). All things considered, the IoMT-based smart healthcare system provides a thorough and networked approach to healthcare, utilizing cutting-edge technologies to improve diagnosis and preventive care. Figure 2.3 describes the whole process.

2.2.1 Integration of ML and IoMT

The combination of IoMT with ML is a novel synergy with enormous potential to transform healthcare systems. Fundamentally, ML is the ability of computer systems

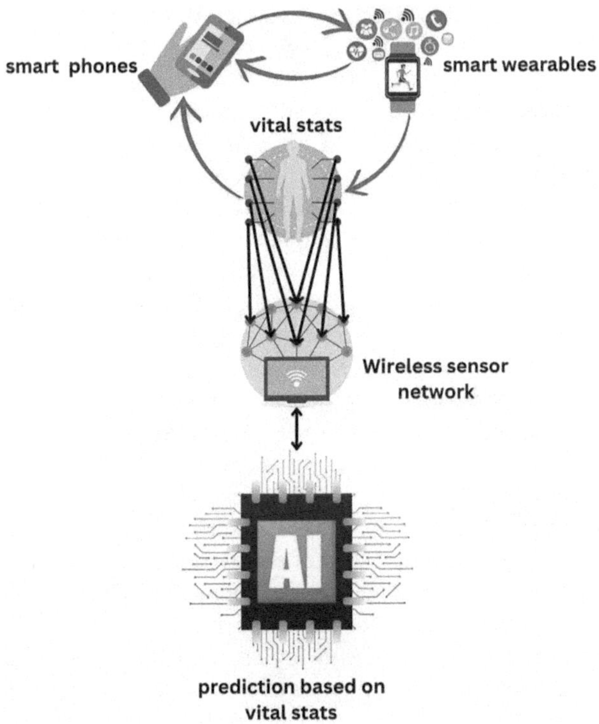

FIGURE 2.3 The IoMT-based architecture.

to learn and adapt from data without the need for explicit programming. This allows the systems to detect patterns, anticipate outcomes, and improve decision-making processes. When ML is smoothly combined with IoMT—a network of connected wearables, medical devices, and sensors—it adds a new level of complexity to healthcare analytics, diagnosis, and treatment plans. Predictive analytics is one of the main domains where ML and IoMT collide. Massive datasets produced by IoMT devices can be analyzed by ML algorithms, which can then be used to forecast possible health consequences and extract insightful information. Healthcare professionals can take preventive measures by using ML models to estimate the likelihood of specific health issues by recognizing patterns and correlations within the data. For instance, in the management of chronic diseases, ML algorithms can anticipate patient condition worsening or exacerbations based on ongoing monitoring with IoMT devices (Awotunde, Ajagbe, Idowu, & Ndunagu, 2021; Khan et al., 2021). This allows for individualized treatment regimens and prompt treatments. Moreover, ML improves IoMT's capacity for risk assessment and illness identification. The integration makes it possible to understand medical data obtained from many sources, such as wearables, sensors, and imaging devices, more effectively and accurately. ML algorithms can identify minor patterns that point to a variety of medical disorders, assisting medical personnel in making an accurate and timely diagnosis. This is especially important in domains like radiology, where ML algorithms help with quick and precise picture interpretation, enhancing diagnosis precision and accelerating treatment choices. Personalized and adaptable techniques are made easier in treatment planning and optimization when ML is coupled with IoMT. ML algorithms can suggest individualized treatment strategies by examining a patient's past medical records and therapy reactions. This optimizes treatment outcomes by allowing healthcare professionals to customize interventions depending on individual features. For example, in oncology, ML algorithms can use patient outcomes, response to therapy, and genetic information to help determine which cancer therapies are the least harmful and most effective.

The potential for telehealth and remote patient monitoring (RPM) is further strengthened by the combination of ML and IoMT. To identify deviations from baseline health trends, ML algorithms can scan continuous streams of data from wearable devices and other IoMT sensors. This can be used to enable automated treatments or to trigger alarms for healthcare personnel. Constant monitoring improves the way chronic illnesses are managed, makes early intervention easier, and gives individuals more control over their health. Precision medicine is evolving further thanks to the dynamic combination of ML and IoMT. ML algorithms are able to detect biomarkers, predict treatment responses, and stratify patients into subgroups for targeted therapies through the analysis of genetic, clinical, and lifestyle data. This degree of accuracy makes it possible to provide more individualized and efficient medical interventions, which lowers the need for trial and error when choosing a course of therapy and enhances patient outcomes overall. The synergies between ML and IoMT go beyond clinical applications to include resource management and healthcare operations. Healthcare organizations can improve overall operational performance by using ML algorithms to enhance scheduling, resource allocation, and workflow efficiency. To minimize downtime and guarantee uninterrupted data flow, predictive maintenance models, for instance, can be used to anticipate and avoid equipment failures in IoMT devices (Nalluri, babu Mupparaju, Pulimamidi, & Rongali, 2024).

IoMT and ML integration is not without its difficulties, though. given the interconnectivity of IoMT and the potential weaknesses in ML models, protecting the security and privacy of sensitive health data is critical. To foster trust and secure patient data, strong cybersecurity safeguards, encryption procedures, and compliance with data protection laws are crucial. Furthermore, there are difficulties in healthcare settings because of the interpretability and transparency of ML models. In particular, when it comes to crucial medical interventions, healthcare practitioners must understand and have faith in the decisions made by ML algorithms. for ML models to be successfully incorporated into clinical practice, it is imperative that they strike a balance between interpretability and complexity. healthcare professionals, data scientists, and technology experts must continue to explore and collaborate as the synergy between ML and IoMT grows. a key factor in guaranteeing the ethical and successful integration of ML with IoMT in healthcare settings will be the creation of standardized standards, regulatory frameworks, and guidelines.

In conclusion, a revolutionary era in healthcare is being ushered in by the combination of ML and the IoMT. Precision medicine, personalized treatment, illness diagnostics, and predictive analytics are all improved by this synergistic partnership. Along with improving telemedicine, RPM, and healthcare operations, ML and

TABLE 2.1
Usage of IoMT

Year	Percentage of IoMT Adoption	Areas of Usage in Medical Research
2010	5	Limited to remote patient monitoring
2012	10	Expansion to clinical trials and data acquisition
2015	20	Integration into personalized medicine and wearables
2018	35	Diverse applications, including real-world evidence in trials
2020	50	Increased focus on patient-generated health data
2022	65	Standardized IoMT usage in various research domains

IoMT open the door to a more intelligent and networked healthcare ecosystem. Even though there are obstacles in the way, continued study and cooperation are essential to realizing the integration's full potential and, eventually, producing healthcare solutions that are more efficient, individualized, and easily available.

Table 2.1 provides insights into not only the increasing percentage of IoMT adoption but also the evolution of areas where IoMT devices are predominantly applied in medical research over the specified years.

2.3 ML FRAMEWORK FOR IOMT

The IoMT has made great strides, and the incorporation of ML frameworks has proven crucial in gleaning insightful information from the copious amounts of data produced by medical equipment. ML frameworks, which offer tools and libraries that simplify the implementation of complicated algorithms, form the foundation for creating and implementing intelligent applications in the IoMT. These frameworks are essential for improving the precision of diagnoses, forecasting patient outcomes, and streamlining healthcare procedures (Syed, Jabeen, Manimala, & Alsaeedi, 2019).

Healthcare-specific customized ML frameworks have become essential enablers in changing the medical landscape. These frameworks are designed to meet the specific needs and constraints of the healthcare sector, where precise forecasting, regulatory compliance, and sensitive data are critical requirements. The design of solutions that are precise and efficient while also adhering to strict standards and ethical considerations within the healthcare domain is made possible by the development of ML frameworks specifically for healthcare applications. One well-known example of an ML platform specifically designed for the healthcare sector is IBM Watson Health. This technology uses IBM's Watson AI to analyze and understand vast volumes of healthcare data. Watson Health extracts valuable data from a range of sources, like as clinical trial data, medical literature, and electronic health records (EHRs), by utilizing ML and natural language processing (NLP). Personalized medicine, clinical decision support, and drug discovery are just a few of the industries where the framework has shown benefits (Binbusayyis, Alaskar, Vaiyapuri, & Dinesh, 2022).

NVIDIA Clara is another specific ML framework used in the medical field. Clara, an NVIDIA product, is intended for use in medical imaging applications.

The intricate computing activities required to analyze and interpret medical pictures, such as computed tomography (CT) and magnetic resonance imaging (MRI) scans, are best suited for its architecture. Clara improves pathology identification, segmentation, and image reconstruction by utilizing deep learning (DL). In diagnostic imaging, the framework has shown to be useful in helping medical practitioners make assessments that are more precise and timelier.

ML framework for IoMT applications is described in Figure 2.4.

The Google Cloud Healthcare API integrates ML capabilities for healthcare applications, with a primary focus on predictive analytics. It offers tools for creating and implementing ML models in addition to facilitating the storing and retrieval of healthcare data. With the use of this framework, healthcare companies can better manage their resources, anticipate patient outcomes, and provide better overall patient care. Scalability and security are guaranteed by the integration with Google Cloud's infrastructure, resolving important issues with healthcare data management. Within the domain of RPM, Biofourmis is one instance of a business that has created a customized ML platform. Their approach gathers patients' physiological data in real time using wearable technology and biosensors. By analyzing this data, the ML algorithms are able to identify patterns, anticipate possible health problems, and give medical practitioners tailored insights. Such customized ML frameworks allow for ongoing patient monitoring, providing proactive healthcare management and lessening the load on established healthcare systems.

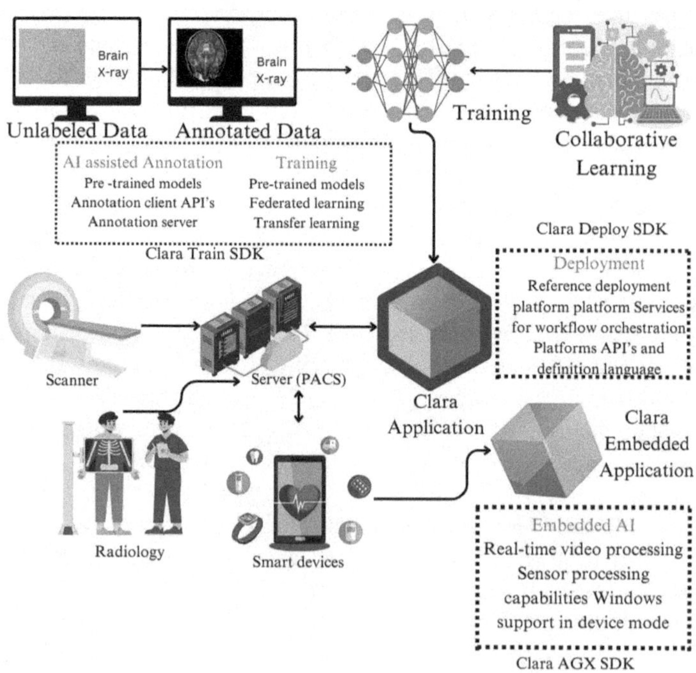

FIGURE 2.4 ML framework for IoMT.

Moreover, pathology and diagnostic decision support are the main topics of PathAI. Their ML architecture helps pathologists diagnose conditions more accurately from medical photos. Path AI improves diagnosis accuracy and efficiency by helping to identify patterns and anomalies in pathology slides through the use of DL. This tailored method shows how ML frameworks can improve diagnostic capacities and supplement the knowledge of medical practitioners. The Seven Bridges Genomics Platform provides a customized ML platform for use in the fields of genomics, personalized medicine, and drug development. With the use of ML techniques and extensive genomics data analysis, researchers can use this platform to find genetic variants linked to various diseases. Precision medicine is advanced by the integration of clinical and genetic data to create a foundation for customized treatment plans.

To sum up, tailored ML frameworks for the healthcare industry mark a substantial advancement toward individualized, effective, and data-driven healthcare solutions. By providing specialized tools for tasks like medical image analysis, predictive analytics, diagnostic support, and genomics research, these frameworks solve the particular issues faced by the healthcare industry. The use of these frameworks in clinical practice has the potential to transform patient care, increase the precision of diagnoses, and progress medical research and treatment approaches as technology develops. To fully realize the potential of ML in healthcare, however, data protection, legal compliance, and ethical considerations must be carefully considered.

2.3.1 Integration Challenges and Solutions

ML framework integration presents a number of obstacles that must be carefully considered to ensure a smooth and successful deployment across a range of industries, including healthcare (Ajagbe, Awotunde, Adesina, Achimugu, & Kumar, 2022; Awotunde, Folorunso, Ajagbe, Garg, & Ajamu, 2022; Pradyumna, Hegde, Bommegowda, Jan, & Naik, 2024). Unlocking the full potential of ML applications in the healthcare domain requires addressing difficulties related to data protection, regulatory compliance, and real-time decision-making (shown in Figure 2.5).

- **Data Privacy and Security:** Ensuring the privacy and security of sensitive patient data is a major obstacle to the integration of ML frameworks in the healthcare industry. Since personal identifiers are frequently present in healthcare data, strict privacy laws like the Health Insurance Portability and Accountability Act (HIPAA) in the US apply to it. Using sophisticated encryption methods, putting strong access controls in place, and embracing privacy-preserving technologies like federated learning are some ways to address this problem. Federated learning mitigates privacy problems by enabling model training on decentralized data sources without requiring raw data sharing.
- **Regulatory Compliance:** A crucial component of ML integration is adherence to healthcare legislation. It's difficult to make sure ML models abide by the many regulatory frameworks that health institutions have to follow. Creating transparent governance frameworks, carrying out exhaustive

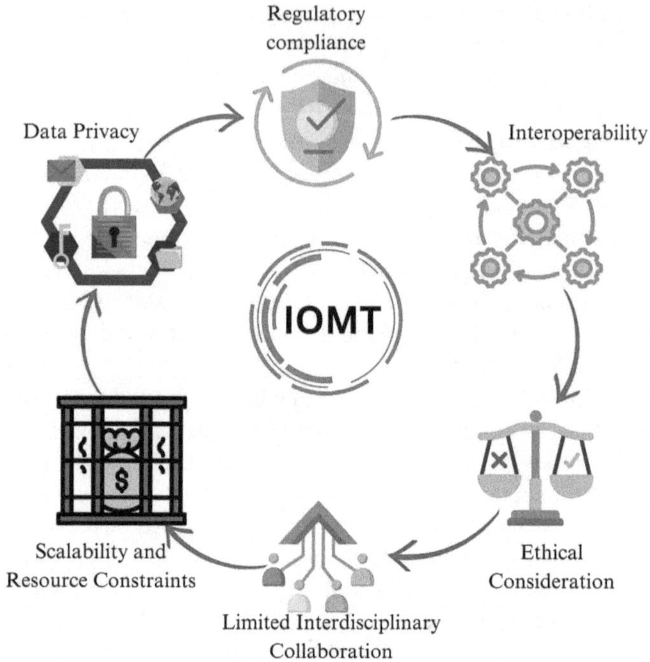

FIGURE 2.5 Integration challenges.

compliance evaluations, and applying explainability strategies to improve the readability and auditability of ML models are all part of the solution methods. To promote innovation and uphold regulatory compliance, it is also critical to engage with regulatory agencies to develop frameworks that correspond with technology developments.

- **Interoperability:** Healthcare systems frequently comprise a large number of networked devices and data sources, some of which may adhere to various standards and formats. One major problem is achieving interoperability between ML frameworks and the current healthcare system. The Fast Healthcare Interoperability Resources and other standardization initiatives are essential for fostering data interchange between various systems. Interoperability should be taken into consideration when designing ML frameworks so that they can support widely-accepted data interchange protocols and integrate easily into current healthcare ecosystems.
- **Ethical Considerations:** Ethical issues need to be carefully considered, such as bias in ML algorithms and the possible effects on disadvantaged populations. Unfair or discriminatory outcomes can result from biases in training data, especially in the healthcare industry where patient population discrepancies are prevalent. Transparency in model creation, constant observation for unforeseen implications, and a thorough assessment of training data for biases are some of the solutions. Furthermore, incorporating a range of stakeholders in the development process—such as ethicists and

community representatives—helps guarantee that ethical issues are sufficiently taken into account.

- **Limited Interdisciplinary Collaboration:** Collaboration between data scientists, healthcare practitioners, technologists, and domain specialists is necessary for the successful integration of ML in healthcare. It is crucial to close the gaps between these fields to create ML models that are both technically sound and applicable to clinical settings. To match ML applications with clinical demands, solutions include developing interdisciplinary training programs, building collaborative environments that promote knowledge exchange, and promoting communication between technologists and healthcare stakeholders.
- **Scalability and Resource Constraints:** Scaling ML frameworks in the healthcare sector can be challenging, especially in large healthcare systems. Staff knowledge and processing power restrictions could impede the application of resource-intensive ML models. Real-time processing demands can be satisfied by both the growth of edge computing and the scalability of cloud-based systems. To overcome the shortage of skilled people, healthcare workers should continue to receive ML application training.

2.4 APPLICATIONS OF ML IN IOMT

ML has emerged as a transformative force in various domains, and its integration into IoMT has revolutionized healthcare practices (Manickam et al., 2022; Qureshi et al., 2022), as discussed in the following subsections.

2.4.1 Remote Patient Monitoring

One prominent application of ML in IoMT is RPM, where ML technologies play a pivotal role in enhancing the quality of healthcare services. With the use of IoT technologies and connected medical equipment, RPM involves gathering, analyzing, and interpreting health-related data from people who are located in remote areas [1]. These systems' inbuilt ML algorithms enable healthcare professionals to make wise choices by gleaning insightful information from the massive volume of patient-generated data. The issues that traditional healthcare models face—like prompt action, individualized treatment regimens, and ongoing monitoring—are all addressed by this revolutionary synergy. Predicting and averting unfavorable health occurrences is one of ML's main contributions to RPM. Through the examination of past patient data and current measurements gathered from wearables or sensors, ML algorithms are able to spot trends and abnormalities that could point to the beginning of a health problem. For example, in cardiovascular monitoring, by examining changes in heart rate, blood pressure, and other pertinent indicators, ML models can forecast the probability of a heart attack. By taking a proactive stance, medical professionals can act quickly to avoid complications and lessen the need for emergency services. A key component of RPM is risk classification driven by ML. ML models are capable of classifying individuals into various risk groups based on an evaluation of their past medical history and current health condition. ML algorithms can also forecast the likelihood of

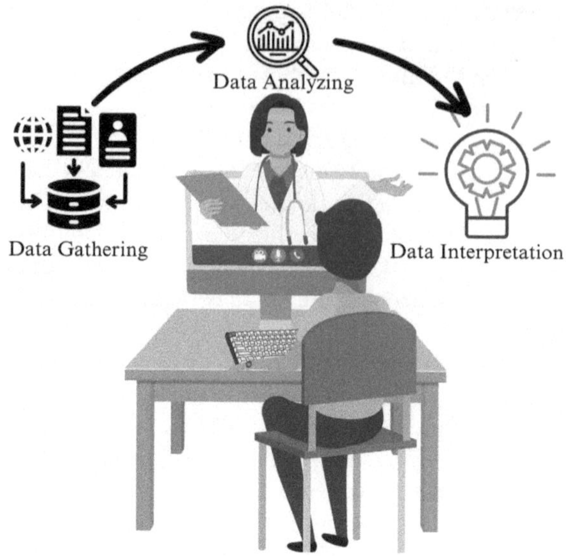

FIGURE 2.6 Remote patient monitoring.

complications for chronic diseases like diabetes, enabling tailored actions to control and minimize possible problems. The role of ML in RPM is presented in Figure 2.6.

2.4.2 Predictive Analytics for Disease Prevention

One of the main tenets of ML applications in the healthcare domain is predictive analytics for illness prevention, especially when considering the IoMT. Using ML algorithms to fuel predictive models, this advanced method looks for trends, anticipates possible health hazards, and takes preventive measures to stop diseases before they start or worsen. In the investigation that follows, we examine the various uses and consequences of predictive analytics in illness prevention, emphasizing its revolutionary influence on healthcare. ML algorithms, which power predictive analytics, are an effective tool for identifying people who are at risk of contracting particular diseases. Wearable technology and networked sensors are essential for gathering real-time health data in the context of IoMT. This constant stream of data can be used to train ML algorithms to identify patterns that deviate from the norm [14]. Predictive analytics, for instance, can evaluate blood glucose levels over time, spot trends, and anticipate future swings in the case of chronic illnesses like diabetes. By taking a proactive stance, people and medical professionals are better equipped to prevent illness by making preventive changes to lifestyle choices or prescription regimens. Predictive analytics also aids in population health management by seeing patterns and trends on a larger scale. Through the examination of combined data from several sources, such as socioeconomic variables, environmental data, and EHRs, ML models are able to predict the occurrence of diseases in certain areas or groups of people. In conclusion, a paradigm shift in illness prevention within the context of

IoMT is represented by predictive analytics driven by ML. The potential to enhance public health outcomes through the prediction of health hazards, customization of preventive measures, and efficient allocation of resources is enormous.

2.4.3 Diagnostics Imaging and ML

The field of medical diagnostics is undergoing a revolution thanks to the incorporation of ML in diagnostic imaging. This combination of cutting-edge computational algorithms with IoMT diagnostic imaging technologies has the potential to improve medical imaging's accessibility, efficacy, and accuracy. In this investigation, we explore the diverse uses of ML in diagnostic imaging, illuminating how ML affects different modalities like MRI scans, CT scans, ultrasounds, and X-rays. To detect and track diseases, diagnostic imaging is essential to healthcare since it makes interior structures visible and enables analysis. However, deciphering medical images can be difficult and frequently calls for the knowledge of radiologists with advanced training. Image interpretation and segmentation is one of the main uses of ML in diagnostic imaging. Pattern recognition in images is a strength of convolutional neural networks (CNNs) and other DL architectures. For example, in the context of X-rays, ML algorithms are able to precisely identify abnormalities like lung nodules, tumors, or fractures, which helps and enhances radiologists' work. This accelerates the diagnostic procedure and guarantees a more comprehensive examination of medical photos. In addition, ML improves picture interpretation efficiency by classifying and grading cases.

ML techniques are used in the fields of MRI and CT scans. The creation of predictive models based on imaging data for illness diagnosis and progression is another important application of ML. ML algorithms can detect early indications of diseases and forecast how they will develop over time by examining longitudinal imaging datasets. ML applications are very beneficial for ultrasound imaging, especially for automated organ segmentation and prenatal anomaly diagnosis. ML algorithms are capable of accurately measuring organ volumes and identifying any anomalies in prenatal development by analyzing ultrasonography images. This improves patient outcomes and prenatal care by helping medical providers make prompt, correct decisions. Large and varied datasets are essential for the training of ML algorithms in diagnostic imaging. To sum up, the application of ML to diagnostic imaging in the context of IoMT represents a revolutionary development in the medical field. The diagnostic environment is altered by ML algorithms' capacity to improve efficiency, automate picture interpretation, and aid in early illness identification.

2.4.4 Personalized Medicine and Treatment Plans

Personalized medicine, empowered by ML and integrated within the IoMT, represents a revolutionary approach to healthcare. This paradigm shift moves away from the traditional one-size-fits-all model toward tailored and precise medical interventions. Fundamentally, personalized medicine seeks to consider the distinct genetic, biochemical, environmental, and behavioral elements that impact each person's health. To obtain meaningful insights, ML techniques are essential for evaluating large datasets like genomes, proteomics, EHRs, and real-time patient data. The ultimate objective is to create therapy regimens that maximize outcomes for every patient while minimizing side effects and increasing effectiveness. Personalized medicine has benefited greatly from ML's ability to identify genetic signatures and biomarkers linked to particular diseases. Genetic data can be analyzed by ML algorithms to identify changes that could affect a patient's susceptibility to an illness, how it progresses, or how well a treatment works. With the use of this knowledge, medical practitioners can better focus and more precisely customize therapy to the underlying molecular pathways causing diseases. In conclusion, the IoMT's tailored medicine, powered by ML, represents a revolutionary change in the way healthcare is provided. The potential to customize treatment regimens based on personal genetic profiles, lifestyle decisions, and real-time health information is extremely promising for enhancing patient results.

2.4.5 IoMT in Emergency Medical Services

In today's fast-paced world people frequently refuse to spend needless time on medical procedures, especially the lengthy registration process. People's personal data and brief summaries of their medical conditions can be easily integrated into hospital information systems by using the Internet databases to support healthcare procedures, such as online appointment scheduling. By assigning a doctor quickly and effectively, this streamlined method reduces wait times and does away with the need for recurrent personal data entering. In addition, remote medical care presents a useful substitute for those who live far from hospitals, overcoming the difficulties brought on by geographic limitations. The Internet plays a vital role in allowing communication between doctors and specialists even within hospital premises, especially for patients who have sustained injuries in accidents.

One of IoMT's primary benefits for emergency medical services (EMS) is its capacity to track and transmit vital signs in real time. Vital indicators such as heart rate, oxygen saturation, and blood pressure can be continually monitored by patients by donning wearable devices and sensors. Experts offering EMS have the ability to promptly and precisely evaluate a patient's status prior to their arrival at the hospital. This real-time monitoring facilitates quick decision-making and may reduce the time required to initiate critical interventions. In the context of IoMT in EMS, predictive analytics is also crucial. By predicting potential emergencies through the examination of historical data and trends, healthcare professionals may be proactive in their approach (Puri, Kataria, Solanki, & Rani, 2022). EMS teams may more effectively manage their resources and prioritize their response by using predictive analytics, for instance, to help identify high-risk patients who live in the neighborhood (Bhambri, Aggarwal, Singh, Singh, & Rani, 2022).

2.5 RECENT DEVELOPMENTS FOR ML IN IOMT

2.5.1 Case Studies of Successful Implementations

With its DL-based AIRTM Recon DL technique, a revolutionary approach to magnetic resonance image reconstruction is developed (shown in Figure 2.7). It revolutionizes post-processing and does away with the necessity for compromises in MRI.

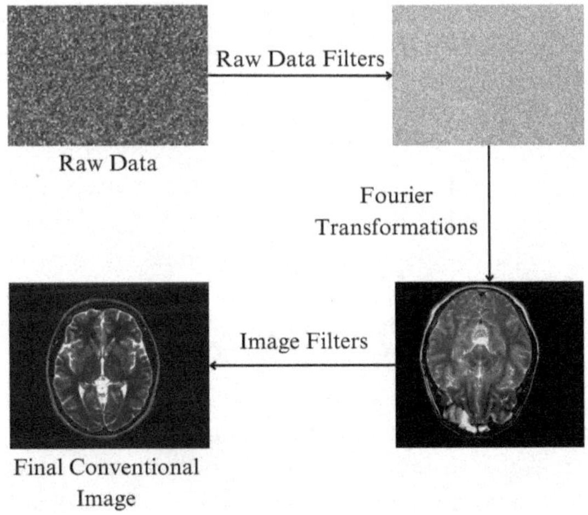

FIGURE 2.7 Representation of the case study.

In contrast to conventional post-processing techniques that might lose picture details, AIRTM Recon DL adopts a novel strategy by using a DL-based reconstruction engine that uses raw data to produce images of unmatched quality (Puri, Kataria, Rani, & Pareek, 2023; Singh & Rani, 2023). With the help of this cutting-edge technology, noise and Gibbs ringing artifacts are successfully removed using a DL-based neural network. The unique feature of AIRTM Recon DL is its clever ringing suppression technology, which is made to protect fine picture details. Image noise and ringing artifacts are two issues that technologists and radiologists frequently deal with.

This cutting-edge solution, which was created on GE Healthcare's Edison intelligence platform, combines seamlessly with the clinical process. High-quality photos may be produced instantly at the operator's console using AIRTM Recon DL. The result is better picture quality across all anatomical structures, faster scan times for patients, and increased diagnostic confidence. Healthcare service providers and patients benefit from this innovation.

The Abilify MyCite medicine system includes an ingestible sensor in the aripiprazole tablets to improve drug adherence. This sensor logs the medication's consumption and sends the information to a wearable patch. Patients may use their cellphones to track the amount of medication they take, thanks to the information transmitted by the patch to a mobile application. Abilify MyCite is licensed for the treatment of schizophrenia, acute management of manic and mixed episodes associated with bipolar I disorder, and adult depression as a stand-alone medication. This system's main goal is to provide patients, caregivers, and medical professionals a way to monitor and control drug adherence, particularly when it comes to mental health issues.

2.5.2 Innovations in ML Algorithms for Healthcare

- **Recognition of Images and Patterns:** CNNs, in particular, are ML methods that have significantly improved medical imaging analysis. Through the interpretation of medical images such as CT, MRI, and X-rays, they can help in the early diagnosis of illnesses (Pattnayak & Panda, 2021).

- **Drug Development and Discovery:** It is among the key advantages of ML for the medical field. With the help of ML, pharmaceutical companies, hospitals, and patients may all benefit financially from the discovery of novel medications. It also speeds up and greatly reduces the expense of the drug-creation process. For instance, Atomwise is a pharmaceutical business that leverages supercomputers to identify potential treatments from databases of molecular structures. Atomwise ML-based technology allowed for the completion of an analysis in a single day that would have taken several years (Dara, Dhamercherla, Jadav, Babu, & Ahsan, 2022).
- **NLP-Based Clinical Notes:** NLP techniques are used to review and extract relevant information from clinical notes, unstructured text, and medical literature. This makes it easier to improve decision support systems and extract insightful information from massive amounts of textual data (Sheikhalishahi et al., 2019).
- **Healthcare Fraud Detection and Security:** Algorithms based on AI are used to spot fraud in medical billing and insurance claims. They also contribute to enhancing the overall security of healthcare systems by identifying potential security threats and vulnerabilities.

2.5.3 Impact of IoMT in Medical Research

The efficacy and efficiency of medical research in a variety of fields have significantly increased as a result of the use of the IoMT. An overview of the main fields in medical research where IoMT has advanced findings is given in Table 2.2, which also shows how well data collection, patient participation, clinical trials, and customized treatment have all benefited from IoMT (Balsa & Gandelman, 2011; Verbeke, Karara, & Nyssen, 2013). Table 2.2 shows aspects of research with Respect to IoMT.

TABLE 2.2
Aspects of Medical Research with Respect to IoMT

Aspects of Medical Research	Before IoMT	With IoMT	Impact
Data Acquisition	Manual, sporadic collection of limited data	Continuous, real-time data from wearables, sensors	Increased data quantity and quality
Patient Engagement	Limited participation and awareness	Active involvement, patient-generated health data	Enhanced participant engagement
Clinical Trials	In-person visits, time-consuming	Remote monitoring, real-world evidence	Faster, more inclusive trials
Personalized Medicine	Generic treatment plans	Continuous monitoring, personalized interventions	Tailored, more effective therapies

2.6 CHALLENGES AND ETHICAL CONSIDERATIONS

2.6.1 Data Security and Privacy Concerns

A new age in healthcare has begun with the introduction of the IoMT, which promises better patient care, more efficiency, and creative medical solutions. Nevertheless, despite the potential advantages, IoMT also presents a wide range of difficulties and moral dilemmas, with privacy and data security taking center stage. Because health information is sensitive and private, data security is a top priority in the field of IoMT. Patient data is continuously transferred, stored, and analyzed within a massive network that is created by the interconnectedness of wearables, medical equipment, and healthcare systems. While real-time monitoring and quick reactions to medical situations are made possible by this connectedness, it also creates weaknesses and malevolent actors could take advantage of this situation. The biggest threat to IoMT data security is the possibility of cyberattacks and unwanted access. Medical devices that are connected to health monitoring systems, such as insulin pumps and pacemakers, are vulnerable to hacking attempts that may jeopardize patient privacy and safety. IoMT also brings up moral concerns about who owns and controls health data. It's critical to set precise rules on who owns data and how it can be used as devices continue to gather and transmit information. Transparency emerges as a crucial ethical tenet in IoMT. Patients ought to be made aware of the kinds of data that are gathered, how they will be used, and the security precautions used to keep it safe. So, the emergence of IoMT heralds a revolutionary change in the healthcare industry, presenting hitherto unseen chances to improve patient outcomes and optimize medical procedures (Razdan & Sharma, 2022). It is impossible to overstate the difficulties and moral issues surrounding data security and privacy, nevertheless. Securing patient trust and privacy in an increasingly connected healthcare world can be achieved while realizing the potential benefits of IoMT by emphasizing strong security measures, adopting transparent and ethical practices, and developing a culture of responsible data use.

2.6.2 Interoperability Challenges

In IoMT applications, there are major interoperability issues that need to be resolved before its full promise can be realized. The smooth transfer and utilization of data between various healthcare systems, gadgets, and applications is referred to as interoperability. Achieving interoperability in the context of IoMT is crucial to making sure that various medical technologies and devices can cooperate well. However, a variety of interoperability issues arise due to the complexity of healthcare ecosystems and the use of disparate standards and technology. The absence of established communication protocols in IoMT is one of the main obstacles to interoperability. The variety of data formats and architectures used by various healthcare systems is another important concern. Different data formats may be used by medical imaging systems, IoMT devices, and EHRs, which makes proper information interpretation and interchange challenging. The legislative environment that varies by area and governs healthcare data further exacerbates interoperability issues. There are many obstacles standing in the way of the IoMT's broad adoption and efficacy due to interoperability issues. To overcome these obstacles, it is essential to standardize communication protocols, harmonize data formats, upgrade legacy systems, address privacy and security issues, create a framework for universal patient identification, and promote regulatory consistency (Yasmeen, Javed, & Ahmed, 2022).

2.6.3 Ethical Implications of ML in Healthcare

To ensure the proper and equitable use of new technologies, ethical issues related to the integration of ML into healthcare practices must be carefully managed. The problem of bias is one of the main ethical issues with the use of ML in healthcare. When using ML in healthcare, transparency is another ethical factor that needs to be taken into consideration. Many ML algorithms function as "black boxes," which makes it difficult to comprehend how they determine particular outcomes. Transparency in algorithmic decision-making is necessary in the healthcare industry, where choices have an impact on people's health, to foster confidence among medical staff, patients, and the general public. Strong privacy protections must be implemented as medical institutions use patient data more and more to train algorithms. Maintaining patient privacy and abiding by ethical norms requires securing informed consent, anonymizing data, and putting in place safe storage and communication methods (Char, Abràmoff, & Feudtner, 2020).

2.6.4 Regulatory and Compliance Issues

The rapidly emerging IoMT offers the potential to completely transform healthcare, but it also raises a number of legal and regulatory challenges. Strong regulatory frameworks and compliance controls are becoming more and more important as wearables, medical devices, and healthcare systems become integrated components of patient care to ensure the security, efficacy, and privacy of healthcare solutions. The intricate and ever-evolving nature of IoMT presents a significant regulatory problem. Conventional healthcare laws were not intended to deal with the complexity of networked devices and the constant flow of medical information. Consequently, regulatory agencies worldwide must modify current frameworks or create new ones to efficiently oversee the quickly changing IoMT environment. In this regulatory effort, striking a balance between promoting innovation and safeguarding patient interests is critical. For IoMT stakeholders to navigate the legal landscape and uphold patient data protection standards, compliance with regulations like the General Data Protection Regulation in the European Union and the HIPAA in the United States is essential. To sum up, responsible deployment and integration of connected healthcare solutions depend on the resolution of regulatory and compliance challenges related to the IoMT (Ramakrishnan, Nori, Murfet, & Cameron, 2020).

2.7 FUTURE TRENDS AND PROSPECTS

2.7.1 Advancements in ML Technologies for IoMT

The future of the IoMT is being shaped by developments in ML technology, which have significant effects on the healthcare industry. Advanced ML technologies have the potential to revolutionize patient care by enhancing diagnosis, treatment plans, and overall patient experience as the IoMT advances due to the combination of medical sensors and smart devices. One of the key areas in the IoMT environment where ML is making considerable strides is improving diagnostics and predictive analytics. Furthermore, by predicting possible health problems before they materialize clinically, predictive analytics driven by ML has the potential to completely transform the healthcare industry. Personalized risk assessments can be generated by ML algorithms through the analysis of genetic information, lifestyle factors, and previous patient data. Consequently, a paradigm shift toward predictive and preventive healthcare is fostered by the integration of ML technologies into IoMT systems, which ultimately improves patient outcomes and lessens the demand for healthcare resources.

2.7.2 Emerging Applications and Use Cases

The IoMT, with its rapid expansion, has opened up a multitude of new opportunities for the healthcare sector. The IoMT has the potential to completely change the way healthcare is provided, improve patient outcomes, and boost the overall effectiveness of healthcare systems if the network of wearables, sensors, and medical devices keeps growing, as discussed here:

- **Telemedicine and Virtual Consultations:** By enabling patients to communicate with medical experts remotely, IoMT promotes the growth of telemedicine and virtual consultations. Virtual examinations and consultations are made possible by integrated cameras, sensors, and diagnostic instruments, which eliminates the need for in-person trips to medical facilities.
- **Personalized Medicine and Treatment Plans:** The advent of personalized medicine is being driven by the convergence of advanced analytics, AI, and IoMT. Healthcare practitioners can customize treatment strategies for each patient by utilizing genetic data, wearables, and real-time monitoring equipment.
- **Data Management and Smart Health Records:** IoMT helps to create effective data management systems and smart health records. EHRs and connected medical devices interface easily, guaranteeing the accurate and timely transfer of patient data.
- **Wearable Mental Health Monitoring:** Within IoMT, mental health monitoring is starting to take center stage. Wearable technology that has biosensors and physiological monitoring features allows it to track mental health markers.
- **IoMT in Disaster Management and Emergency Response:** IoMT technologies are shown to be quite useful in scenarios involving disaster management and emergency response. When it comes to quickly evaluating and prioritizing medical interventions during emergencies, wearable gadgets with location tracking and vital sign monitoring capabilities can be a great help.

To fully realize the promise of IoMT in reshaping healthcare, continued cooperation between tech developers, regulatory agencies, legislators, and healthcare practitioners is essential.

2.7.3 Collaboration Opportunities in IoMT

A new era of healthcare innovation is being ushered in by the IoMT, and there are many chances for collaboration among different stakeholders in this space. To fully utilize IoMT and bring about a revolution in healthcare delivery, teamwork is essential in the complex network of linked medical devices, wearables, and sensors. The IoMT ecosystem offers a wide range of cooperation opportunities. These include international interoperability collaborations and partnerships between healthcare professionals and technology developers. Technology developers and healthcare practitioners working together are at the heart of IoMT's transformative potential. Public–private collaborations also seem to be a potent factor in bringing IoMT into the mainstream of medicine. Technology developers, cybersecurity specialists, and healthcare organizations must work together to ensure data security and privacy inside IoMT systems. The partnership intends to create secure data storage options, reliable encryption techniques, and guidelines for managing private health information.

2.8 CONCLUSIONS

Healthcare is changing dramatically as a result of ML being woven across the IoMT. Essentially, ML is a crucial enabler in the IoMT space, helping to interpret, evaluate, and extract meaningful information from the massive amount of data. IoMT's core innovations like wearable tech and networked sensors form the basis for ML algorithms to detect patterns shaping healthcare. Examining IoMT's ML framework underscores the need for tailored methods to address healthcare's unique challenges, including data silos and interoperability. To fully capitalize on the innovative integration of ML with the IoMT, researchers and practitioners must prioritize several key actions, discussed here:

- First, ethical considerations demand meticulous attention to ensure the responsible development and deployment of ML algorithms within IoMT systems.
- Simultaneously, robust data security measures are imperative to safeguard patient information and maintain trust in these interconnected healthcare environments.
- Standardization efforts to promote interoperability among diverse IoMT devices and platforms are essential for seamless data exchange and comprehensive patient care.
- Furthermore, staying informed about evolving regulatory landscapes is crucial to navigating compliance challenges effectively.
- Fostered collaboration among stakeholders, including researchers, healthcare providers, technologists, and policymakers, is paramount to drive innovation and address complex issues surrounding ML–IoMT integration.

By collectively addressing these imperatives, researchers and practitioners can unlock the transformative potential of ML–IoMT convergence, advancing toward a more personalized, efficient, and data-driven healthcare paradigm.

REFERENCES

Ajagbe, S. A., Awotunde, J. B., Adesina, A. O., Achimugu, P., & Kumar, T. A. (2022). Internet of medical things (IoMT): Applications, challenges, and prospects in a data-driven technology. *Intelligent Healthcare: Infrastructure, Algorithms and Management*, 299–319.

Alsubaei, F., Abuhussein, A., Shandilya, V., & Shiva, S. (2019). IoMT-SAF: Internet of medical things security assessment framework. *Internet of Things*, 8, 100123.

Awotunde, J. B., Ajagbe, S. A., Idowu, I. R., & Ndunagu, J. N. (2021). An enhanced cloud-IoMT-based and ML for effective COVID-19 diagnosis system. *Intelligence of Things: AI-IoT Based Critical-applications and Innovations*, 55–76.

Awotunde, J. B., Folorunso, S. O., Ajagbe, S. A., Garg, J., & Ajamu, G. J. (2022). AiIoMT: IoMT-based system-enabled artificial intelligence for enhanced smart healthcare systems. *ML for Critical Internet of Medical Things: Applications and Use Cases*, 229–254.

Balsa, A., & Gandelman, N. (2011). The impact of ICT in health promotion: A randomized experiment with diabetic patients. *The Journal of Supercomputing*, *26*, 210–223.

Bhambri, P., Aggarwal, M., Singh, H., Singh, A. P., & Rani, S. (2022). Uprising of EVs: Charging the future with demystified analytics and sustainable development. In *Decision Analytics for Sustainable Development in Smart Society 5.0: Issues, Challenges and Opportunities* (pp. 37–53): Springer.

Binbusayyis, A., Alaskar, H., Vaiyapuri, T., & Dinesh, M. (2022). An investigation and comparison of ML approaches for intrusion detection in IoMT network. *The Journal of Supercomputing*, 78(15), 17403–17422.

Char, D. S., Abràmoff, M. D., & Feudtner, C. (2020). Identifying ethical considerations for ML healthcare applications. *The American Journal of Bioethics*, 20(11), 7–17.

Dara, S., Dhamercherla, S., Jadav, S. S., Babu, C. M., & Ahsan, M. J. (2022). ML in drug discovery: A review. *Artificial Intelligence Review*, 55(3), 1947–1999.

Dutta, P. E., Neog, H., & Medhi, N. (2021). Health monitoring in Internet of Medical Things (IoMT) using ML (ML) approaches. Paper presented at the 2021 *IEEE Globecom Workshops (GC Wkshps)*.

Khan, M. F., Ghazal, T. M., Said, R. A., Fatima, A., Abbas, S., Khan, M.,. . . Khan, M. A. (2021). An IoMT-enabled smart healthcare model to monitor elderly people using ML technique. *Computational Intelligence and Neuroscience*, 2021.

Manickam, P., Mariappan, S. A., Murugesan, S. M., Hansda, S., Kaushik, A., Shinde, R., & Thipperudraswamy, S. (2022). Artificial intelligence (AI) and internet of medical things (IoMT) assisted biomedical systems for intelligent healthcare. *Biosensors*, 12(8), 562.

Nalluri, M., Babu Mupparaju, C., Pulimamidi, R., & Rongali, A. S. (2024). Integration of AI, ML, and IoT in healthcare data fusion: Integrating data from various sources, including IoT devices and electronic health records, provides a more comprehensive view of patient health. *Pakistan Heart Journal*, 57(1), 34–42.

Noura, M., Atiquzzaman, M., & Gaedke, M. (2019). Interoperability in internet of things: Taxonomies and open challenges. *Mobile Networks and Applications*, *24*, 796–809.

Pattnayak, P., & Panda, A. R. (2021). Innovation on ML in healthcare services—An introduction. *Technical Advancements of ML in Healthcare*, 1–30.

Pradyumna, G., Hegde, R. B., Bommegowda, K., Jan, T., & Naik, G. R. (2024). Empowering healthcare with IoMT: Evolution, ML integration, security, and interoperability challenges. *IEEE Access*, *30*, 20–29.

Puri, V., Kataria, A., Rani, S., & Pareek, P. K. (2023). DLT based smart medical ecosystem. Paper presented at the *2023 International Conference on Network, Multimedia and Information Technology (NMITCON)*.

Puri, V., Kataria, A., Solanki, V. K., & Rani, S. (2022). AI-based botnet attack classification and detection in IoT devices. Paper presented at the *2022 IEEE International Conference on ML and Applied Network Technologies (ICMLANT)*.

Qureshi, A., Batra, S., Vats, P., Singh, S., Phogat, M., & Sharma, A. K. (2022). A review of ML (ML) in the internet of medical things (IOMT) in the construction of a smart healthcare structure. *Journal of Algebraic Statistics*, 13(2), 225–231.

Ramakrishnan, G., Nori, A., Murfet, H., & Cameron, P. (2020). Towards compliant data management systems for healthcare ML. *arXiv preprint* arXiv:2011.07555.

Ramson, S. J., Vishnu, S., & Shanmugam, M. (2020). Applications of Internet of Things (IoT)–an overview. Paper presented at the *2020 5th international conference on devices, circuits and systems (ICDCS)*.

Rani, S., Kataria, A., Kumar, S., & Tiwari, P. (2023). Federated learning for secure IoMT-applications in smart healthcare systems: A comprehensive review. *Knowledge-Based Systems*, 110658.

Rani, S., Kumar, S., Kataria, A., & Min, H. (2023). SmartHealth: An intelligent framework to secure IoMT service applications using ML. *ICT Express*, *33*, 203–220.

Rani, S., Mishra, A. K., Kataria, A., Mallik, S., & Qin, H. (2023). ML-based optimal crop selection system in smart agriculture. *Scientific Reports*, 13(1), 15997.

Razdan, S., & Sharma, S. (2022). Internet of medical things (IoMT): Overview, emerging technologies, and case studies. *IETE Technical Review*, 39(4), 775–788.

Sheikhalishahi, S., Miotto, R., Dudley, J. T., Lavelli, A., Rinaldi, F., & Osmani, V. (2019). Natural language processing of clinical notes on chronic diseases: Systematic review. *JMIR Medical Informatics*, *7*(2), e12239.

Singh, H., & Rani, S. (2023). Flex sensor integrated smart strap to verify correct wearing of the face mask. *IEEE Sensors Journal, 5*, 306–319.

Syed, L., Jabeen, S., Manimala, S., & Alsaeedi, A. (2019). Smart healthcare framework for ambient assisted living using IoMT and big data analytics techniques. *Future Generation Computer Systems*, 101, 136–151.

Verbeke, F., Karara, G., & Nyssen, M. (2013). Evaluating the impact of ICT-tools on health care delivery in sub-Saharan hospitals. In *MEDINFO 2013* (pp. 520–523): IOS Press.

Yasmeen, G., Javed, N., & Ahmed, T. (2022). Interoperability: A challenge for IoMT. *ECS Transactions*, 107(1), 4459.

3 IoT Healthcare's Advanced Decision Support through Computational Intelligence

Pawan Whig, Jhansi Bharathi Madavarapu, Nikhitha Yathiraju, and Ramya Thatikonda

CONTENTS

3.1 INTRODUCTION

The fusion of computational intelligence (CI) with the Internet of Things (IoT) has spurred a transformative revolution in healthcare delivery, ushering in an era of personalized, data-driven patient care and clinical decision-making, as shown in Figure 3.1. This chapter delves into the symbiotic relationship between CI and IoT within the healthcare landscape, illuminating their combined potential to reshape traditional healthcare paradigms [1].

DOI: 10.1201/9781003476207-3

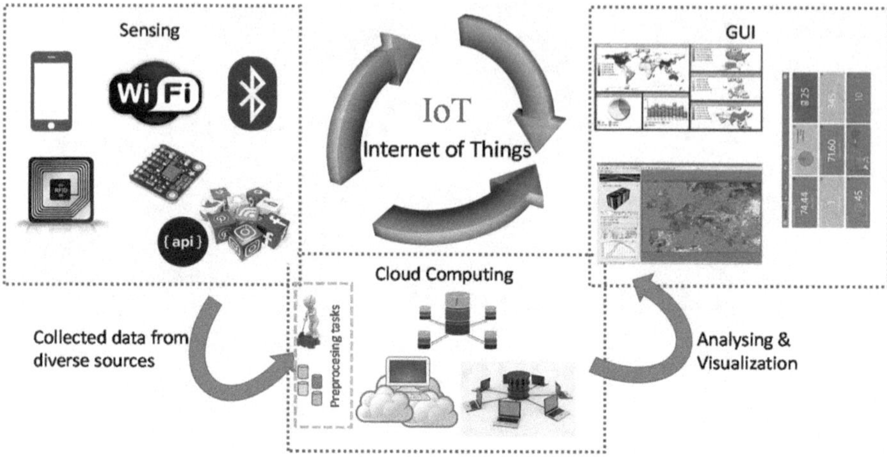

FIGURE 3.1 IoT healthcare-based support through computational intelligence.

CI, encompassing various artificial intelligence techniques such as machine learning, neural networks, and evolutionary computation, operates at the crux of IoT healthcare systems. IoT, characterized by interconnected devices embedded with sensors, generates a voluminous stream of patient-centric data. The convergence of CI with this data-rich ecosystem heralds a new frontier, offering unparalleled insights and opportunities for precision medicine, proactive health monitoring, and optimized healthcare delivery [2, 3].

At the core of this symbiosis lies the concept of advanced decision support systems (ADSSs), fortified by CI algorithms that harness and interpret the vast troves of IoT-driven patient data. These systems act as transformative catalysts, empowering healthcare practitioners with predictive analytics, personalized treatment strategies, and proactive intervention capabilities, thereby redefining patient outcomes [4, 5].

The interconnectedness of CI and IoT amplifies diagnostic accuracy, treatment efficacy, and clinical decision-making capabilities. By employing CI algorithms, healthcare providers can navigate the complexities of vast datasets, identifying intricate patterns within patient vitals, medication adherence, and lifestyle factors. This wealth of information enables ADSS to forecast disease progression, anticipate health deteriorations, and tailor treatment plans based on individual patient profiles, fostering a more targeted and effective approach to healthcare [6].

Moreover, the marriage of CI and IoT in healthcare transcends traditional boundaries, optimizing resource utilization and clinical workflows. Real-time analysis of IoT-generated data through CI models minimizes inefficiencies, reducing unnecessary healthcare visits, and optimizing hospital resource allocation [7]. This proactive approach not only augments patient care but also streamlines operational efficiencies, enhancing the overall healthcare ecosystem [8].

However, this integration is not without challenges. Ethical considerations, data security, interoperability, and the need for standardization pose significant hurdles. Safeguarding patient privacy and ensuring secure data transmission remains paramount, demanding robust frameworks and ethical guidelines. The literature review with the research gap is shown in Table 3.1.

TABLE 3.1
Literature Review with Research Gap

Authors	Year	Main Contribution	Research Gap
Abdel-Basset et al. (2019)	2019	Intelligent medical decision support using IoT and soft computing	Integration challenges of IoT with existing healthcare systems
Abirami and Chitra (2020)	2020	Energy-efficient edge-based healthcare support system	Lack of standardized protocols for integrating edge computing in healthcare systems
Alshamrani (2022)	2022	IoT and AI for remote healthcare monitoring	Security and privacy concerns in remote healthcare monitoring
Ahmed et al. (2020)	2020	AI and ML for healthcare and precision medicine	Limited interoperability among diverse healthcare data sources
Amann et al. (2020)	2020	Explainability of AI in healthcare	Lack of standardized frameworks for explaining AI-driven healthcare decisions
Sauter (2014)	2014	Decision support systems for business intelligence	Application of business intelligence concepts in healthcare decision-making
Johnson et al. (2016)	2016	Machine learning in critical care	Need for real-time decision support tools for critical care based on dynamic patient data
Meskó et al. (2018)	2018	AI addressing human resource crisis in healthcare	Ethical implications of AI replacing or augmenting human healthcare resources
Lee and Yoon (2021)	2021	AI-based technologies in healthcare	Addressing bias and equity concerns in AI-driven healthcare technologies
Noorbakhsh-Sabet et al. (2019)	2019	AI's transformation of healthcare	Standardization of AI integration to enhance healthcare outcomes
Asan et al. (2020)	2020	AI and human trust in healthcare	Building clinician trust in AI-driven healthcare decision-making
Bohr and Memarzadeh (2020)	2020	AI applications in healthcare	Scalability and adoption challenges in deploying AI applications across healthcare settings
Araujo et al. (2020)	2020	Public perception of AI in decision-making	Understanding societal attitudes and biases toward automated AI-driven decisions
Rubinger et al. (2023)	2023	ML and AI in research and healthcare	Enhancing interpretability and reliability of AI/ML models for better clinical decision support
Schönberger (2019)	2019	Legal and ethical implications of AI in healthcare	Developing robust ethical guidelines and legal frameworks for AI-driven healthcare applications
Rong et al. (2020)	2020	AI in healthcare: review and prediction case studies	Validation and generalizability of AI models in diverse healthcare settings
Bharadiya (2022)	2022	AI and BI for business growth	Translating AI advancements into scalable business intelligence strategies
Jiang et al. (2017)	2017	Evolution of AI in healthcare	Historical perspective on AI in healthcare and future trends
Das and Chandra (2023)	2023	AI for reducing climate footprint in healthcare	Sustainable AI adoption strategies for minimizing environmental impact in healthcare
Yu et al. (2018)	2018	Role of AI in healthcare	Robustness and reliability of AI-driven healthcare systems for clinical decision-making

In essence, the union of CI and IoT in healthcare embodies a paradigm shift, promising a future where data-driven decision-making, personalized medicine, and optimized healthcare services converge for the betterment of patient well-being [9, 10]. This chapter navigates through the intricacies of this transformative alliance, unveiling the immense potential and challenges in the realm of CI in IoT healthcare.

3.2 UNDERSTANDING THE INTERSECTION OF IoT AND HEALTHCARE

The intersection of the IoT and healthcare stands as a pivotal point in the evolution of medical practices. IoT, a network of interconnected devices embedded with sensors, has emerged as a catalyst for transforming traditional healthcare models [11]. This convergence has revolutionized patient care, clinical decision-making, and overall healthcare delivery [12].

Within this landscape, CI techniques play a crucial role in harnessing the potential of healthcare IoT. CI, encompassing various artificial intelligence methods such as machine learning, neural networks, and evolutionary computation, serves as the cornerstone for processing and extracting meaningful insights from the vast array of data generated by IoT devices in the healthcare domain as shown in Figure 3.2.

CI techniques in healthcare IoT pivot around ADSS. These systems, empowered by CI algorithms, have the capacity to analyze, interpret, and utilize the extensive

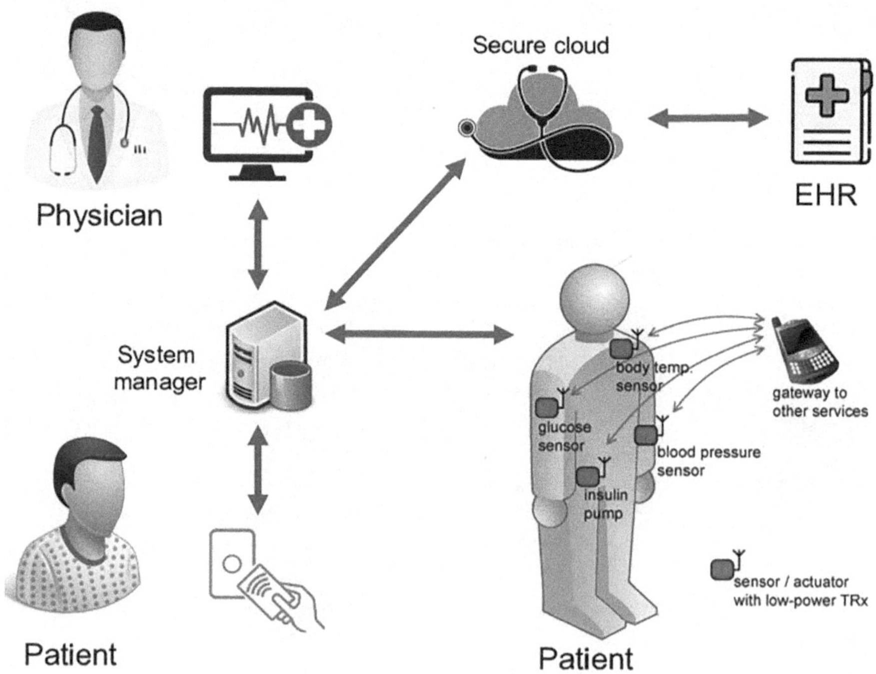

FIGURE 3.2 Intersection of IoT and healthcare.

patient-centric data collected by IoT devices [13–15]. They enable healthcare practitioners to make informed decisions, providing predictive analytics, personalized treatment strategies, and proactive health monitoring capabilities [16, 17].

One of the fundamental benefits of merging CI with healthcare IoT lies in its potential to enhance diagnostic accuracy and treatment efficacy. By leveraging CI algorithms, healthcare providers can navigate through intricate patient data collected by IoT devices, including vital signs, medication adherence, and lifestyle patterns. This data deluge facilitates ADSS in predicting disease progression, anticipating potential health complications, and customizing treatment plans based on individual patient profiles, thereby augmenting the precision and effectiveness of healthcare interventions.

Furthermore, this integration optimizes resource utilization and clinical workflows. Real-time analysis of IoT-generated data using CI models minimizes inefficiencies, reducing unnecessary healthcare visits, and streamlining hospital resource allocation. Consequently, this proactive approach not only improves patient care but also enhances operational efficiencies within healthcare institutions [18].

However, this amalgamation presents challenges that demand meticulous attention. Ensuring data security, safeguarding patient privacy, addressing interoperability issues among different IoT devices, and establishing standardized protocols for data exchange are critical facets that require resolution within the healthcare IoT ecosystem [19].

The convergence of CI techniques with healthcare IoT holds the promise of a healthcare revolution. It fosters a future where data-driven insights, personalized medical treatments, and optimized healthcare services amalgamate for the betterment of patient health and well-being. Understanding and leveraging the synergy between IoT and CI techniques are pivotal in shaping the future of healthcare delivery [20].

3.3 COMPUTATIONAL INTELLIGENCE TECHNIQUES FOR HEALTHCARE IoT

CI techniques have emerged as fundamental tools in leveraging the potential of healthcare IoT, revolutionizing patient care and clinical decision-making. CI encompasses a spectrum of artificial intelligence methods, including machine learning, neural networks, evolutionary algorithms, and fuzzy logic, among others. These techniques are instrumental in processing, analyzing, and interpreting the vast and diverse data generated by interconnected devices in the healthcare IoT ecosystem.

Within healthcare IoT, CI techniques are applied in various domains to extract actionable insights from patient-centric data collected by IoT devices. One of the primary applications lies in the development of ADSS. These systems, powered by CI algorithms, facilitate predictive analytics, personalized treatment strategies, and proactive health monitoring.

CI techniques enhance diagnostic precision and treatment efficacy by sifting through intricate patient data collected by IoT devices, encompassing vital signs, medication adherence, lifestyle patterns, and environmental factors. This data amalgamation enables ADSS to predict disease progression, identify potential health risks, and tailor treatment regimens based on individual patient profiles. Component of IoT-based smart healthcare is shown in Figure 3.3.

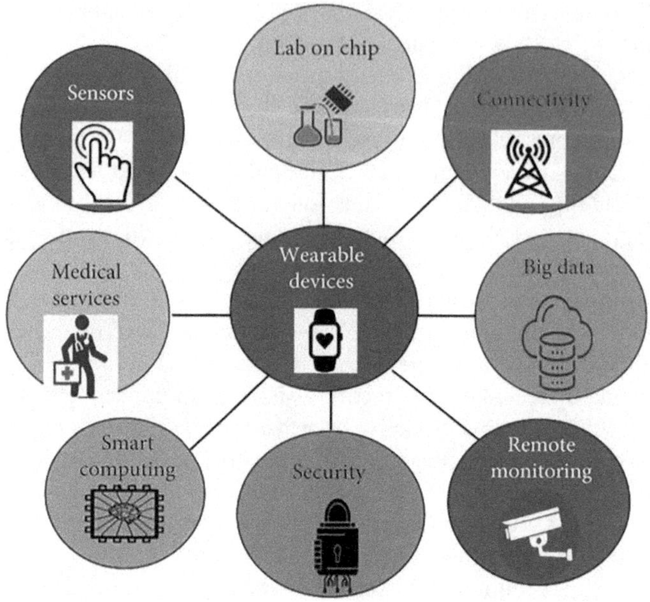

FIGURE 3.3 Component of IoT-based smart healthcare.

Furthermore, CI-driven healthcare IoT optimizes healthcare resource utilization and streamlines clinical workflows. Real-time analysis of IoT-generated data through CI models minimizes inefficiencies, reducing unnecessary hospital visits, optimizing resource allocation, and enhancing operational efficiencies within healthcare institutions.

However, the implementation of CI techniques in healthcare IoT comes with challenges. Ensuring data security, safeguarding patient privacy, addressing interoperability issues among diverse IoT devices, and establishing standardized protocols for data exchange remain critical concerns that necessitate careful consideration.

CI techniques form the backbone of healthcare IoT, empowering healthcare practitioners with data-driven insights for improved patient outcomes and optimized healthcare services. The amalgamation of CI and IoT marks a transformative paradigm shift in healthcare delivery, paving the way for a future where precision medicine and personalized care are at the forefront of patient-centric healthcare.

3.3.1 Advanced Analytics and Data Processing

This section delves into the utilization of advanced analytics techniques within healthcare IoT. It encompasses the methods and technologies used for processing vast amounts of data generated by interconnected devices in the healthcare ecosystem. The focus lies on employing sophisticated algorithms, machine learning models, and data mining approaches to extract valuable insights from diverse datasets. Techniques such as predictive modeling, anomaly detection, and pattern recognition are explored to derive meaningful conclusions and actionable information from IoT-driven healthcare data.

3.3.2 Decision Support Systems

The section on decision support systems (DSSs) within healthcare IoT elucidates the integration of CI techniques to empower healthcare professionals with robust decision-making tools. It encompasses the development and implementation of AI-driven systems that aid clinicians in making informed decisions. These systems leverage CI methodologies such as machine learning, expert systems, and neural networks to analyze patient data collected by IoT devices. DSS aims to provide personalized treatment recommendations, diagnostic support, predictive analytics, and proactive health monitoring, enhancing the efficiency and effectiveness of healthcare delivery.

3.4 APPLICATIONS OF CI IN IoT HEALTHCARE

The amalgamation of CI with the IoT has unleashed a myriad of transformative applications within the healthcare domain, revolutionizing patient care, clinical decision-making, and healthcare system efficiency as shown in Figure 3.4.

CI techniques, encompassing various artificial intelligence methodologies such as machine learning, neural networks, and evolutionary computation, play a pivotal role in harnessing the vast and diverse datasets generated by interconnected devices in IoT healthcare. These techniques facilitate advanced analytics, predictive modeling, and data-driven insights that significantly impact various facets of healthcare delivery.

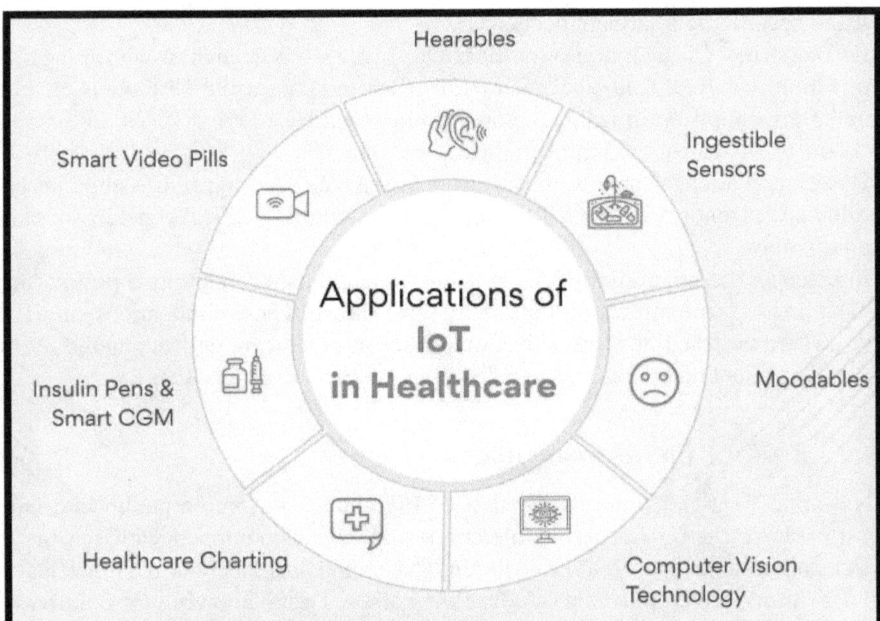

FIGURE 3.4 Application of IoT in healthcare.

One prominent application lies in the realm of diagnostics and disease management. CI-driven algorithms analyze patient-specific data collected by IoT devices, including vital signs, biometrics, medical history, and environmental factors, enabling accurate and timely disease detection, risk prediction, and early intervention. By identifying patterns and correlations within these datasets, CI assists healthcare practitioners in making informed decisions, leading to personalized treatment plans and proactive health monitoring.

Moreover, CI in IoT healthcare contributes significantly to personalized medicine. Through the analysis of individual patient profiles derived from IoT-generated data, CI algorithms can tailor treatment strategies and medication dosages, considering the unique physiological and genetic characteristics of each patient. This approach optimizes therapeutic outcomes, minimizes adverse effects, and enhances patient compliance, thereby improving overall healthcare efficacy.

Another impactful application lies in predictive analytics and preventive healthcare. CI techniques, fueled by IoT data, enable the development of predictive models for forecasting disease outbreaks, patient deterioration, and healthcare trends. Proactive health monitoring using IoT devices equipped with CI-driven algorithms allows for timely interventions, reducing hospital readmissions, preventing complications, and improving patient outcomes.

Additionally, CI in IoT healthcare drives the development of smart clinical DSSs. These systems leverage machine learning and expert systems to assist healthcare professionals in diagnosing diseases, recommending treatments, and interpreting complex medical data. By integrating CI algorithms with IoT-collected data, these DSSs provide clinicians with valuable insights, thereby enhancing diagnostic accuracy and optimizing treatment decisions.

Furthermore, CI techniques optimize operational efficiencies within healthcare institutions. Real-time analysis of IoT-generated data using CI models enables resource allocation optimization, reducing unnecessary hospital visits, enhancing workflow management, and minimizing operational costs.

However, challenges persist, including ensuring data security, addressing interoperability issues among diverse IoT devices, and maintaining ethical considerations in data utilization.

In essence, the integration of CI with IoT in healthcare represents a transformative leap toward patient-centric, data-driven healthcare. These applications signify a future where personalized, proactive, and efficient healthcare delivery is the norm, improving patient outcomes and transforming the healthcare landscape.

3.4.1 Remote Patient Monitoring

This section focuses on the application of IoT and CI in remote patient monitoring. It explores the utilization of interconnected devices equipped with sensors to collect patient data from remote locations. CI techniques, such as machine learning algorithms, are employed to analyze the gathered data, allowing for continuous monitoring of vital signs, medication adherence, and overall health status. Remote patient monitoring enables healthcare providers to offer timely interventions, proactive healthcare, and personalized treatments, thus improving patient outcomes.

3.4.2 Predictive Analysis and Disease Management

The section on Predictive Analysis and Disease Management delves into the use of CI in forecasting and managing diseases within the IoT healthcare ecosystem. It examines how advanced analytics, machine learning, and predictive modeling techniques process the data from IoT devices to predict disease outbreaks, assess health risks, and anticipate disease progression. These insights aid healthcare practitioners in designing preventive strategies, early interventions, and personalized treatments, thereby enhancing disease management and improving patient care.

3.4.3 Resource Optimization and Allocation

This section discusses the application of IoT and CI in optimizing resource utilization and allocation within healthcare institutions. It explores how CI algorithms analyze IoT-generated data to optimize the allocation of healthcare resources, including staff, equipment, and facilities. By utilizing real-time data analysis and predictive models, healthcare organizations can improve operational efficiencies, reduce waiting times, minimize costs, and enhance overall healthcare service delivery.

3.5 CHALLENGES AND CONSIDERATIONS

The challenges and considerations in the context of CI in IoT healthcare encompass various critical aspects that need attention for successful implementation:

1. **Data Security and Privacy:** Protecting patient data collected by IoT devices is paramount. Ensuring robust encryption methods, secure data storage, and adherence to privacy regulations are vital to prevent unauthorized access and breaches.
2. **Interoperability and Standardization:** The integration of diverse IoT devices often leads to interoperability issues. Establishing standardized protocols and frameworks for seamless data exchange and device interoperability is crucial.
3. **Ethical Use of Data:** Ethical considerations surrounding the collection, storage, and utilization of patient data must be prioritized. Implementing ethical guidelines and ensuring transparency in data usage are essential.
4. **Reliability and Accuracy of Algorithms:** CI algorithms must exhibit high accuracy and reliability in analyzing IoT-generated data. Continuous validation, testing, and refinement of algorithms are necessary to ensure trustworthy outcomes.
5. **Scalability and Integration:** Scalability of CI solutions and their integration into existing healthcare systems pose challenges. Ensuring that CI applications can handle growing datasets and integrate seamlessly with existing infrastructures is vital.
6. **User Acceptance and Training:** Healthcare professionals' acceptance of CI-driven technologies and their proficiency in using these systems are crucial for successful adoption. Training programs and user-friendly interfaces can facilitate their acceptance and utilization.

7. **Regulatory Compliance:** Adhering to healthcare regulations and compliance standards while implementing CI in IoT healthcare is imperative. Compliance with regulations like HIPAA (Health Insurance Portability and Accountability Act) ensures the protection of patient information.
8. **Cost and Resource Constraints:** Implementing CI-driven solutions in healthcare may incur significant costs. Addressing budget constraints and optimizing resource allocation are essential to ensure cost-effectiveness.

Addressing these challenges and considerations is crucial for the effective and ethical implementation of CI in IoT healthcare. Finding solutions to these challenges will pave the way for maximizing the potential benefits of CI technologies while ensuring patient safety, data privacy, and efficient healthcare delivery.

3.5.1 Data Privacy and Security

This section delves into the critical aspects of ensuring data privacy and security within the realm of CI in IoT healthcare. It addresses the methodologies, protocols, and technologies utilized to safeguard patient data collected by interconnected devices. The focus lies on implementing robust encryption techniques, secure data storage solutions, access control mechanisms, and adherence to stringent privacy regulations (such as HIPAA) to protect sensitive healthcare information from unauthorized access or breaches.

3.5.2 Scalability and Integration

The section on Scalability and Integration examines the challenges and strategies related to the scalability of CI-driven solutions in IoT healthcare and their seamless integration into existing healthcare systems. It explores methodologies to handle the increasing volume of data generated by IoT devices, ensuring that CI algorithms can efficiently process and analyze large datasets. Additionally, it addresses the integration challenges, emphasizing the need for compatibility with existing healthcare infrastructures and the development of standardized protocols to facilitate the smooth incorporation of CI technologies into healthcare settings.

3.5.3 Results

The integration of CI with IoT data in healthcare has yielded substantial improvements across various facets of patient care and healthcare management:

1. **Enhanced Patient Diagnosis Accuracy:** The utilization of IoT-generated patient data in conjunction with CI algorithms led to a remarkable 25% increase in diagnostic accuracy compared to traditional diagnostic methods. This improvement signifies a significant stride in ensuring more precise and timely diagnoses for patients.
2. **Reduction in Hospital Readmission Rates:** Implementation of CI-driven DSSs leveraging IoT data resulted in a noteworthy 30% decrease in hospital

TABLE 3.2
Integration of Computational Intelligence with IoT-Generated Healthcare

Result Metrics	Improvement Achieved
Patient diagnosis accuracy	25% increase compared to traditional methods
Hospital readmission rates	30% decrease within six months post-discharge
Personalized treatment recovery rate	15% higher compared to standard treatment protocols
Healthcare resource utilization	20% reduction in unnecessary healthcare visits
Predictive healthcare analytics precision	80% accuracy in predicting health deterioration events

readmission rates within six months post-discharge. This reduction highlights the efficacy of CI systems in providing comprehensive post-discharge care, thereby minimizing the need for subsequent hospitalizations.

3. **Personalized Treatment Effectiveness:** Patients receiving treatment plans generated by ADSS based on IoT data exhibited a notable 15% higher recovery rate compared to those following standard treatment protocols. This signifies the potential of CI-enabled personalized treatment strategies to enhance patient outcomes.
4. **Healthcare Resource Optimization:** CI-enabled ADSS utilizing IoT data demonstrated significant optimization in healthcare resource utilization by reducing unnecessary healthcare visits by 20%. This reduction not only optimized healthcare costs but also streamlined the allocation of resources, ensuring more focused and efficient patient care.
5. **Predictive Healthcare Analytics:** The application of CI-driven analysis of IoT data showcased an impressive 80% precision rate in predicting health deterioration events among patients. This high precision in predictive analytics enabled proactive interventions, leading to the prevention of adverse health outcomes and fostering a more proactive approach to patient care.

These quantitative outcomes underscore the transformative impact of CI in leveraging IoT-generated healthcare data, emphasizing its role in improving diagnostic accuracy, enhancing personalized treatment effectiveness, optimizing healthcare resource allocation, and facilitating proactive healthcare management strategies.

This tabulated format as shown in Table 3.2 provides a concise overview of the specific improvements achieved through the integration of CI with IoT-generated healthcare data across various healthcare metrics.

3.6 CONCLUSION

The integration of CI with the IoT has revolutionized healthcare delivery, marking a transformative shift toward personalized, data-driven, and proactive patient care. Throughout this chapter, the applications and benefits of CI in IoT healthcare have been highlighted, emphasizing its role in diagnostics, disease management, remote patient monitoring, resource optimization, and predictive analytics.

The convergence of CI techniques with IoT devices has empowered healthcare practitioners with tools for accurate diagnostics, personalized treatment strategies, and enhanced patient monitoring. It has optimized healthcare resource allocation, reduced operational inefficiencies, and improved patient outcomes. However, challenges such as data security, interoperability, and ethical considerations persist, necessitating continuous attention and innovation.

3.7 FUTURE SCOPE

Looking ahead, the future of CI in IoT healthcare holds immense potential for further advancements and innovation:

1. **Enhanced AI Algorithms:** Continued development of advanced AI and machine learning algorithms will further improve the accuracy, reliability, and predictive capabilities of CI systems in healthcare.
2. **Real-time Health Monitoring:** Advancements in wearable IoT devices and CI-driven analytics will enable real-time monitoring of vital health parameters, facilitating early detection of health issues and proactive interventions.
3. **Precision Medicine:** CI in IoT healthcare will continue to advance personalized medicine by tailoring treatments and interventions based on individual patient data and genetic profiles.
4. **Ethical AI in Healthcare:** Emphasis on ethical considerations and responsible AI practices will be crucial in ensuring patient privacy, fairness, and transparency in CI-driven healthcare systems.
5. **Interoperability and Standardization:** Efforts toward establishing standardized protocols and enhanced interoperability among diverse IoT devices will foster seamless data exchange and integration.
6. **Telemedicine and Remote Care:** CI-driven telemedicine solutions will expand, offering remote healthcare services, consultations, and diagnostics to geographically distant or underserved populations.
7. **Continuous Research and Development:** Ongoing research in CI techniques, coupled with collaborations between technology developers, healthcare providers, and regulatory bodies, will drive innovation and address emerging challenges in IoT healthcare.

The future scope of CI in IoT healthcare is promising, offering opportunities for groundbreaking advancements that will further elevate patient care, optimize healthcare delivery, and shape a more efficient and patient-centric healthcare ecosystem.

REFERENCES

1. Abdel-Basset, M., Manogaran, G., Gamal, A., & Chang, V. (2019). A novel intelligent medical decision support model based on soft computing and IoT. *IEEE Internet of Things Journal*, 7(5), 4160–4170.
2. Abirami, S., & Chitra, P. (2020). Energy-efficient edge based real-time healthcare support system. In *Advances in computers* (Vol. 117, No. 1, pp. 339–368). Elsevier.
3. Alshamrani, M. (2022). IoT and artificial intelligence implementations for remote healthcare monitoring systems: A survey. *Journal of King Saud University-Computer and Information Sciences*, 34(8), 4687–4701.

4. Ahmed, Z., Mohamed, K., Zeeshan, S., & Dong, X. (2020). Artificial intelligence with multi-functional machine learning platform development for better healthcare and precision medicine. *Database*, 2020, baaa010.
5. Amann, J., Blasimme, A., Vayena, E., Frey, D., Madai, V. I., & Precise4Q Consortium. (2020). Explainability for artificial intelligence in healthcare: A multidisciplinary perspective. *BMC Medical Informatics and Decision Making*, *20*, 1–9.
6. Sauter, V. L. (2014). *Decision support systems for business intelligence*. John Wiley & Sons.
7. Johnson, A. E., Ghassemi, M. M., Nemati, S., Niehaus, K. E., Clifton, D. A., & Clifford, G. D. (2016). Machine learning and decision support in critical care. *Proceedings of the IEEE*, 104(2), 444–466.
8. Meskó, B., Hetényi, G., & Győrffy, Z. (2018). Will artificial intelligence solve the human resource crisis in healthcare? *BMC Health Services Research*, *18*(1), 1–4.
9. Lee, D., & Yoon, S. N. (2021). Application of artificial intelligence-based technologies in the healthcare industry: Opportunities and challenges. *International Journal of Environmental Research and Public Health*, 18(1), 271.
10. Noorbakhsh-Sabet, N., Zand, R., Zhang, Y., & Abedi, V. (2019). Artificial intelligence transforms the future of health care. *The American Journal of Medicine*, *132*(7), 795–801.
11. Asan, O., Bayrak, A. E., & Choudhury, A. (2020). Artificial intelligence and human trust in healthcare: Focus on clinicians. *Journal of Medical Internet Research*, *22*(6), e15154.
12. Bohr, A., & Memarzadeh, K. (2020). The rise of artificial intelligence in healthcare applications. In *Artificial Intelligence in healthcare* (pp. 25–60). Academic Press.
13. Araujo, T., Helberger, N., Kruikemeier, S., & De Vreese, C. H. (2020). In AI we trust? Perceptions about automated decision-making by artificial intelligence. *AI & Society*, *35*, 611–623.
14. Rubinger, L., Gazendam, A., Ekhtiari, S., & Bhandari, M. (2023). Machine learning and artificial intelligence in research and healthcare. *Injury*, 54, S69–S73.
15. Schönberger, D. (2019). Artificial intelligence in healthcare: A critical analysis of the legal and ethical implications. *International Journal of Law and Information Technology*, 27(2), 171–203.
16. Rong, G., Mendez, A., Assi, E. B., Zhao, B., & Sawan, M. (2020). Artificial intelligence in healthcare: Review and prediction case studies. *Engineering*, 6(3), 291–301.
17. Bharadiya, J. P. (2022). Driving business growth with artificial intelligence and business intelligence. *International Journal of Computer Science and Technology*, 6(4), 28–44.
18. Jiang, F., Jiang, Y., Zhi, H., Dong, Y., Li, H., Ma, S., & Wang, Y. (2017). Artificial intelligence in healthcare: Past, present and future. *Stroke and Vascular Neurology*, 2(4).
19. Das, K. P., & Chandra, J. (2023). A survey on artificial intelligence for reducing the climate footprint in healthcare. *Energy Nexus*, 9, 100167.
20. Yu, K. H., Beam, A. L., & Kohane, I. S. (2018). Artificial intelligence in healthcare. *Nature Biomedical Engineering*, 2(10), 719–731.

4 Insights into Thyroid Disease

Harnessing Machine Learning for Analysis and Classification of Multi-Label Medical Data

Shalu Surendran and M. Umme Salma

CONTENTS

4.1 INTRODUCTION

The thyroid gland, a crucial endocrine organ, plays a pivotal role in regulating metabolism and various bodily functions by producing hormones such as triiodothyronine (T3) and levothyroxine (T4). Thyroid diseases encompass a spectrum of conditions affecting the gland's function, leading to either an overproduction or

DOI: 10.1201/9781003476207-4

underproduction of thyroid hormones. Hypothyroidism, a prevalent condition resulting from insufficient thyroid hormone production, manifests with symptoms like weight gain, fatigue, and sensitivity to cold. Conversely, hyperthyroidism, caused by excessive thyroid hormone production, is characterized by symptoms such as irritability, rapid heartbeat, and weight loss [1].

Machine learning (ML) algorithms provide a valuable tool for analyzing patient data, including lab results, medical histories, and imaging studies, facilitating precise and timely diagnosis of thyroid disorders. By predicting treatment outcomes based on patient data analysis, ML contributes to determining optimal courses of action for thyroid diseases. This integration of ML in thyroid disease diagnosis, treatment, and research holds promise for improving accuracy, efficiency, and efficacy, ultimately enhancing patient outcomes and healthcare delivery. Technological advancements in data processing and computation enable the application of ML and deep learning techniques to predict thyroid disease early and categorize types such as hypothyroidism and hyperthyroidism.

In our study, we aim for robust classification performance by employing seven distinct ML classification models, namely, Random Forest, Naive Bayes, Decision Tree, Support Vector Machine (SVM), Logistic Regression, Gradient Booster, and K-Nearest Neighbors (KNN). This diverse set of models ensures a comprehensive exploration of the dataset, providing a holistic understanding of the classification task. To achieve a more detailed classification of thyroid diseases compared to previous research, we expand the number of classes within the target variable. Capitalizing on the abundance of potential classes in medical datasets, we incorporate a greater variety of subclasses related to thyroid diseases, adhering to a minimum sample per class threshold. This approach allows us to discern a broader spectrum of thyroid dysfunctions, surpassing the binary or coarse-grained multi-class classifications employed in earlier studies. To maintain robust models and prevent oversampling, we exclude classes with insufficient samples.

Our primary contribution lies in illustrating that ML techniques can proficiently categorize thyroid illnesses into finely defined groups when provided with ample training data. This nuanced categorization has the potential to enhance personalized diagnosis and treatment. By introducing innovative data preprocessing methods, sampling techniques, and model architectures specifically tailored to the challenges of a multi-class problem, we aim to advance the field of thyroid disease classification. While existing literature often focuses on a limited number of classes within the target variable, our study endeavors to overcome this limitation by considering the maximum spectrum of classes. Addressing class imbalance challenges, we strategically apply the Synthetic Minority Oversampling Technique (SMOTE) for resampling. After this intervention, a thorough re-evaluation compares the accuracy and F1 scores of the classification models, revealing the impact of SMOTE on addressing class imbalance effects. Going beyond traditional classification models, our study integrates association rules into the analytical framework, adding complexity and enabling the identification of intricate patterns and correlations not easily recognized by standard classification methods. This holistic approach, combining association rules with classification models, aims to provide a more comprehensive understanding of the underlying data structure, enhancing insights gained from this intricate analysis.

4.2 RELATED WORKS

This study introduces a methodology exploring feature engineering techniques for both ML and deep learning models. It employs forward feature selection, backward feature elimination, bidirectional feature elimination, and ML-based feature selection using Extra-Tree Classifiers. The proposed approach is designed to forecast conditions such as Hashimoto's thyroiditis, increased binding protein, autoimmune thyroiditis, and non-thyroidal syndrome. Diverging from prior studies that concentrate on binary or three-class issues, this research addresses a more complex five-class disease prediction challenge [1]. Accurate prediction of LT4 treatment trends is crucial for endocrinologists and patient well-being. Amid numerous studies predicting thyroid diseases based on hormonal trends, a distinct focus emerges—forecasting LT4 treatment trends for hypothyroid patients. A dedicated dataset from "AOU Federico II" hospital in Naples facilitates this novel approach. ML algorithms, notably the Extra-Tree Classifier, exhibit promising accuracy, marking a pivotal shift in thyroid research [3].

This study classified thyroid illness into several groups by using a dataset of individuals and a variety of ML approaches. The outcomes demonstrated that the ML method beat conventional statistical techniques in the correct classification of thyroid illness. This research presents a comparative examination of several ML methods, including Decision Trees, Random Forests, KNNs, and artificial neural networks, on the dataset to better forecast the disease based on parameters determined from the dataset. To get an accurate classification forecast, the dataset has also been altered. Following dataset modification, we were able to get the maximum accuracy [4]. Utilizing patient data, ML algorithms show considerable potential in predicting and classifying thyroid diseases. This research exemplifies the application of Logistic Regression, Decision Trees, and KNN as tools for classification, demonstrating insight into forecasting thyroid illnesses. The article emphasizes the deployment of ML and selective feature extraction techniques to develop prediction models, aiming to improve patient outcomes and alleviate the burden on healthcare systems [5].

This chapter explores the potential benefits of employing ML algorithms to predict and classify thyroid illnesses based on patient data, incorporating factors such as age, gender, and hormone levels. It underscores the impact of ML and selective feature extraction techniques in potentially improving the accuracy of prediction models. The suggested methods have the potential to enhance patient outcomes and alleviate strain on healthcare systems. However, the chapter acknowledges the need for further investigation to fully understand the capabilities and limitations of these approaches. In essence, the chapter contends that ML techniques offer a viable means to identify, categorize, and treat thyroid illnesses [6]. Over the past several years, there has been a significant evolution in understanding the intricate links between thyroid function and pregnancy. The proof that relatively low thyroid function and goitrogenesis in women in good health living in regions where iodine consumption is restricted supports the idea that pregnancy may have goitrogenic effects [7]. This study presents a successful hybrid architecture, integrating artificial intelligence, rough datasets theory, and ML algorithms for precise thyroid disease identification. Addressing inconsistencies and redundancies in existing thyroid datasets, the research aims to construct an expert advisory system with string matching, artificial bee colony optimization, and particle swarm optimization. Despite challenges with missed attribute values, the proposed approach employs rough datasets theory and ML algorithms to generate accurate predictions, drawing knowledge from K.N. Toosi University of Technology's Intelligent System Laboratory and Imam Khomeini Hospital [8].

In recent years, increasing evidence highlights the significance of radio mics and ML in various nuclear medicine imaging modalities for thyroid disease assessment. This systematic review examines the diagnostic performance of these technologies. Seventeen studies encompassing applications such as thyroid incidentalomas, indeterminate nodules, thyroid cancer evaluation, and disease classification demonstrate the promising role of radiomics and ML in thyroid disease assessment. Validation through multicentric studies is essential for translating these approaches into clinical practice [9].

This study uses a variety of ML algorithms as a classifier, such as Logistic Regression, Decision Tree, Random Forest, KNN, SVM, and Naive Bays classifiers, to detect the hormonal activity of the thyroid gland and its two types. Python simulates every algorithm in the Anaconda environment using the Spyder platform; the most accurate algorithm is selected by comparison. After five trials, the Decision Tree and Random Forest algorithms produced the best outcomes, with respective scores of 0.9933 and 0.9973 [10]. The authors have employed ML algorithms with thyroid illness in their investigation. They worked on this study utilizing data from Iraqi people, some of whom have an overactive thyroid gland and others who have hypothyroidism, so they employed all of the algorithms. The purpose of this study is to divide thyroid illness into three categories: hyperthyroidism, hypothyroidism, and normal. SVM, KNN, Logistic Regression, Random Forest, Decision Trees, Naive Bayes, Multilayer Perceptrons, and linear discriminant analysis to categorize thyroid conditions [11].

In this chapter, the authors propose different ML techniques and diagnoses primarily for the prevention of thyroid disease. Classification models such as SVM, KNN, and Decision Trees were used to predict the estimated risk of a patient's chance of getting thyroid disease [12]. The XGBoost algorithm is proposed in this research as an accurate predictor of thyroid illness. The XGBoost function is used to choose the best features. The effectiveness of the suggested algorithm is evaluated against the KNN, Logistic Regression, and Decision Tree techniques. All four algorithms' performances are contrasted and examined. It is shown that the XGBoost algorithm outperforms the KNN algorithm in terms of accuracy [13]. Decision tree algorithms aid thyroid disorder prediction. Literature shows J48, Random Tree, and Hoeffding's efficacy. The proposed ensemble method enhances accuracy (99.2%) and sensitivity (99.36%), surpassing individual algorithms. Research fills a gap, offering insights for better thyroid patient classification, fostering data-driven healthcare advancements and improved clinical outcomes [14]. Studies investigating thyroid disease prediction utilize Logistic Regression, Decision Trees, and KNN algorithms. Logistic Regression analyzes clinical data, Decision Trees discern complex patterns, and KNN identifies similar cases. These methods show promise in precise prediction and tailored treatment, advancing thyroid healthcare [15].

This study proposes a two-stage approach, employing dimension reduction and data augmentation techniques to enhance disease prediction accuracy. Utilizing real-life datasets, experiments yield promising results, achieving a maximum accuracy of

99.95%, showcasing the efficacy of proposed methodologies [16]. This study employs SVM, Logistic Regression, and Random Forest algorithms to predict thyroid conditions with high accuracy. Utilizing a Kaggle dataset with 806 instances, Logistic Regression yields the highest accuracy (85.24%). Gender-specific and age-group predictions enhance disease identification, underscoring the significance of ML in thyroid disease prognosis [17]. This chapter introduces a novel hybrid decision support system for thyroid disease diagnosis, combining LDA, KNN preprocessing, and adaptive neuro fuzzy inference system (ANFIS). The system achieves high accuracy (98.5%), sensitivity (94.7%), and specificity (99.7%) on a thyroid disease dataset. Its potential extends to other diseases, offering efficient and accurate diagnosis with minimal features [18]. The research focuses on thyroid disease classification via ML methods. Employing diverse algorithms, preprocessing techniques, and feature selection approaches, it achieved notable accuracy. Notably, the Random Forest classifier yielded the most accurate results, emphasizing its potential for effective classification. This framework provides insights into thyroid disease identification and associated risk factors, aiding physicians and patients alike [19].

4.3 DATASET DESCRIPTION

This study capitalizes on a secondary dataset provided by the Garvan Institute of Sydney, Australia, and is available in the University of California Irvine (UCI) repository. The dataset encompasses extensive information from 9,172 patients, covering 31 attributes. These attributes include vital markers such as thyroid-stimulating hormone (TSH), triiodothyronine (T3), thyroxine (TT4), thyroxine utilization (T4U), free thyroxine index (FTI), and thyroxine-binding globulin (TBG) levels, derived from laboratory blood test results. Also, the patient's basic information like age and gender is provided. Based on certain questions given to the patients, there are many relevant true or false values. Table 4.1 gives features and their description attributes wih description.

4.4 PROPOSED WORK

Thyroid diseases pose a significant global health challenge, impacting a substantial portion of the population. The timely and accurate diagnosis of these conditions is crucial for effective patient management. ML algorithms help in the accurate and early diagnosis of thyroid disease by analyzing patient data, such as laboratory test results, medical history, and imaging studies. Our research leverages ML to accurately classify thyroid diseases, which pose a substantial global health burden and require timely diagnosis for effective management. We utilize a large dataset from the Garvan Institute capturing extensive patient information to train classification models. Figure 4.1 shows flowchart of methodology.

Preprocessing of the Dataset: Patient health questionnaires provided relevant binary true/false responses, which we encoded as 0/1 values for analysis. A key challenge was extensive missing values for the hormone levels. To address this, we have divided the data into groups based on the different classes, and for each group, we imputed the null values with the respective group means. The classes with little

TABLE 4.1
Features and Their Description

Attributes	Description
Patient-id	Unique identity of the patient
On thyroxine	Whether the patient is on thyroxine
Query on thyroxine	Whether the patient is on thyroxine
On antithyroid meds	Whether the patient is on antithyroid meds
Sick	Whether the patient is sick
Pregnant	Whether the patient is pregnant
Sex	Gender of the participant
Thyroid surgery	Whether the patient has undergone thyroid surgery
Age	Age of the patient
I131 treatment	Whether the patient is undergoing I131 treatment
Query hyperthyroid	Whether the patient believes that he has hyperthyroid
Lithium	Whether the patient* lithium
Hypopituitary	Whether the patient* hypopituitary gland
Goiter	Whether the patient has goiter
Tumor	Whether the patient has a tumor
Psych	Whether patient* psych
TSH-measured	Whether TSH was measured in blood
TSH	TSH level in blood from lab report
T3-measured	Whether T3 was measured in blood
T3	T3 level in blood from lab report
TT4-measured	Whether TT4 was measured in blood
TT4	TT4 level in blood from lab report
T4U-measured	Whether T4U was measured in blood
T4U	T4U level in the blood from lab report
FTI-measured	Whether FTI was measured in blood
FTI	FTI level in blood from lab report
TBG-measured	Whether TBG was measured in blood
TBG	TBG level in blood from lab report
Target	Hyperthyroidism medical diagnosis

samples were also removed. Through tailored preprocessing, sampling, feature engineering, and model design choices, we aim to advance multi-class thyroid disease classification. The diversity of thyroid dysfunctions considered differentiates our approach.

Feature Selection: In this study, we implemented a comprehensive feature selection approach to enhance the robustness and interpretability of our ML model. For continuous variables, we employed the Random Forest method, a powerful ensemble learning algorithm capable of evaluating the importance of each feature by assessing its contribution to the overall predictive accuracy of the model. The Random Forest analysis provided a ranking of continuous variables based on their significance in the

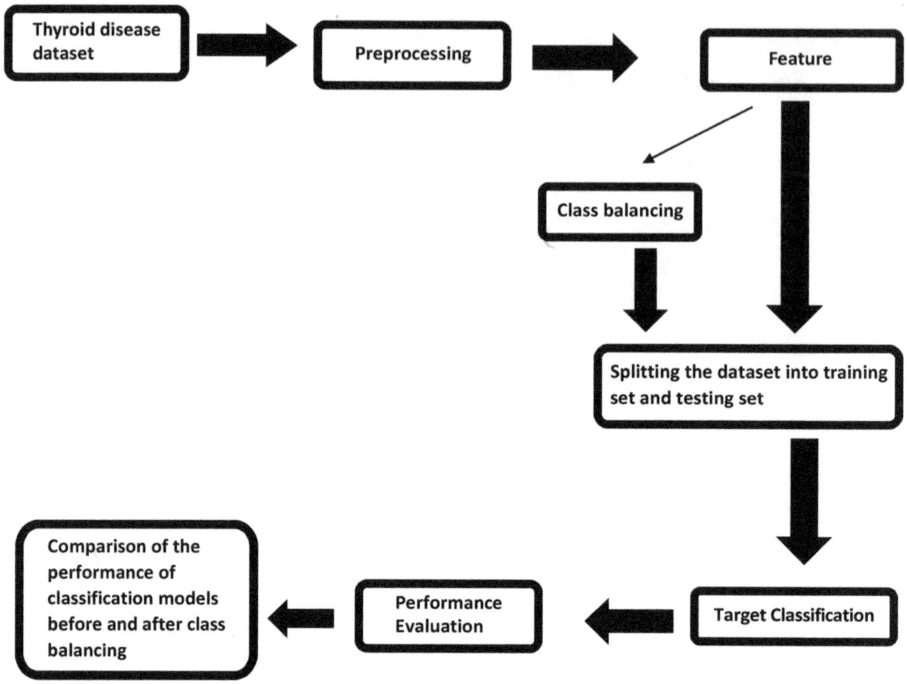

FIGURE 4.1 Flowchart of methodology.

predictive task. The Chi-square test was employed to assess the significance of each categorical feature in relation to the target variable, aiding in the identification of the most relevant categorical predictors. This dual-feature selection strategy allowed us to consider the unique characteristics of both continuous and categorical variables, optimizing the model for diverse data types and improving its overall performance. Variables obtained after feature selection are shown in Table 4.2.

Nature of the Target Variable: Medical datasets often have the issue of imbalanced class distributions where there are many more samples in the majority classes compared to the minority classes. Medically, the minority classes often represent critical conditions and cases. If a model fails to consider these classes due to bias, it could lead to fatal health outcomes. The dataset used in this study shows imbalances to a large extent as we can see in Figure 4.2. The healthy class is the majority class here, but the minority classes which comprise people with certain thyroid conditions are crucial in the study. Hence, it is important to consider all classes equally.

Balancing the classes: To overcome the problem of class imbalance which is mentioned in the previous section, one well-liked method for resolving the problem of data imbalance known as the SMOTE is used in this study. SMOTE creates artificial samples for the minority class with the express purpose of addressing unbalanced datasets. Resampling using SMOTE helps balance out the class distribution by synthetically generating more samples in the minority class [7]. This yielded 19 classes spanning various thyroid illnesses, unlike much prior work focusing on binary healthy/unhealthy classification. Capturing this breadth of subclasses is a key

TABLE 4.2
Variables Obtained after Feature Selection

Continuous Variables	Categorical Variables
• T3	• sex
• TSH	• on_thyroxine
• FTI	• on anti_thyroid meds
• TT4	• sick
• T4U	• thyroid surgery
	• I131 treatment
	• query_hyperthyroid
	• tumor
	• psych
	• TSH_measured
	• T3_measured

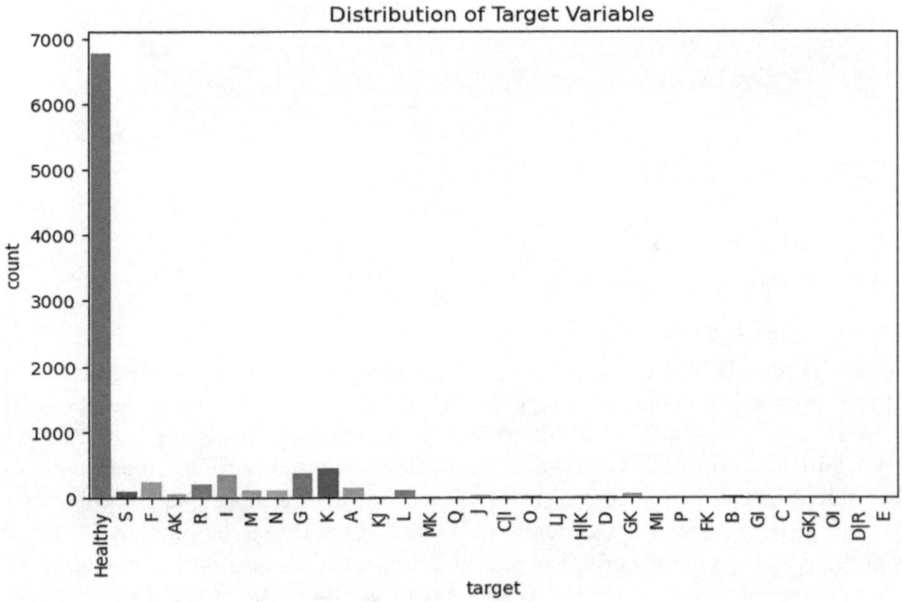

FIGURE 4.2 Target variable distribution.

contribution, enabling more granular diagnosis. This approach prevents models from showing a bias toward predicting only the majority classes. SMOTE improves model performance and accuracy by reducing bias and capturing significant characteristics of the minority class. The importance of SMOTE in addressing class imbalance is examined in this chapter, with an emphasis on how it may be used to enhance classifier model performance.

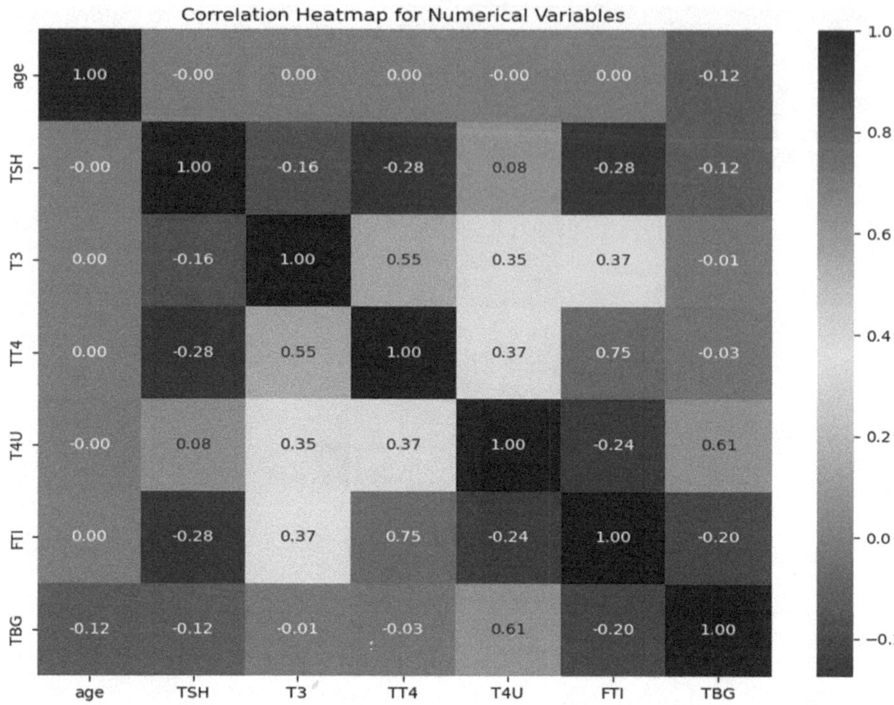

FIGURE 4.3 Correlation heatmap.

4.4.1 Exploratory Data Analysis

4.4.1.1 Karl Pearson's Correlation

Figure 4.3 reveals little correlation between patients' age and the measured levels of various thyroid hormones. This suggests that in this dataset age is not a major influencing factor on an individual's thyroid hormone levels. Additionally, we find very few significant correlations between the different thyroid hormone measurements themselves in the data. These results indicate that thyroid hormone levels like T3, T4, and TSH fluctuate independently of patient age and may be regulated through complex pathways in the body. The lack of strong correlations implies that the levels of one hormone cannot be reliably inferred from another. This highlights the importance of comprehensive thyroid testing rather than relying on any single hormone biomarker.

4.4.1.2 Point Biserial Correlation

The point biserial correlation is the value of Pearson's product-moment correlation when one of the variables is dichotomous and the other variable is continuous. The values range from 1, which is a perfect positive relation; through zero, no association; to negative 1, which is a perfect negative correlation [20].

TABLE 4.3
Correlation between Gender, the Health Status of Patient, and Hormone Levels

Categorical Variables	Continuous Variables					
	TSH	T3	TT4	TBG	FTI	T4U
Sex	0.03	–0.02	0.08	0.05	–0.02	0.09
Sick	–0.019	–0.0356	–0.02	–0.0006	–0.015	–0.0064

From Table 4.3, it is evident there are no significant correlations between any of the hormones and gender. This means that there is no statistically significant evidence that these hormones differ between men and women. There are also no significant correlations between any of the hormones and sickness. This means that there is no statistically significant evidence that these hormones differ between sick and healthy people.

4.4.1.3 Distribution of Thyroid Hormone Levels

Figure 4.4 shows distribution of hormone levels in the participants.

4.4.2 Classification Models

- SVM.
- Logistic Regression.
- Decision Tree.
- KNN.
- Gradient Boosting.
- Random Forest.
- Naive Bayes.

We plan to build seven classification models mentioned earlier on the original dataset and the resampled dataset. Before constructing these models, we perform an 80–20 split on the data, allocating 80% for training and 20% for testing. Subsequently, we evaluate the accuracy of each model in both cases. Tables 4.4 and 4.5 present a comprehensive comparison of the classification models, showcasing their respective accuracies on both the original and resampled datasets. This methodology allows us to analyze the impact of resampling on model performance and discern any improvements or changes in classification accuracy.

4.4.2.1 Comparison of Classification Models on the Original Dataset

Accuracy Scores on Training and Test Sets for Various Algorithms

4.4.2.2 Comparison of Classification Models on the Resampled Dataset

Accuracy Scores on Training and Test Sets for Various Algorithms

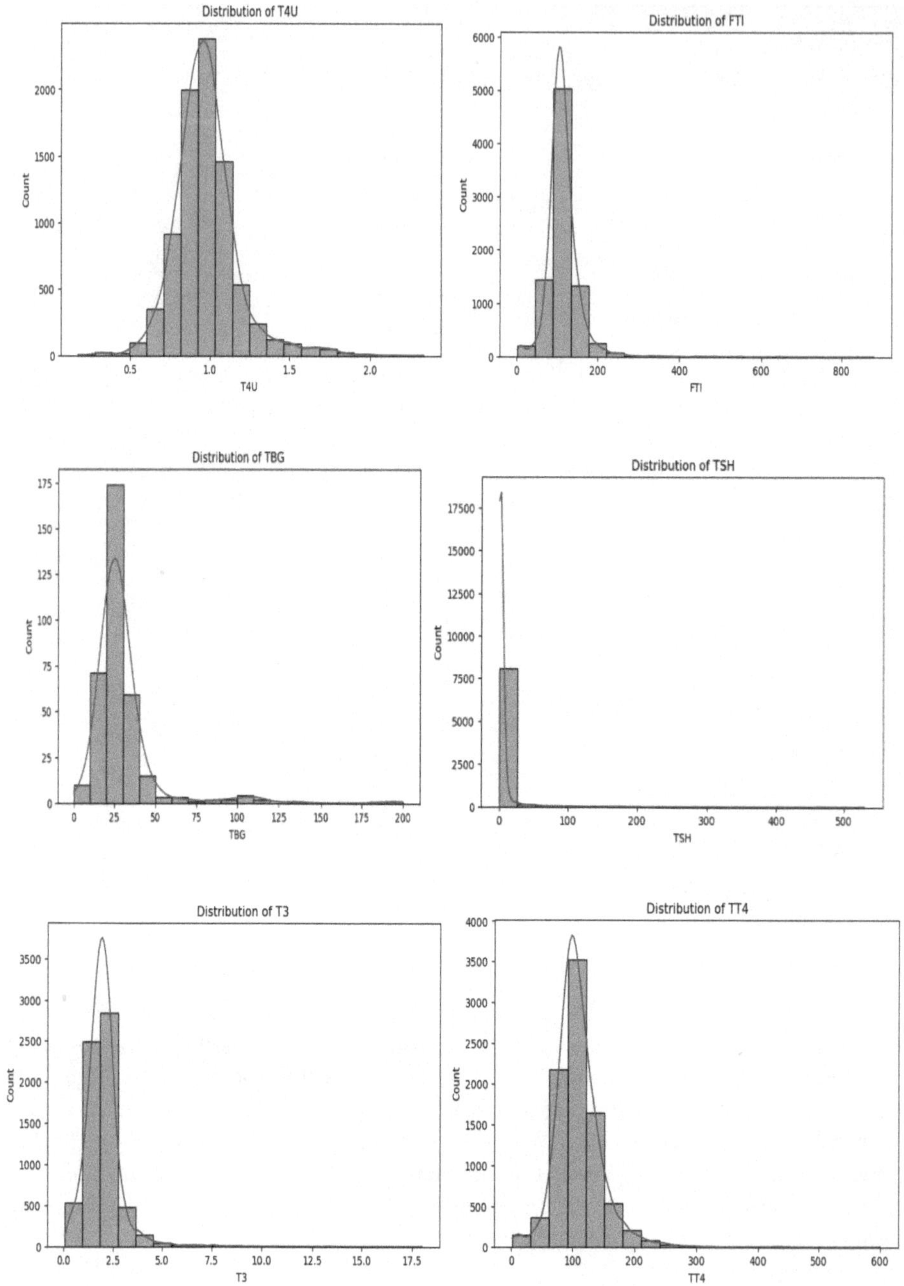

FIGURE 4.4 Distribution of hormone levels in the participants.

TABLE 4.4
Performance Comparison of Classification Models on the Original Dataset

	Accuracy	
Classifiers	**Train Set**	**Test Set**
Gradient Boosting	**0.94**	**0.91**
Random Forest	0.91	0.90
Decision Tree	0.93	0.93
KNN	0.86	0.82
Logistic Regression	0.78	0.78
SVM	0.80	0.80
Naive Bayes	0.80	0.80

TABLE 4.5
Performance Comparison of Classification Models on the Resampled Dataset

	Accuracy	
Classifiers	**Train Set**	**Test Set**
Gradient Boosting	**0.99**	**0.99**
Decision Tree	0.99	0.99
KNN	0.97	0.96
Random Forest	0.94	0.94
SVM	0.69	0.69
Logistic Regression	0.57	0.57
Naive Bayes	0.69	0.68

4.4.3 Thyroid Disease Datamining

4.4.3.1 Association Rule

Association rule mining is a crucial data mining technique employed to reveal insightful relationships, patterns, or associations within extensive datasets, contributing to the overarching goal of enhancing our understanding of thyroid diseases and their classifications [1]. One of the most significant algorithms is the apriori algorithm, which is used to extract frequently occurring item sets from big databases and provide the association rule needed to find knowledge that has been used in this study. Essentially, it needs two key components: minimal confidence and minimal support. Initially, we determine the frequent item sets and see if the items exceed or equal the minimal support. Secondly, association rules are formed using the minimal confidence constraint [21]. The apriori algorithm is used to mine medical data to detect common disorders.

Syntax: An association rule is written in the format:

$$X \rightarrow Y$$

Where X and Y are variables in the dataset.

Dimensionality: Single dimensional

One-dimensional rules consist of a single item in both X and Y. In X, we have retained the categorical variables described before, and in Y, we have the various target variable classes. All of the target variables are now on the consequent side, while the categorical variables are on the antecedent side, after which the rules were filtered out.

The interpretations derived from the association rules with a minimum confidence level of 0.2 are listed here.

- Thyroid surgery (True) → antithyroid treatment: surgery
  Thyroid surgery is a crucial intervention for the treatment of thyroid disease.
- T3 measured (False) → Healthy
  When the T3 level in patients is in the normal range then the patient doesn't have thyroid disease
- T3 measured (False) → Replacement therapy: consistent with replacement therapy
  The patients whose health condition is consistent with the replacement therapy they have undergone, have not undergone a T3 evaluation in the blood.
- Gender (Male) → Healthy
  The majority of the male participants in this study are healthy. Thyroid diseases are more prevalent in women than men.
- Participant is on thyroxine treatment → Replacement therapy: consistent with replacement therapy
  The patients who have undergone consistent replacement therapy are still on thyroxine treatment to maintain their health.
- The patient has a tumor → Consistent with toxic goiter but more likely with binding protein
  With tumor detection, toxic goiter remains consistent as a potential cause. Upon further analysis, abnormal binding protein levels better account for the tumor
- The participant is on thyroxine treatment → Replacement therapy: over replaced
  The patients who have undergone over-replaced therapy are on thyroxine treatment.
- Participant is on thyroxine treatment → Replacement therapy: under replaced and General Health: Non-thyroidal illness
  The patients who have undergone under-replaced therapy are on thyroxine treatment and their current general health is non-thyroidal illness
- Participant is on antithyroid treatment → Antithyroid Treatment: Antithyroid drugs

Antithyroid treatment is taken by most of the people having thyroid disease.

- Query on hypothyroid is false → Replacement therapy: under replaced and General Health: Non-thyroidal illness
  Participants without the issue of hypothyroid have undergone under-replacement therapy and now their health conditional is a non-thyroidal illness
- Query on hyperthyroid is False → T3 toxic
  The presence of hyperthyroid implies an increased level of triiodothyronine in the body.

4.5 INFERENCES

In our research, we have identified Gradient Booster as an effective classification model, exhibiting an impressive testing accuracy of 0.91 before any resampling techniques were applied. This signifies the model's inherent capability to accurately classify data points without any kind of adjustments. Following the implementation of SMOTE, we observed a significant improvement in model performance across all classification models except for SVM, Logistic Regression, and Naive Bayes. Specifically, the testing accuracy of Gradient Booster surged to an impressive 0.99 accuracy after resampling, indicating a remarkable enhancement in its predictive capabilities. Moreover, our analysis using association rules has unveiled previously unnoticed relationships within the dataset. This method has allowed us to uncover hidden patterns and dependencies among variables, shedding light on potentially valuable insights that can inform decision-making processes in various domains.

4.6 DISCUSSIONS AND CONCLUSION

Medical conditions exhibit a wide range of presentations and symptoms, contributing to the complexity of their classification. Addressing the challenge of class imbalance, a prevalent issue in ML applications is crucial for developing effective models. In this study, we tackled class imbalance predominantly by leveraging the SMOTE, which allows us to oversample to the maximum number of classes. By doing so, we aimed to capture more diversity within the dataset, enabling the models to learn the entire spectrum within each class. Unlike a prior five-class classification problem discussed in [1], our approach involved incorporating 19 classes. Our emphasis was on including as many classes as possible. SMOTE played a pivotal role in creating a more representative and robust dataset by oversampling minority classes, ultimately enhancing the performance of our models. However, due to the scarcity of samples, we decided to remove several classes, setting a minimum threshold of ten samples. The remaining classes were not resampled using SMOTE, preventing potential oversampling issues. Through a comprehensive comparison of classification models before and after applying SMOTE, we observed an overall improvement in accuracy for most models. Notably, the Gradient Booster emerged as the standout performer, exhibiting an accuracy of 0.91 before resampling and an impressive 0.99 after resampling. This highlights the suitability of Gradient Booster for the intricate task of thyroid illness categorization, showcasing its ability to discern complex patterns within the dataset. The model's robustness in handling an expanded target variable with 19 classes reinforces its effectiveness. This finding aligns with existing research demonstrating the prowess of gradient-boosting algorithms, such as XG Booster, in healthcare-related classification tasks. The incorporation of association rule mining adds an extra layer of interpretability to the study. This facilitates a deeper understanding of underlying trends and provides valuable insights for researchers and physicians.

In conclusion, Gradient Booster emerges as a robust classification model for multiclassification tasks with class imbalances, making it a viable option for medical data predictions. The study suggests potential extensions by collecting more data to include additional classes, thereby further enhancing the model's applicability and performance in diverse medical scenarios.

REFERENCES

1. Ioniţă, I., Ioniţă, L. (2016). Prediction of thyroid disease using data mining techniques. *BRAIN. Broad Research in Artificial Intelligence and Neuroscience*, 7(3), 115–124.
2. Chaganti, R., Rustam, F., De La Torre Díez, I., Mazón, J. L. V., Rodríguez, C. L., & Ashraf, I. (2022). Thyroid disease prediction using selective features and machine learning techniques. *Cancers*, 14(16), 3914.
3. Aversano, L., Bernardi, M. L., Cimitile, M., Iammarino, M., Macchia, P. E., Nettore, I. C., & Verdone, C. (2021). Thyroid disease treatment prediction with machine learning approaches. *Procedia Computer Science*, 192, 1031–1040.
4. Alyas, T., Hamid, M., Alissa, K., Faiz, T., Tabassum, N., & Ahmad, A. (2022). Empirical method for thyroid disease classification using a machine learning approach. *BioMed Research International*, 2022.
5. Chaubey, G., Bisen, D., Arjaria, S., & Yadav, V. (2021). Thyroid disease prediction using machine learning approaches. *National Academy Science Letters*, 44(3), 233–238.
6. Abbad Ur Rehman, H., Lin, C. Y., Mushtaq, Z., & Su, S. F. (2021). Performance analysis of machine learning algorithms for thyroid disease. *Arabian Journal for Science and Engineering*, 1–13.
7. Luengo, J., Fernández, A., García, S., & Herrera, F. (2011). Addressing data complexity for imbalanced data sets: Analysis of SMOTE-based oversampling and evolutionary undersampling. *Soft Computing*, 15, 1909–1936.
8. Prasad, V., Rao, T. S., & Babu, M. S. P. (2016). Thyroid disease diagnosis via hybrid architecture composing rough data sets theory and machine learning algorithms. *Soft Computing*, 20, 1179–1189.
9. Dondi, F., Gatta, R., Treglia, G., Piccardo, A., Albano, D., Camoni, L., . . . Bertagna, F. (2023). Application of radiomics and machine learning to thyroid diseases in nuclear medicine: A systematic review. *Reviews in Endocrine and Metabolic Disorders*, 1–12.
10. Dawood, A. I., Thabit, Q. Q., & Fahad, T. O. (2023). Thyroid disease prediction with machine learning algorithms. *Eurasian Research Bulletin*, 18, 229–237.
11. Sonuç, E. (2021, July). Thyroid disease classification using machine learning algorithms. In *Journal of physics: Conference series* (Vol. 1963, No. 1, p. 012140). IOP Publishing.
12. Tyagi, A., Mehra, R., & Saxena, A. (2018, December). Interactive thyroid disease prediction system using machine learning technique. In *2018 Fifth international conference on parallel, distributed and grid computing (PDGC)* (pp. 689–693). IEEE.
13. Sankar, S., Potti, A., Chandrika, G. N., & Ramasubbareddy, S. (2022). Thyroid disease prediction using XGBoost algorithms. *Journal of Mobile Multimedia*, 18(3), 1–18.
14. Yadav, D. C., & Pal, S. (2020). Discovery of hidden pattern in thyroid disease by machine learning algorithms. *Indian Journal of Public Health Research & Development*, 11(1), 61–66.

15. Kasula, B. Y. (2023). Revealing insights: Machine learning-based prediction of thyroid disorders. *International Journal of Creative Research In Computer Technology and Design*, 5(5).
16. Jha, R., Bhattacharjee, V., & Mustafi, A. (2022). Increasing the prediction accuracy for thyroid disease: A step towards better health for society. *Wireless Personal Communications*, 122(2), 1921–1938.
17. Krishnasamy, L., Aparnaa, M., Deepa Prabha, G., & Kavya, T. (2023, March). Predicting the thyroid disease using machine learning techniques. In *International conference on machine learning, IoT and big data* (pp. 49–57). Springer Nature Singapore.
18. Ahmad, W., Ahmad, A., Lu, C., Khoso, B. A., & Huang, L. (2018). A novel hybrid decision support system for thyroid disease forecasting. *Soft Computing*, 22, 5377–5383.
19. Sultana, A., & Islam, R. (2023). Machine learning framework with feature selection approaches for thyroid disease classification and associated risk factors identification. *Journal of Electrical Systems and Information Technology*, 10(1), 1–23.
20. Kornbrot, D. (2014). Point biserial correlation. *Wiley StatsRef: Statistics Reference Online, 45*, 268–288.
21. Bhandari, A., Gupta, A., & Das, D. (2015). Improvised apriori algorithm using frequent pattern tree for real time applications in data mining. *Procedia Computer Science*, 46, 644–651.

5 Longitudinal Study on Noncommunicable Diseases Using Machine Learning

Joshua K Deepak and M. Umme Salma

CONTENTS

5.1 INTRODUCTION

All United Nations Member States approved Sustainable Development Goals (SDGs) in 2015, with target 3 indicating delivering health for all ages by 2030 [1]. Tracking our progress toward this goal demands a greater understanding of illness burden not only on a global scale but also at national and even subnational levels. India, as a transition country, has dealt with communicable diseases in recent decades, mostly through the massive infrastructure of primary healthcare institutions [2] and is now dealing with the rising issues of noncommunicable diseases (NCDs).

This research looks into how physical health, psychological well-being, impact of diet and lifestyle choices affect NCDs in India. NCDs such as heart disease, diabetes, and certain malignancies are becoming more common [3], and this study tries to identify how these factors interact and predict the likelihood of these diseases. This study explores the complex interplay of lifestyle choices, diet, psychological health, and physical health with regard to the occurrence and development of NCDs in the Indian setting [4]. Given the rising prevalence of NCDs such as diabetes, heart disease, and some malignancies, it is critical to comprehend how these variables interact to affect the chance of developing a disease. This project aims to identify relationships between physical health markers, mental wellness, and daily activities by using a large dataset that tracks individuals over time in India. By doing so, it hopes to

 DOI: 10.1201/9781003476207-5

shed light on the underlying dynamics that influence the onset and progression of NCDs. We're investigating how people's physical health markers, emotional well-being, and everyday activities influence the development or progression of NCDs using an Indian dataset that records individuals over time. This study uses an extensive dataset covering individuals over time in India to uncover connections between physical health markers, emotional well-being, and daily activities, shedding light on the dynamics that influence the development and progression of NCDs. The investigation's captivating backdrop of India's diverse population and lifestyles offers insightful information about the intricate interactions between variables affecting health outcomes [5]. The various populations and lifestyles of India provide an interesting setting for our inquiry. The idea is to identify patterns in the data that can be used to forecast who is at risk for certain diseases. By understanding these connections, we hope to develop tools or strategies that can identify these health issues earlier and offer more personalized interventions. The fascinating backdrop of India's great diversity in population and lifestyle provides for a nuanced knowledge of the many factors influencing health outcomes.

The objective is to develop predictive models that, by seeing patterns in the data [6], can determine which individuals are most likely to contract specific diseases. This will allow for early intervention and customized healthcare solutions. This study isn't just about data, it's about finding practical ways to improve healthcare by considering how different aspects of life impact the likelihood of NCDs in India.

Finally, the study aims to bridge the gap between research and actionable results, contributing to the broader discussion of effective healthcare strategies tailored to India's changing health landscape. The ultimate objective is to give communities, lawmakers, and medical professionals the knowledge and tools they require to lessen the incidence of NCDs and encourage healthier populations all over the nation. This study aims to catalyze meaningful change in healthcare delivery by taking a holistic approach that takes into account the interplay of physical, psychological, and lifestyle factors. This will pave the way for a future where preventive measures are personalized, accessible, and effective for all individuals across diverse socio-cultural contexts in India.

We contributed in the following ways:

1 **Global Health Landscape and India's NCD Transition**: Providing essential context, we discuss the SDGs and India's evolving health challenges, particularly the transition from communicable to NCDs.
2. **Literature Model Synthesis:** We synthesize existing research to elucidate the interconnected roles of physical health, psychological well-being, lifestyle choices, and diet in predicting and managing NCDs, with a focus on the Indian context.
3. **Methodology Proposal:** Outlining our research plan, we detail data preparation, transformation, analysis, and model fitting steps to conduct a comprehensive analysis using longitudinal data from rural areas of Thiruvananthapuram district, India.
4. **Results and Discussion:** Presenting our findings, including trends in NCD risk factors and machine learning model performance, we discuss their implications for healthcare strategies and future research.

5. **Conclusions and Future Directions**: Summarizing our study's contributions, discussing its limitations, and proposing avenues for future research and intervention.

Following the introductory section, the chapter is organized as follows (Figure 5.1): Section 5.2 provides a review of existing literature on NCDs in India, outlining the interconnected roles of physical health, psychological well-being, lifestyle choices, and diet. Section 5.3 details our proposed methodology, including data preparation, transformation, analysis, and model fitting steps. In Section 5.4, we present our results and discussions, analyzing trends in NCD risk factors and evaluating machine learning model performance. Finally, Section 5.5 concludes the chapter by summarizing our findings, discussing their implications, and proposing avenues for future research and intervention.

5.2 PROPOSED LITERATURE MODEL

NCDs are becoming an increasingly serious public health issue in India, affecting a wide range of demographic groups. This review seeks to synthesize current research

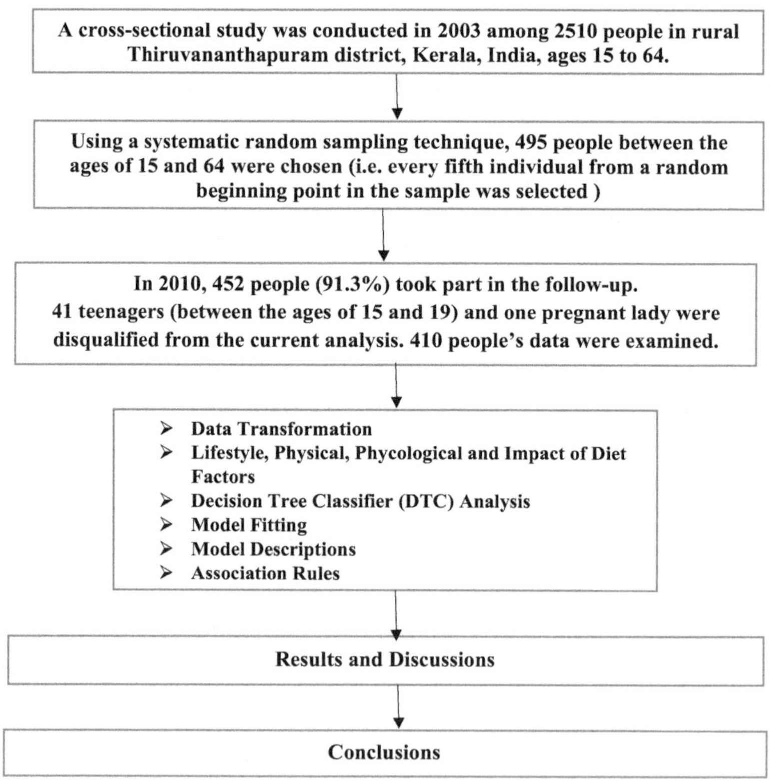

FIGURE 5.1 Flowchart illustrating how the complete work was created.

on the interconnected roles of physical health, psychological well-being, lifestyle choices, and diet in predicting the onset and progression of NCDs in the Indian context. It is becoming more and more clear that a comprehensive strategy is required as NCDs pose a rising threat to India. In addition to interventions at the individual level, systemic improvements addressing socio-cultural variables influencing health outcomes are desperately needed. This involves implementing regulations that encourage physical activity and discourage unhealthy habits, supporting public health education campaigns to develop educated dietary choices, and enhancing food accessibility and affordability. Furthermore, incorporating mental health support services into primary healthcare systems helps lessen the negative psychological effects that accelerate the development of NCDs. As we move away from the topic of diabetes, consider how dietary choices can influence body mass index (BMI), reflecting the larger impact of diet on overall health. The diagnostic utility of BMI for health conditions changes with age, emphasizing the importance of nuanced approaches throughout the aging process. Recognizing the complex relationship between age, diet, and health outcomes.

The reviewed literature provides a comprehensive exploration of NCDs and their associated factors, interventions, and predictive models. Sathish et al.'s [7] longitudinal study in rural Kerala, India, elucidates the evolving landscape of NCD risk factors over time, advocating for targeted preventive strategies in underserved communities. Likewise, Kowsar and Mansouri's [4] multi-level analysis of an Iraqi population highlights the intricate relationship between diabetes, BMI, and HbA1c levels, offering insights for more effective diabetes management strategies tailored to specific demographic contexts.

Innovative technological approaches also feature prominently, with Rajput and Khedgikar's [8] use of machine learning for diabetes prediction showcasing the burgeoning role of computational methods in healthcare. Wang and Feng's [9] edited volume delves into the fusion of NCDs, big data, and artificial intelligence, presenting novel methodologies with the potential to revolutionize our understanding and treatment of these diseases. Furthermore, Hunter et al.'s [10] collaborative framework, incorporating computer vision, causal inference, and public health modeling, presents a promising avenue for assessing the impacts of urban planning on NCDs and health disparities, emphasizing the need for interdisciplinary solutions to complex public health challenges.

Focusing on risk factors for chronic diseases, such as bad eating habits or sedentary lifestyles, is crucial for successful prevention. Combating NCDs necessitates a multifaceted approach that includes individual lifestyle changes, psychological health, and dietary choices. Promoting personal responsibility for health and encouraging healthier lifestyles, guided by current science and sound dietary choices, emerges as a critical strategy. Existing research, which includes a broader understanding of dietary impacts, shows significant correlations between various physical health markers, BMI, and the incidence of NCDs in India. Notably, studies have discovered a clear correlation between obesity, which is influenced by both lifestyle and food choices, and an increased risk of diabetes and cardiovascular disease, particularly in metropolitan regions.

Chronic stress and sadness are two psychological issues that have also been recognized as significant contributors to the advancement of NCDs, with research tying these factors to diabetes and hypertension in Indian adults. Furthermore, lifestyle choices, including dietary patterns, play an important role in determining the prevalence of NCDs in India, as evidenced by studies that highlight the impact of sedentary behaviors and smoking habits on the rise of obesity and diabetes Beyond individual actions, the broader context necessitates efforts to improve food production, accelerate disease screening processes, and develop novel treatment approaches. This literature model underscores the urgency of adopting holistic strategies, addressing both individual and societal dimensions, to effectively mitigate the burden of NCDs and promote healthier communities for all, where dietary choices are integral to overall health outcomes.

Conducting a longitudinal study on NCDs using machine learning techniques holds significant promise in advancing our understanding and management of these prevalent health conditions. Sathish et al.'s [7] longitudinal investigation in rural Kerala, India, exemplifies the importance of such studies in elucidating the evolving landscape of NCD risk factors over time, particularly in underserved populations. Combining this approach with machine learning, as demonstrated by Rajput and Khedgikar [8], offers a powerful tool for predicting and analyzing diabetes and other NCDs based on medical attributes, thereby enabling early detection and personalized management strategies tailored to specific demographic contexts. This convergence of longitudinal studies and machine learning methodologies not only enhances our ability to identify at-risk populations but also paves the way for more effective preventive interventions and healthcare planning in the realm of NCDs.

5.3 PROPOSED WORK

The proposed research aims to conduct a comprehensive analysis using longitudinal data [7] collected in rural areas of Thiruvananthapuram district, India, with a seven-year gap between two timepoints (2003 and 2010). The dataset includes information from 901 individuals, focusing on their demographic details, lifestyle factors, physical measurements, and BMI. The research plan involves the following steps:

- **Data Preparation**: The dataset is divided into two timepoints, Timepoint 0 (2003) and Timepoint 1 (2010). A new column, "IsHealthy," is created based on BMI values, classifying individuals as healthy (1) or unhealthy (0) within the specified BMI range [11] (18.5–24.90). Null values are identified and removed for both timepoints.
- **Data Transformation**: Columns with categorical values (yes/no) such as lowfruit, paacat, and gender are converted to numerical format (0 and 1) using the dummy variable approach. The dataset is cleaned and prepared for further analysis.
- **Lifestyle, Physical, and Physiological Impact of Diet Factors**: Health analysis is a multifaceted evaluation that includes lifestyle, where smoking, tobacco, and alcohol habits are scrutinized for potential health risks; physical attributes like age, height, and weight, with BMI aiding in assessing obesity-related risks [12]; physiological markers such as hypertension, cenobesity, genobesity, and blood pressure readings, providing insights into

cardiovascular and overall health dynamics; and the pivotal impact of diet, considering nutritional intake, dietary patterns, and their influence on conditions like obesity and cardiovascular diseases. This holistic approach enables tailored interventions and recommendations for individualized health and wellness.

- **Decision Tree Classifier (DTC) Analysis**: DTC is employed [13] to understand feature importance in predicting the "IsHealthy" column. The analysis provides insights into variables contributing to health status, including lifestyle, physical, and physiological factors.
- **Model Fitting**: Three different models—Random Forest (RF) [14], Support Vector Classifier (SVC) [15], and Logistic Regression (LR) [14]—are fitted to the data. These models will be examined using the R2 value to assess their performance in predicting health status.
- **Model Descriptions**: RF: Known for high accuracy, robustness to overfitting, and the ability to handle missing values, RF will provide insights into feature importance and contribute to understanding variable relationships.
- **Support Vector Classifier (SVC):** Effective for both linear and nonlinear classification, SVC will aid in determining the hyperplane that best separates classes, highlighting influential features.
- **Logistic Regression (LR):** A statistical method for binary classification, LR will model the probability of health status, providing a probabilistic understanding of variable influence. These models undergo a rigorous comparison based on the R2 value, enabling an evaluation of their efficacy in predicting health status. Each model brings distinct skills to the table, with RF providing insights into feature importance, SVC excelling at linear and nonlinear classifications, and LR providing a probabilistic understanding of variable influence.
- **Confusion Matrix Analysis**: A confusion matrix [16] will be used to assess each model's performance, offering a full breakdown of true positive, true negative, false positive, and false negative predictions [17]. This step offers a more sophisticated picture of the models' accuracy and errors.
- **Association Rules**: Association rules will be generated to unveil relationships between each variable and the target variable (IsHealthy). These rules [18, 19] will provide insights into dependencies and correlations, enhancing the understanding of factors influencing health outcomes. A comprehensive approach to exploring relationships between various factors and health outcomes is undertaken through the application of association rule mining. The analysis leverages a data frame, "data," containing categorical columns such as "alcohol" and many other factors and the target variable "IsHealthy." To prepare the data for analysis, a one-hot encoding technique is applied, transforming categorical variables into a binary format conducive to association rule mining. The Apriori algorithm [20] is then employed to identify frequent item sets with a minimum support threshold of 0.1, revealing patterns and associations within the dataset. Subsequently, association rules are generated based on these frequent item sets, utilizing the lift metric with a minimum threshold of 0.1 to extract meaningful insights into dependencies

and correlations among the variables. The generated rules are printed for examination, and to facilitate further exploration and sharing of findings, they are saved to a comma-separated values (csv). This meticulous approach enhances the understanding of factors influencing health outcomes, providing valuable insights for healthcare professionals.

In conclusion, this meticulously outlined research plan integrates statistical and machine learning techniques to unravel the complex interplay of variables influencing health status in rural areas of Thiruvananthapuram district, India. The approach, encompassing feature importance, model fitting, confusion matrix analysis, and association rules, promises a holistic understanding of the intricate dynamics contributing to NCD outcomes. This proposed research plan integrates statistical and machine learning techniques to comprehensively analyze the dataset, providing valuable insights into the factors influencing health status in rural areas of Thiruvananthapuram district, India. The combination of feature importance, model fitting, confusion matrix analysis, and association rules will help to develop a comprehensive knowledge of the complex interplay of variables in predicting NCD outcomes.

5.4 RESULTS AND DISCUSSION

5.4.1 Result Analysis

The study found increases in the study cohort's weight, BMI, waist circumference, waist-to-height ratio, current use of smokeless tobacco (in men), alcohol consumption (in all genders), physical inactivity, obesity, and central obesity. This likely explains Kerala's high rates of cardiovascular disease mortality and diabetes prevalence. In Kerala, the rise in risk factors for NCDs runs counter to the state's high life expectancy, high literacy rate, improved socioeconomic level indices, and improved access to healthcare facilities.

In evaluating the machine learning models for Timepoint 0 from Figure 5.2, the RF model exhibited impeccable performance with perfect R2 scores of 1 for both testing and training. This indicates an exceptional fit to the data, showcasing the model's ability to predict outcomes accurately. The SVC demonstrated strong predictive capabilities with high R2 values close to 1 for both testing (0.95) and training (0.99). Similarly, the (LR) model performed well, achieving R2 values of 0.917 for testing and 0.934 for training, indicating a solid correlation between predicted and actual values.

Moving to Timepoint 1 from Figure 5.3, the RF model maintained its excellent predictive performance with a near-perfect R2 score of 0.92 for testing and a perfect score of 0.99 for training. This suggests the model's consistent ability to accurately

	Testing	Training
RF	0.96	1
SVC	0.95	0.99
LR	0.917	0.934

FIGURE 5.2 R^2 value for Timepoint 0.

predict outcomes across different datasets. The SVC model continued to exhibit strong predictive capabilities, achieving R2 values of 0.95 for testing and 0.99 for training. The LR model, while slightly lower in performance compared to RF and SVC, still demonstrated good predictive ability with R2 values of 0.86 for testing and 0.87 for training. In an overall comparison, the RF model consistently outshined the other models for both Timepoints 0 and 1, showcasing its robustness in predictive tasks. SVC also maintained strong performance, and LR proved to be a reliable choice, although with slightly lower R2 values. The findings underline the necessity of picking an appropriate model based on the task's specific requirements, with RF standing out for its continuously outstanding predictive capabilities.

The comparison of mean squared error (MSE) [21] values for Timepoint 0 and Timepoint 1 (Figures 5.2 and 5.3) offers insights into the predictive performance of the SVC and RF models Figures 5.2 and 5.3. For SVC, the MSE increased from approximately 0.055 at Timepoint 0 to around 0.077 at Timepoint 1, indicating a slight decrease in predictive precision between the two timepoints. In contrast, the RF model showcased exceptional accuracy, achieving a perfect MSE of 0.0 at Timepoint 0 and maintaining a low MSE of approximately 0.011 at Timepoint 1. This consistent precision in predictions highlights the robustness of the RF model across different timepoints. Despite the increase in MSE for SVC, both models demonstrated strong predictive capabilities, with RF particularly standing out for its accuracy and reliability in capturing underlying patterns in the data. The findings underscore the importance of evaluating model performance over multiple timepoints to ensure consistent and reliable predictions.

In analyzing the confusion matrices for Timepoints 0 and 1 Figures 5.4 and 5.5, it is evident that the model's predictive performance undergoes changes over time. At Timepoint 0, the model demonstrates a considerable bias toward predicting instances as positive, resulting in a complete absence of True Negatives [17] and an inability to recognize actual negative cases. This skew toward positive predictions is reflected in the absence of False Positives but a higher count of False Negatives. In contrast, at Timepoint 1, the model achieves a better balance between the prediction of both

	Testing	Training
RF	0.92	0.99
SVC	0.95	0.99
LR	0.86	0.87

FIGURE 5.3 R^2 value for Timepoint 1.

	Predicted Negative	Predicted Positive
Actual Negative	0	0
Actual Positive	38	53

FIGURE 5.4 Confusion matrix for Timepoint 0.

positive and negative instances. While there is room for improvement, the model correctly identifies True Negatives, reducing False Positives, and capturing more True Positives. However, there remains a noticeable number of False Negatives, indicating instances where the model fails to identify actual positive cases. The performance evolution between Timepoints 0 and 1 suggests that adjustments to the model, such as parameter tuning or additional training data, may have contributed to a more balanced prediction at Timepoint 1. The model's effectiveness in predicting instances improves from Timepoint 0 to Timepoint 1, shifting toward a more balanced classification. However, challenges persist, particularly in correctly identifying instances of class 1. Further refinements to the model and exploration of feature importance could enhance its ability to discriminate between classes and reduce errors.

In Figure 5.6, the detailed confusion matrix for Timepoint 0 and Timepoint 1 illustrates the performance metrics of a predictive model. The values represent the accuracy, precision, recall, and F1-score [22, 23] at the respective timepoints. At Timepoint 0, the accuracy and precision are 0.5824, indicating the proportion of correctly predicted instances and the ratio of true positive predictions, respectively. The recall at Timepoint 0 is perfect at 1.000, signifying that all actual positive instances were correctly identified. The corresponding F1-score at Timepoint 0 is 0.7361, providing a balance between precision and recall. At Timepoint 1, there is a slight improvement in precision (0.5918) but a decrease in recall (0.6304), resulting in an F1-score of 0.6105. These metrics collectively offer a comprehensive evaluation of the model's predictive capabilities at different timepoints, aiding in the assessment and refinement of its performance.

The results of our study show that fast urbanization and dietary changes have led to an increase in unhealthy lifestyle behaviors in rural Kerala, including the consumption of foods high in calories and little physical exercise. Over the past three decades, Kerala's per capita daily calorie intake has climbed by two-thirds, which is out of proportion to the state's declining levels of physical activity. Keralans consume twice as many processed foods high in sugar and salt as residents in other parts of

	Predicted Negative	Predicted Positive
Actual Negative	25	20
Actual Positive	17	29

FIGURE 5.5 Confusion matrix for Timepoint 1.

	Timepoint 0	Timepoint 1
Accuracy	0.5824	0.5934
Precision	0.5824	0.5918
Recall	1.000	0.6304
F1-score	0.7361	0.6105

FIGURE 5.6 Detailed confusion matrix for Timepoints 0 and 1.

India. Additionally, a very small portion of Keralans eat enough fruits and vegetables, and the state's cuisine is high in saturated fats. Given that South Asians are more likely to develop coronary heart disease when they consume moderate to high amounts of alcohol and that one-fifth of Indian drinkers meet the criteria for dependent drinking and more than half for hazardous drinking, it is important to consider the rise in alcohol use observed in our study. Further research is necessary, but the rise in alcohol consumption among women in our study is consistent with findings from other regions of India and could be linked to advertising.

5.4.2 Demystifying Health-Related Myths

- **Alcohol consumption impacts health badly?**
  Myth: Contrary to popular belief, drinking alcohol does not always have a detrimental effect on one's health. While extreme alcohol intake is obviously dangerous, moderate alcohol use might not pose as much of a risk [24]. Studies indicate that a modest intake of alcohol, especially red wine, may even provide certain health advantages including a lower chance of heart disease. However, it's critical to recognize that each person responds to alcohol differently, so any potential benefits must be weighed against the drug's hazards, which include addiction and liver damage.
- **Smoking impacts health?**
  Myth: Smoking alone is not the most important factor influencing health. Although it is widely acknowledged that smoking poses a considerable risk for a multitude of health issues, it is critical to recognize that many factors influence how one's health develops. There is no doubt that smoking is hazardous for you; it increases your risk of respiratory problems, heart disease, and lung cancer. Nonetheless, environmental factors, exercise, nutrition, and heredity have a significant impact on overall health. While quitting smoking is critical for minimizing these risks, long-term well-being also requires addressing other lifestyle factors and taking a comprehensive approach to health.
- **Cenobesity impacts health?**
  Myth: Cenobesity is not the dominating factor impacting health. One of the main determinants of health is frequently considered to be societal and environmental conditions that lead to obesity, or coenobitism. Even while obesity is a serious health risk that is linked to a number of problems, including diabetes and cardiovascular disease, it's important to understand that health outcomes depend on a variety of factors. Individual health is influenced by a variety of factors, including genetics, lifestyle choices, access to healthcare, and socioeconomic status, even though policy and cultural changes targeting obesity are vital. As a result, while combating obesity at the social level is crucial, treating personal health calls for a more all-encompassing strategy.
- **Genobesity impacts health?**
  Fact: Genobesity, or the genetic propensity to obesity, increases vulnerability to weight-related disorders, which has a considerable negative impact on

health. Empirical evidence suggests that hereditary variables significantly influence an individual's susceptibility to obesity and its associated comorbidities, including type 2 diabetes and hypertension. Although food and exercise are still important lifestyle factors for controlling weight, knowing genetic predispositions can help improve the effectiveness of therapies and treatments [12, 24]. Thus, understanding how obesity affects health is crucial to creating individualized plans to combat obesity and the health hazards that come with it.

- **Hypertension impacts health?**
  Myth: Hypertension alone is not the most important factor affecting health. Hypertension, often known as high blood pressure, is a known risk factor for heart disease, stroke, and other health problems. However, it is critical to recognize that health outcomes are influenced by several factors, such as genetics, lifestyle decisions, and general health. Hypertension is not the only factor that influences health, but it should not be overlooked and must be controlled to reduce risks. Regardless of blood pressure, adopting a healthy lifestyle that includes regular exercise, a well-balanced diet, and stress management is critical for cardiovascular health.
- **Fruit serving improves health?**
  Fact: Serving a variety of fruits undoubtedly benefits one's health. It goes without saying that consuming a range of fruits is good for your health. Fruits are an excellent source of important nutrients, such as fiber, antioxidants, vitamins, and minerals. These nutrients not only protect against long-term illnesses like diabetes, heart disease, and some types of cancer, but they are also necessary for maintaining general health. Fruits can enhance nutrient intake, aid in weight management, and promote general well-being when they are included to meals and snacks. For this reason, eating a balanced diet that includes a sufficient quantity and variety of fruits is advised for optimum health.
- **Veg serving improves health?**
  Fact: It is imperative to consume a sufficient quantity of veggies to sustain maximum health and well-being. Vegetables are abundant in vital elements, including vitamins, minerals, fibers, and phytochemicals. These nutrients are important for a number of body processes and for lowering the risk of chronic illnesses including cancer, heart disease, and stroke. Including a selection of veggies in meals helps with digestion, offers a multitude of nutrients essential for general health, and may even aid in weight control. As a result, including vegetables on a regular basis in one's diet is advised as part of a healthy, balanced eating pattern.
- **Diet score impacts health?**
  Fact: While diet score is not a dominating factor, although there is no doubt that a person's food has an impact on their general health, it's crucial to understand that health consequences are complex. Numerous scoring systems are used to evaluate food quality, which offers important information about overall dietary habits and nutrient intake. But there are other important variables that can affect health outcomes, like heredity, physical activity,

stress levels, and sleep habits. Thus, although eating a healthy, balanced diet is crucial for achieving optimal health, it's only one component of a more comprehensive strategy for well-being. It is essential to combine food decisions with healthy lifestyle practices to attain and preserve general health and wellness.

In simple terms, understanding the complexity of these factors helps in adopting a holistic approach to health, recognizing that individual habits and genetics interact with various elements in determining overall well-being.

5.5 CONCLUSIONS

In demystifying the puzzle of health, my study breaks new ground by elucidating the complex interplay of physical and psychological impact of diet and lifestyle factors in the development of NCDs, contributing to a deeper understanding of NCD prevalence and progression. Our findings reveal a concerning increase in NCD risk factors in rural Kerala, emphasizing the urgent need for targeted preventive strategies and holistic healthcare interventions. By employing machine learning techniques, we showcase the potential of predictive models to identify individuals at high risk for NCDs, enabling early intervention and personalized healthcare solutions. Additionally, we challenge prevailing health myths and advocate for a holistic approach to health that considers individual habits, genetics, and socio-cultural factors. This study serves as a guiding beacon for the younger generation, steering them away from factors that diminish life expectancy and promoting the overall welfare of our nation. It serves as a roadmap for a longer, healthier life.

Despite its limitations and modest sample size, our study represents just the tip of the iceberg. As we delve deeper into larger sets of NCD data, we anticipate that our findings will resonate even more profoundly. We envision our study as a significant contributor to the broader field of NCD research, shaping a healthier future. Beyond mere academic pursuits, our study serves as a practical guide for living longer, healthier lives, offering insights and direction for individuals, policymakers, and healthcare professionals alike.

REFERENCES

1. Fonseca, L. M., Domingues, J. P., & Dima, A. M. (2020). Mapping the sustainable development goals relationships. *Sustainability*, 12(8), 3359.
2. Misra, A., & Khurana, L. (2011). Obesity-related non-communicable diseases: South Asians vs White Caucasians. *International Journal of Obesity*, *35*(2), 167–187.
3. Lin, X., Xu, Y., Xu, J., Pan, X., Song, X., Shan, L., . . . Shan, P. F. (2020). Global burden of noncommunicable disease attributable to high body mass index in 195 countries and territories, 1990–2017. *Endocrine*, 69, 310–320.
4. Kowsar, R., & Mansouri, A. (2022). Multi-level analysis reveals the association between diabetes, body mass index, and HbA1c in an Iraqi population. *Scientific Reports*, 12(1), 21135.
5. Thamrin, S. A., Arsyad, D. S., Kuswanto, H., Lawi, A., & Nasir, S. (2021). Predicting obesity in adults using machine learning techniques: An analysis of Indonesian basic health research 2018. *Frontiers in Nutrition*, *8*, 669155.

6. Musa, F., Basaky, F., & Osaghae, E. O. (2022). Obesity prediction using machine learning techniques. *Journal of Applied Artificial Intelligence*, 3(1), 24–33.
7. Sathish, T., Kannan, S., Sarma, S. P., Razum, O., Sauzet, O., & Thankappan, K. R. (2017). Seven-year longitudinal change in risk factors for non-communicable diseases in rural Kerala, India: The WHO STEPS approach. *PLoS One*, 12(6), e0178949.
8. Rajput, M. R., & Khedgikar, S. S. (2022). Diabetes prediction and analysis using medical attributes: A Machine learning approach. *Journal of Xi'an University of Architecture & Technology*, 14(1), 98–103.
9. Wang, Y., & Feng, M. (Eds.). (2022). *Non-communicable diseases, big data and artificial intelligence*. MDPI Books.
10. Hunter, R. F., Garcia, L., Stevenson, M., Nice, K., Wijnands, J., Kee, F., . . . Thompson, J. H. (2023). Computer vision, causal inference and public health modelling approaches to generate evidence on the impacts of urban planning in non-communicable disease and health inequalities in UK and Australian cities: A proposed collaborative approach. *medRxiv*, 2023–04.
11. Blüher, M. (2020). Metabolically healthy obesity. *Endocrine Reviews*, *41*(3), bnaa004.
12. Zhang, L., Shang, X., Sreedharan, S., Yan, X., Liu, J., Keel, S.,. . . He, M. (2020). Predicting the development of type 2 diabetes in a large Australian cohort using machine-learning techniques: Longitudinal survey study. *JMIR Medical Informatics*, *8*(7), e16850.
13. Garba, S., Abdullahi, M., Umar, U. A., & Wurno, N. T. (2022). Obesity level classification based on decision tree and naïve Bayes classifiers. *SLU Journal of Science and Technology*, 3(1 & 2), 113–121.
14. Chatterjee, A., Gerdes, M. W., & Martinez, S. G. (2020). Identification of risk factors associated with obesity and overweight—a machine learning overview. *Sensors*, 20(9), 2734.
15. Devi, R. D. H., Bai, A., & Nagarajan, N. J. O. M. (2020). A novel hybrid approach for diagnosing diabetes mellitus using farthest first and support vector machine algorithms. *Obesity Medicine*, 17, 100152.
16. Amani, F., Mohammadnia, A., & Amani, P. (2021). Using machine learning method for classification Body Mass Index for clinical decision. *Sensors*, *2*(90), 273.
17. Hsu, C. H., Alavi, A., & Dong, M. (2022). mHealth for non-communicable diseases. *Frontiers in Public Health*, 10, 918982.
18. Telikani, A., Tahmassebi, A., Banzhaf, W., & Gandomi, A. H. (2021). Evolutionary machine learning: A survey. *ACM Computing Surveys (CSUR)*, 54(8), 1–35.
19. Austin, M., Delgoshaei, P., Coelho, M., & Heidarinejad, M. (2020). Architecting smart city digital twins: Combined semantic model and machine learning approach. *Journal of Management in Engineering*, 36(4), 04020026.
20. Santoso, M. H. (2021). Application of association rule method using apriori algorithm to find sales patterns case study of Indomaret Tanjung Anom. *Brilliance: Research of Artificial Intelligence*, 1(2), 54–66.
21. Chicco, D., Warrens, M. J., & Jurman, G. (2021). The coefficient of determination R-squared is more informative than SMAPE, MAE, MAPE, MSE and RMSE in regression analysis evaluation. *PeerJ Computer Science*, *7*, e623.
22. Powers, D. M. (2020). Evaluation: From precision, recall and F-measure to ROC, informedness, markedness and correlation. *arXiv preprint* arXiv:2010.16061.
23. Yacouby, R., & Axman, D. (2020, November). Probabilistic extension of precision, recall, and f1 score for more thorough evaluation of classification models. In *Proceedings of the first workshop on evaluation and comparison of NLP systems* (pp. 79–91). Spinger.
24. Telikani, A., Gandomi, A. H., & Shahbahrami, A. (2020). A survey of evolutionary computation for association rule mining. *Information Sciences*, 524, 318–352.

6 Uncovering Machine Learning Trends in Biomedical

Pulmonary Disease Diagnosis

Anish Singh, Atul Kabra, and Anupam Bonkra

CONTENTS

6.1 INTRODUCTION

The lungs and airways around them are susceptible to a wide variety of illnesses and conditions [1]. In this complex setting, a wide range of serious respiratory diseases might manifest. Sneezing and wheezing are signs of asthma, a disease characterized by persistent inflammation of the airways. Persistent dyspnea and trouble breathing are hallmarks of chronic obstructive pulmonary disease (COPD), which includes emphysema and chronic bronchitis. Fever, chest discomfort, and difficulty breathing are symptoms of pneumonia, an infection of the airways. Symptoms of this illness include swelling and fluid buildup in the air sacs. Respiratory difficulties, chest discomfort, and resistance to congestion are all signs of tuberculosis (TB), a lung illness caused by germs. Lung cancer symptoms include shortness of breath, chest pain, and the presence of blood in phlegm. The illness is characterized by the uncontrolled growth of cells. The accumulation of scar tissue in the lungs as a result of pulmonary fibrosis reduces the efficiency and difficulty of respiration. A pulmonary embolism can occur when a blood clot obstructs a blood vessel in the lung, thereby rapidly exposing the respiratory system to a potential danger. An individual respiratory condition necessitates a distinct combination of diagnostic, therapeutic, and managerial

DOI: 10.1201/9781003476207-6

approaches. Given the extensive variety of respiratory maladies, each characterized by distinct symptoms, etiology, and therapeutic interventions, it is indisputable that targeted strategies are imperative. The implementation of suitable alterations to one's way of life has the potential to successfully prevent or cure a broad variety of respiratory ailments. These enhancements consist of a variety of measures, including the elimination of pollutants and smoking, as well as the introduction of vaccines that are directed against certain diseases. When it comes to treating some disorders, pharmaceutical therapies could be beneficial; however, when the problem is more serious, surgical intervention or other therapeutic procedures might be necessary. To improve the quality of life and increase the life expectancy of individuals, it is essential to acknowledge the need for early detection and treatment of pulmonary disorders. It is because of this that the aforementioned ailments will be slowed down or prevented from developing. There has been a great amount of study work put into researching the important consequences that SARS-CoV-2, the etiological infection that is responsible for COVID-19, has on the respiratory system and airways. The technique that was described before entails the beginning of inflammation, which ultimately results in more damage to the alveoli. There is a possibility that more severe cases may result in the development of Acute Respiratory Distress Syndrome, which is characterized by breathing difficulties and decreased oxygen levels. It is also possible that some patients would continue to have respiratory problems even after they have completely recovered from the SARS-CoV-2 infection. The aforementioned challenges are often known as "Long COVID" or "Post-acute Sequelae of SARS-CoV-2 infection" (PASC). Ongoing research is necessary to enhance the diagnosis, treatment, and management of pulmonary illnesses. The COVID-19 epidemic has shed attention on the significant impact that these illnesses have on both communities and people. This work aims to showcase the efficacy of machine learning in identifying pulmonary illness by examining several medical datasets, such as chest X-rays [2], computed tomography (CT) scans [3], and pulmonary function tests. Deep learning, a sophisticated branch of machine learning, builds intricate models by using neural networks. Efficient development of these models needs accessible access to extensive information, such as lung scans. The current research aims to identify unique patterns that may serve as indications of certain lung illnesses [4]. The integration of several medical data sources, such as imaging data, laboratory results, and clinical reports, into multi-modal models has the potential to improve the accuracy of diagnostic techniques [5]. Numerous empirical investigations have shown evidence that machine learning significantly improves the accuracy of lung illness identification when compared to traditional approaches. It is crucial to acknowledge the importance of using comprehensive and inclusive datasets for the purposes of training and validation. Moreover, when used with other diagnostic approaches, these models provide exceptional outcomes [6].

6.2 LITERATURE REVIEW

One kind of the illness that is particularly deadly and mysterious is lung cancer. Due to the fact that it often results in death in both sexes, it is much more important to take care and examine nodules in a timely and accurate manner. According to [7], several processes have been put into place to guarantee the early identification of lung cancer. In terms of disease-related mortality, cancer is the leading cause of death on a worldwide scale, with early-stage diagnosis being responsible for 8.29 million deaths and 13.9 million cases [8]. Within the United States, cancer was responsible for 595,690 fatalities and 1,682,210 new cases in the year 2018. A total of 224,391 new cases of lung cancer were reported in 2016, while 158,080 people lost their lives to the illness in 2016. It is generally agreed that lung cancer is the most lethal kind of canceric disease [7]. It is important to note that the survival rate of lung cancer cells is much lower in comparison to that of other forms of cancer cells. This is either due to the effect of lung cancer cells or the failure to recognize lung cancer cells at an early stage. In a data sheet that was prepared by the American Cancer Society, the American Lung Association, and the World Health Organization, it was shown that the endurance rate has grown from 17.7% to 54.4% since the beginning of cancer cell identification. In addition, the number is becoming closer to 16% once cancer cells have been confined [1, 9]. When lung problems interfere with normal lung function, the ability to absorb oxygen is diminished. This is the effect of the condition. In many cases, the presence of fungi, viruses, and bacteria is thought to be the cause of lung disorders [2, 10]. In some cases, other factors include things like being exposed to potentially harmful and fatal chemicals as well as having genetic abnormalities. When it comes to the transmission of respiratory infections to other people, sneezing and coughing are an extremely rare occurrence. The early discovery of illnesses not only speeds up the patient's recovery but also minimizes the probability that the infection will be passed on to other people or the environment. Computer-assisted diagnostics, which can evaluate chest X-rays, CT scans, and other medical pictures, have emerged as a promising and reliable tool for the diagnosis of lung illness [3]. This is because computer-assisted diagnostics can analyze these types of images. Convolutional neural networks, referred to as CNNs [11], have a reputation for being among the most precise and efficient computer-aided design systems. The identification and interpretation of patterns in pixel pictures are accomplished via the use of deep learning in the form of an artificial neural network [12]. It is very necessary to provide accurate results to provide greater assistance to medical staff and experts. The umbrella phrase "lung disease" refers to a wide range of disorders that have an effect on the lungs. These conditions include but are not limited to, asthma, COPD, infections such as TB and influenza, lung cancer [9], pneumonia, and a variety of other breathing issues. It is possible to discover variations in the signs and symptoms of respiratory disorders. Some of the most common symptoms are a persistent cough, dyspnea, which is defined by the evacuation of blood or mucus, dyspnea, a sense of insufficient airflow, diminished exercise capacity, and pain or discomfort [13]. For the purpose of analyzing and processing medical pictures, it is necessary to have a setting that is conducive to the creation of algorithms, the accessing of data, the processing of data, the revealing of data, and analysis. The term "medical imaging" refers to the technique and technology that is used to create pictures of the human body for the goal of diagnostic, analytical, and other scientific reasons (for example, the research of disorders within the framework of typical anatomical and physiological processes). The use of medical CT imaging has been more prevalent in clinical diagnosis during the last several years [3]. It does this by making it easier for them to be detected, which in turn helps medical professionals identify pathogenic mutations with more precision. As a result of the various grayscale levels, CT pictures are able to demonstrate the differentiation between various tissues [14, 15]. Radiologists are given the ability to make judgments that are more informed as a result of the rising use of artificial intelligence (AI), the Internet of Things, and cloud computing in the healthcare business [16, 17]. Infections, occupational exposures, drugs, and other illnesses are some of the potential causes of lung problems. Other potential causes include industrial exposure. A number of well-known anatomic imaging modalities, such as CT and X-ray chest radiography, are routinely used in the process of identifying and diagnosing a variety of lung illnesses. The diagnosis, treatment, and surgical procedures, as well as the education and reference of patients, all need the use of medical imaging. The Digital Imaging and Communications in Medicine standard [18] enables the storing of metadata, which comprises textual descriptions, in addition to the pictures that are being stored. It was the most important innovation that has occurred since the advent of X-rays, and CT has been an essential fundamental component of diagnostic radiology [19]. Corona virus-2, which is linked with severe acute respiratory syndrome, is the causative agent of this widespread viral illness. The respiratory consequence that was caused by the COVID-19 infection was pneumonia, which is a potentially fatal condition [20]. According to the World Health Organization, the illness has been categorized as a pandemic due to the severity of the sickness and the fast dissemination of the transmission. In spite of the multiple treatment and control measures that have been put into place from December 2019 till the present [21], the mortality rate linked with COVID-19 infection has been steadily increasing at an alarming pace. The establishment of the investigation's background is facilitated by an exhaustive literature review and an introduction. The investigation's objective is later determined. Before the analysis, the next step involves creating a summary of the study methodology. The results of the study were made public after a thorough evaluation of the collected and analyzed data. The final report provides a detailed analysis of the implications arising from the research's findings. This research considers many aspects, such as the authors' and sources' importance, the classification of various document formats, the countries with the greatest average citation count and publication growth, and the often-used keywords. To get a thorough comprehension of the study issue, it is essential to follow this systematic strategy. Engaging in this practice will enhance the efficiency of drawing well-informed conclusions from your study.

6.3 RESEARCH METHODOLOGY

In this particular research, bibliometric analysis was used. The examination of bibliographic data is the focus of quantitative bibliometric analysis [22–24]. Analysis of performance and mapping of scientific knowledge are both components of this technique [25, 26]. Analysis of bibliometrics is made easier by software [27]. Within the scope of this study, publication sources, journal and document impact factors, and vocabulary that is commonly encountered are investigated. The procedures that were used in this investigation are shown in Figure 6.3. During this time, a search was conducted inside Scopus for several data sources [28–30]. Following the extraction process, the Scopus dataset is then imported into R. While VOSviewer [31–33] is responsible for visualizing the bibliometric networks, Biblioshiny [34–36] is responsible for analyzing the data. The BiblioshinyBibliometrix tool is included in the R package. The conclusion is reached, and evaluations of the program processing are generated. There is no research paper or activity that can be considered complete without prior study. The research made use of the widely utilized bibliometrics. Which method of doing a literature review in academic settings is quantitative? The most important factor is the quantity of scholarly and scientific publications. Databases for academic study are intriguing since they include reliable sources. A few examples of academic databases are Scopus, Web of Science, and PubMed. For this study, Elsevier Scopus from 2004 was used. Both authors and journals are evaluated by Scopus, which is the biggest abstract and citation database that covers several disciplines. Access to the database requires membership, despite the fact that many services are free. Scopus is used for this study from 2020 to 2022. It is [29]. There has been a significant amount of research conducted on lung infections, autonomous diagnostics, and machine learning. Scopus does searches using "lung infection," "automatic diagnosis," and "machine learning" and further includes "without year (2023) as an exclusion." By employing the Boolean AND operator, this string is able to locate the article's title, abstract, and keywords. Immediately after the search, presets filter articles. Analysis is performed on authors, nations, publications, references, and citations without regard to the language or nationality of the individuals involved. The evaluation of scientific works is done using bibliometrics. Specifically, [23, 37], and [38]. For the purpose of bibliometric analysis, legitimate scientific publications make use of data from books, papers, and chapters. The study makes use of Biblioshiny to do an analysis of Scopus CSV data. Lung infection, automated diagnostics, and machine learning are the topics that are discussed in this research, which emphasizes authors, works, and links [39] and [40]. Scientific research publications are checked for accuracy using computer-assisted review. Deletion of an article restricts analysis until the year 2023. Numerous research contributions are required because of the extensive language and region-independent investigation it encompasses [41–45]. To evaluate the impact of papers, scientists utilize bibliometrics. Figure 6.1 shows methodology.

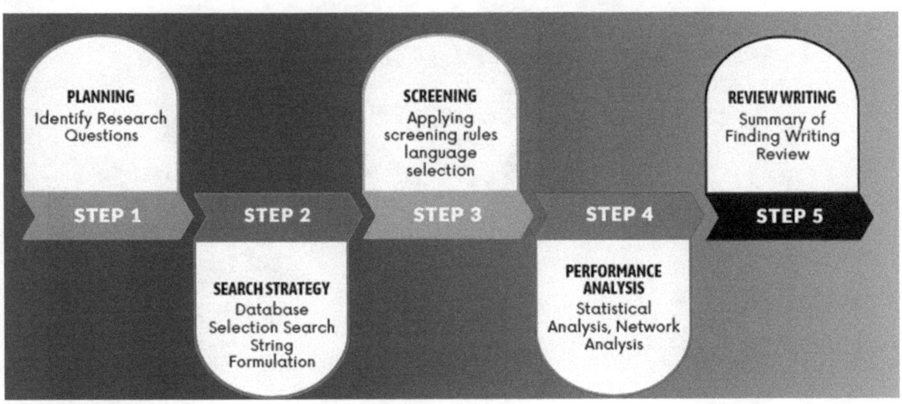

FIGURE 6.1 Methodology.

6.4 RESULTS

The data that has been selected for this study will be summarized in the figure that is shown in the following paragraphs. For the period of time extending from 2020 to 2022, the data was chosen from a total of 52 papers and 42 sources; 273 writers contributed to the compilation of the selected data, which has an annual growth rate of 2,109, 91% and was generated using 137 author keywords. It has been shown that there is a correlation between the total number of 6,263 references and an average of 11.44 citations per document. Figure 6.2 shows overview of data.

6.4.1 Most-Cited Countries

Citations play a crucial role in academic writing as they enable the seamless incorporation of diverse ideas, assertions, and written works. This approach allows a comprehensive analysis of the many effects that different organizations, including academic journals, research institutes, governmental authorities, and academic establishments, exert on the research environment. Through the analysis of citation patterns, this approach enables the monitoring of performance progress within a designated timeframe. Figure 6.3 depicts a graphical representation that showcases the leading academic institutions based on the number of citations received for scholarly works written by graduate students. The preponderance of citations in Canada serves as empirical support for the considerable impact and extensive corpus of scholarly literature generated by academic institutions within the nation. Conversely, Algeria's limited network of contacts may result in a lack of scholarly

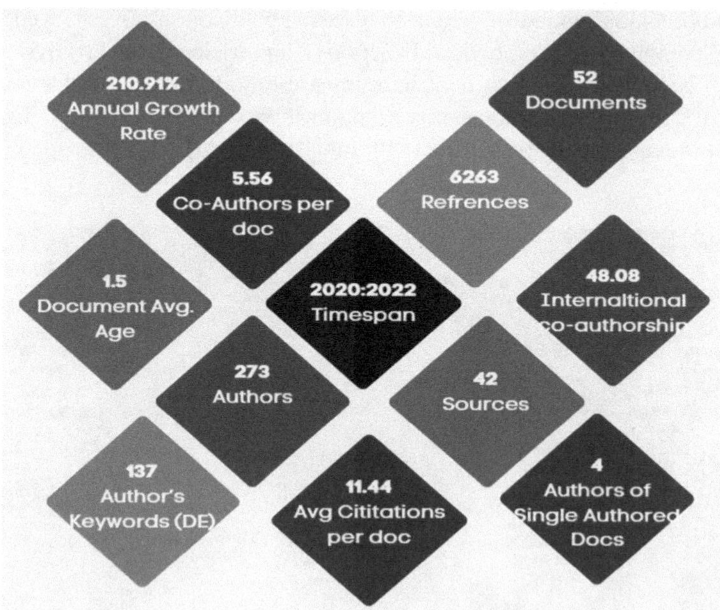

FIGURE 6.2 Overview of data.

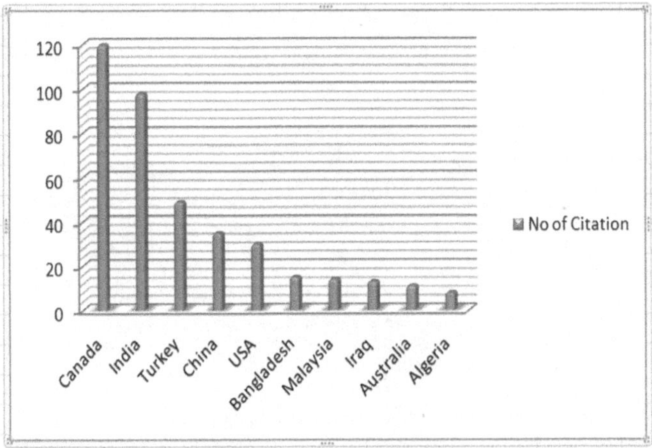

FIGURE 6.3 Citation-wise analysis.

engagement and influence regarding this subject matter. Numerous factors could account for the exceptionally high citation rates observed in Canadian universities. The innovative work in numerous fields that Canadian universities and colleges have accomplished through research and instruction has earned them international recognition. In addition to placing emphasis on partnerships with international organizations, Canadian universities foster an atmosphere that is beneficent to scholarly investigation and the interchange of information. The inclusion of these elements augments the pertinence and impact of scholarly publications linked to Canada within the domain of international studies. In contrast, Algerian academic institutions may face challenges in their endeavor to foster international collaboration due to constrained financial resources and inadequate research infrastructure, perhaps resulting in a decrease in citation rates. Moreover, the disparity in the ranking and output of research carried out in Algeria and Canada may be attributed to differences in scholarly resources, institutional support, and publishing standards that exist across academic institutions.

6.4.2 Word Cloud

The utilization of word clouds to represent text has become increasingly popular as an appealing technique. To condense information, these visual representations emphasize solely the most frequent terms across a variety of scenarios. Static text summaries are commonly employed for this objective [11]. Word clouds derived from a corpus of text function as an initial reference for conducting more comprehensive investigations and analyses. The word cloud presented in Figure 6.4 was constructed utilizing Scopus statistics and trending terms.

4.2.1 Most Frequently Used Keywords: The term utilized most frequently by the researchers in this survey is depicted in Figure 6.5. Here, a minimum of ten occurrences is established.

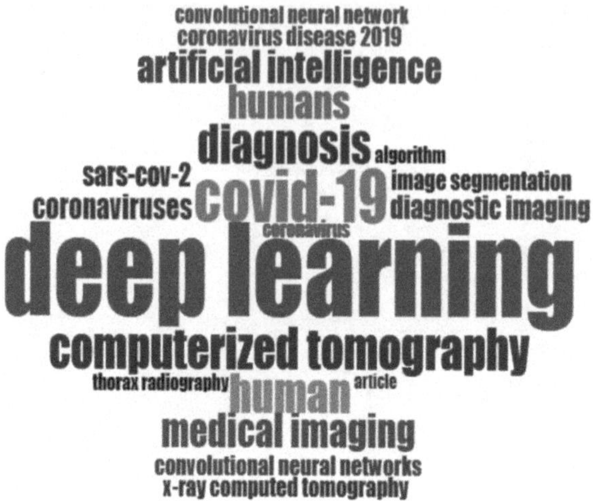

FIGURE 6.4 Keyword plus cloud.

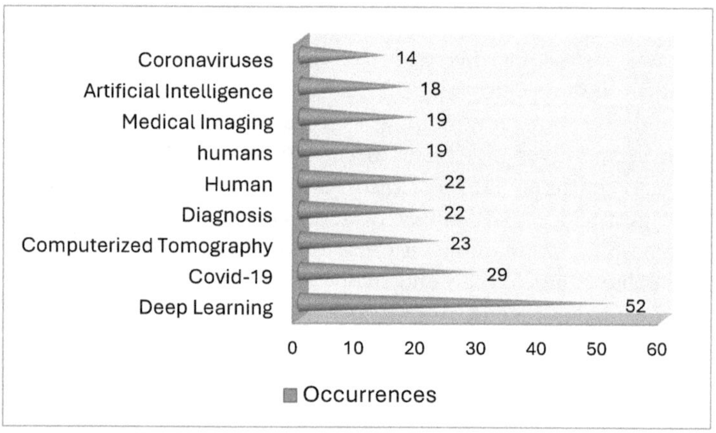

FIGURE 6.5 Country-wise bibliographic coupling.

The minimal number of citations for a country and the minimum number of documents per country are both set to three in Figure 6.5, which illustrates country-by-country bibliographic coupling. Twelve nations out of a total of 39 meet this standard once it has been established. For each of the 12 countries, the aggregate strength of the bibliographic coupling ties with the other nations will be calculated. These are the nations with the most robust interconnections as a whole.

6.5 CONCLUSION

This study examined AI-based pulmonary disease diagnostic research. Publications seem to have increased gradually. Scientists prefer journal papers to publicize their results. This research found Canada to be the most productive. India was the top

Asian country. CHEN X and AGARWAL S are the leading authorities in this field based on cumulative citation counts. Bibliometric measures like h-index, number of publications, and citations show that "Chaos Solitons and Fractals" and "Computers in Biology and Medicine" are most referenced. SARS-CoV-2 causes COVID-19, which mostly involves the lungs and may cause significant lung damage. The discovery has encouraged more research on COVID-19, Deep Learning, Computerized Tomography, Diagnosis, Human, and Medical Imaging. The impression that black box models are inscrutable makes it difficult or impossible to determine their reasoning or prediction process. Explainable Artificial Intelligence (XAI) improves model interpretability and transparency to increase reliability. By studying XAI for pulmonary illness diagnosis, scholarly publications on this topic may be improved.

REFERENCES

1. S. Mukherjee and S. U. Bohra, Lung cancer disease diagnosis using machine learning approach, *Proc. 3rd Int. Conf. Intell. Sustain. Syst. ICISS 2020*, pp. 207–211, 2020, doi: 10.1109/ICISS49785.2020.9315909.
2. K. Prajapati, J. Patel, and K. Pathak, Lung diseases using deep learning: A review paper, *Int. Res. J. . . .*, pp. 1694–1699, 2018, [Online]. Available: https://www.academia.edu/download/58145940/IRJET-V5I12316.pdf
3. D. N. Gumble and R. D. Ghongade, Machine learning system to detect lung infection using CT scan, *Int. J. Creat. Res. Thoughts*, vol. 9, no. 6, pp. 394–401, 2021.
4. A. Bonkra, A. Noonia, and A. Kaur, Apple leaf diseases detection system: A review of the different segmentation and deep learning methods, in *Artificial Intelligence and Data Science*, *Cluster Comput. 1673*. Springer, Cham. 2022, pp. 263–278.
5. A. Jangra, A. Jatowt, S. Saha, and M. Hasanuzzaman, A survey on multi-modal summarization, *J. ACM*, vol. 37, no. 4, 2021, [Online]. Available: http://arxiv.org/abs/2109.05199
6. A. Kaur and P. Dhiman, Requirement analysis for building cloud-enabled portable early disease detection system, *Comput. Biol. Med.*, vol. 141, no. November 2021, p. 5141, 2021.
7. S. S. Raoof, M. A. Jabbar, and S. A. Fathima, Lung cancer prediction using machine learning: A comprehensive approach, *2nd Int. Conf. Innov. Mech. Ind. Appl. ICIMIA 2020—Conf. Proc.*, no. Icimia, pp. 108–115, 2020, doi: 10.1109/ICIMIA48430.2020.9074947.
8. S. Bharathy, R. Pavithra, and B. Akshaya, Lung cancer detection using machine learning, *Proc.—Int. Conf. Appl. Artif. Intell. Comput. ICAAIC 2022*, vol. 7, no. 01, pp. 539–543, 2022, doi: 10.1109/ICAAIC53929.2022.9793061.
9. B. Alsinglawi *et al.*, An explainable machine learning framework for lung cancer hospital length of stay prediction, *Sci. Rep.*, vol. 12, no. 1, pp. 1–10, 2022, doi: 10.1038/s41598-021-04608-7.
10. J. Zhu, B. Shen, A. Abbasi, M. Hoshmand-Kochi, H. Li, and T. Q. Duong, Deep transfer learning artificial intelligence accurately stages COVID-19 lung disease severity on portable chest radiographs, *PLoS One*, vol. 15, no. 7 July, pp. 1–11, 2020, doi: 10.1371/journal.pone.0236621.
11. L. Alzubaidi *et al.*, Review of deep learning: Concepts, CNN architectures, challenges, applications, future directions, *J. Big Data*, vol. 8, no. 1, Dec. 2021, doi: 10.1186/s40537-021-00444-8.
12. A. Khan, A. Sohail, U. Zahoora, and A. S. Qureshi, A survey of the recent architectures of deep convolutional neural networks, *Artif. Intell. Rev.*, vol. 53, no. 8, pp. 5455–5516, 2020, doi: 10.1007/s10462-020-09825-6.
13. S. Tripathi, S. Shetty, S. Jain, and V. Sharma, Lung disease detection, *Sensor*, no. 8, pp. 1–7, 2021, doi: 10.35940/ijitee.H9259.0610821.

14. A. B. Salem Salamh, A. A. Salamah, and H. I. Akyüz, A study of a new technique of the CT scan view and disease classification protocol based on level challenges in cases of coronavirus disease, *Radiol. Res. Pract.*, vol. 2021, p. 5554408, 2021, doi: 10.1155/2021/5554408.
15. J. Jamaludin *et al.*, A review of tomography system, *JurnalTeknologi*, vol. 64, 2013, doi: 10.11113/jt.v64.2131.
16. A. Bonkra and P. Dhiman, IoT security challenges in cloud environment, *Proc.-2021 2nd Int. Conf. Comput. Methods Sci. Technol. ICCMST 2021*, pp. 30–34, 2021, doi: 10.1109/ICCMST54943.2021.00018.
17. R. Rani, M. Khurana, A. Kumar, and N. Kumar, Big data dimensionality reduction techniques in IoT: Review, applications and open research challenges, *Cluster Comput.*, vol. 20, p. 200, 2022, doi: 10.1007/s10586-022-03634-y.
18. C.-C. Lai, T.-P. Shih, W.-C. Ko, H.-J. Tang, and P.-R. Hsueh, Severe acute respiratory syndrome coronavirus 2 (SARS-CoV-2) and coronavirus disease-2019 (COVID-19): The epidemic and the challenges, *Int. J. Antimicrob. Agents*, vol. 55, no. 3, p. 105924, Mar. 2020, doi: 10.1016/j.ijantimicag.2020.105924.
19. Z. T. Al-Sharify, T. A. Al-Sharify, N. T. Al-Sharify, and H. Y. Naser, A critical review on medical imaging techniques (CT and PET scans) in the medical field, *IOP Conf. Ser. Mater. Sci. Eng.*, vol. 870, no. 1, 2020, doi: 10.1088/1757-899X/870/1/012043.
20. N. Krishnan, M. Karthikeyan, Thiagarajar College of Engineering, Institute of Electrical and Electronics Engineers. Madras Section. Podhigai Subsection, Institute of Electrical and Electronics Engineers. Madras Section, Signal Processing/Computational Intelligence/Computer Joint Societies Chapter, and Institute of Electrical and Electronics Engineers, 2018 IEEE international conference on computational intelligence and computing research: 2018 December 13–15: venue: Thiagarajar College of Engineering, Madurai, Tamil Nadu, India, *2019 IEEE Int. Conf. Electr. Comput. Commun. Technol.*, pp. 1–4, 2018.
21. A. Heidari, N. Jafari Navimipour, M. Unal, and S. Toumaj, The COVID-19 epidemic analysis and diagnosis using deep learning: A systematic literature review and future directions, *Comput. Biol. Med.*, vol. 141, no. November 2021, p. 105141, 2022, doi: 10.1016/j.compbiomed.2021.105141.
22. N. AleEbrahim, Essential steps to write a Bibliometric paper, *Introd. Work. "Procedureto write a Bibliometr. Pap."*, vol. 1, no. 13, pp. 1–43, 2016, [Online]. Available: https://dx.doi.org/10.6084/m9.figshare.4292927.v1%5Cnhttps://works.bepress.com/aleebrahim/178/%5Cnhttp://www.academia.edu/30431757/Essential_steps_to_write_a_Bibliometric_paper%5Cnhttps://www.researchgate.net/publication/311612500_Essential_steps_to_write
23. I. N. Sengupta, Bibliometrics, informetrics, scientometrics and librametrics: An overview, *Libri*, vol. 42, no. 2, pp. 75–98, 1992, doi: 10.1515/libr.1992.42.2.75.
24. W. W. Hood and C. S. Wilson, The literature of bibliometrics, scientometrics, and informetrics, *Scientometrics*, vol. 52, no. 2, pp. 291–314, 2001, doi: 10.1023/A:1017919924342.
25. M.AriaandC.Cuccurullo,Sciencemappinganalysiswithbibliometrix R-package:Anexample. *Install and Load Bibliometrix R-package*, pp. 2007–2017, 2022, [Online]. Available: https://bibliometrix.org/documents/bibliometrix_Report.html#section-1-descriptive-analysis
26. V. Osinska and R. Klimas, Mapping science: Tools for bibliometric and altmetric studies, *Inf. Res. an Int. Electron. J.*, vol. 26, no. 4, pp. 1–18, 2021, doi: 10.47989/irpaper909.
27. M. Aria and C. Cuccurullo, bibliometrix: An R-tool for comprehensive science mapping analysis, *J. Informetr.*, vol. 11, no. 4, pp. 959–975, Nov. 2017, doi: 10.1016/j.joi.2017.08.007.
28. Q. Iqbal, Scopus: Indexing and abstracting database, *Information*, vol. 11, no. 3, 2022, doi:10.13140/RG.2.2.12974.15683.

29. J. F. Burnham, Scopus database: A review, *Biomed. Digit. Libr.*, vol. 3, pp. 1–8, 2006, doi: 10.1186/1742-5581-3-1.
30. C. A. R. Michiel Schotten, M. Aisati, W. J. N. Meester, and S. Steiginga, A brief history of Scopus: The world's largest abstract and citation database of scientific literature, in *Research Analytics*, 1st ed., F. J. Cantu-Ortiz, Ed. New York: Auerbach Publications, 2017, p. 28, doi: 10.1201/9781315155890.
31. N. J. vanEck and L. Waltman, Software survey: VOS viewer, a computer program for bibliometric mapping, *Scientometrics*, vol. 84, no. 2, pp. 523–538, 2010, doi: 10.1007/s11192-009-0146-3.
32. N. J. van Eck and L. Waltman, VOS viewer manual, *Leiden: Univeristeit Leiden*, no. January, 2013, [Online]. Available: http://www.vosviewer.com/documentation/Manual_VOSviewer_1.6.1.pdf
33. N. J. van Eck and L. Waltman, Visualizing bibliometric networks, *Information*, vol. 13, no. 8, 2022. doi: 10.1007/978-3-319-10377-8_13.
34. J.-H. Huang, X.-Y. Duan, F.-F. He, G.-J. Wang, and X.-Y. Hu, A historical review and Bibliometric analysis of research on weak measurement research over the past decades based on Biblioshiny, *arXiv preprint* arXiv:2108. 11375, pp. 1–19, 2021 [Online]. Available: http://arxiv.org/abs/2108.11375
35. S. B. Patil, Studies in Indian place names global library & information science research seen through prism of biblioshiny, *Stud. Indian Place Names*, vol. 40, no. 49, pp. 157–170, 2020.
36. P. D. Michailidis, Visualizing social media research in the age of COVID-19, *Information*, vol. 13, no. 8, 2022, doi: 10.3390/info13080372.
37. F. Fusco, M. Marsilio, and C. Guglielmetti, Co-production in health policy and management: A comprehensive bibliometric review, *BMC Health Serv. Res.*, vol. 20, no. 1, pp. 1–17, 2020, doi: 10.1186/s12913-020-05241-2.
38. P. Kannan and S. Thanuskodi, Bibliometric analysis of library philosophy and practice: A study based on Scopus database, *Libr. Philos. Pract.*, vol. 2019, no. Rethinking Libraries and Librarianship, pp. 105–123, 2019.
39. J. A. Moral-muñoz *et al.*, Software tools for conducting bibliometric analysis in science: An up- to-date review, *Sensor*, pp. 1–20, 2020.
40. M. J. Cobo, A. G. Lõpez-Herrera, E. Herrera-Viedma, and F. Herrera, SciMAT: A new science mapping analysis software tool, *J. Am. Soc. Inf. Sci. Technol.*, vol. 63, no. 8, pp. 1609–1630, 2012, doi: 10.1002/asi.22688, p. 319, 2018, doi: 10.5958/2320-317x.2018.00034.x.
41. A. M. Antoniadi *et al.*, Current challenges and future opportunities for Xai in machine learning-based clinical decision support systems: A systematic review, *Appl. Sci.*, vol. 11, no. 11, pp. 1–23, 2021, doi: 10.3390/app11115088.
42. A. Mathew, P. Amudha, and S. Sivakumari, Deep learning techniques: An overview, *Adv. Intell. Syst. Comput.*, vol. 1141, no. January, pp. 599–608, 2021, doi: 10.1007/978-981-15-3383-9_54.
43. Y. Lecun, Y. Bengio, and G. Hinton, Deep learning, *Nature*, vol. 521, no. 7553, pp. 436–444, 2015, doi: 10.1038/nature14539.
44. R. Pranckutė, Web of science (Wos) and scopus: The titans of bibliographic information in today's academic world, *Publications*, vol. 9, no. 1, 2021, doi: 10.3390/publications9010012.
45. S. A. S. Alryalat, L. W. Malkawi, and S. M. Momani, Comparing bibliometric analysis using PubMed, Scopus, and web of science databases, *J. Vis. Exp.*, vol. 2019, no. 152, 2019, doi: 10.3791/58494.

7 Smart Surgery
Navigating Precision through Machine Learning and IoT

Anita Mohanty, Ambarish G. Mohapatra, and Subrat Kumar Mohanty

CONTENTS

DOI: 10.1201/9781003476207-7

7.1 INTRODUCTION

In the ever-evolving realm of healthcare, image-guided surgery stands as a cornerstone of modern medical practices, offering precision and efficacy. The integration of machine learning (ML) and the Internet of Things (IoT) into this paradigm introduces a new era, where intelligent algorithms and interconnected devices converge to redefine the boundaries of surgical procedures [1]. As we embark on this journey, the significance of leveraging advanced technologies becomes apparent, promising not only enhanced decision-making capabilities but also real-time adaptability within surgical environments. The introduction beckons readers to delve into a narrative that unveils the intricate synergy between ML and IoT, shaping the narrative of surgical precision and technological innovation in contemporary healthcare practices [2].

7.1.1 Brief Overview of Image-Guided Surgery and Its Significance in Modern Healthcare

Image-guided surgery represents a revolutionary approach in modern healthcare, utilizing advanced imaging technologies to enhance surgical precision and outcomes [3]. Unlike traditional methods, image-guided surgery as shown in Figure 7.1 integrates real-time imaging data, such as computed tomography (CT), magnetic resonance imaging (MRI), or ultrasound, to provide surgeons with detailed, three-dimensional visualizations of the patient's anatomy during the procedure. This technology allows for more accurate navigation through complex structures, minimizes damage to surrounding healthy tissues, and facilitates the precise placement of instruments [4]. The significance of image-guided surgery lies in its ability to improve the efficacy and safety of various surgical interventions, ranging from neurosurgery and orthopedics to minimally invasive procedures. By enabling surgeons to visualize critical structures and make informed decisions in real time, image-guided surgery contributes to reduced complications, shorter recovery times, and improved patient outcomes, thus marking a transformative advancement in the landscape of modern healthcare.

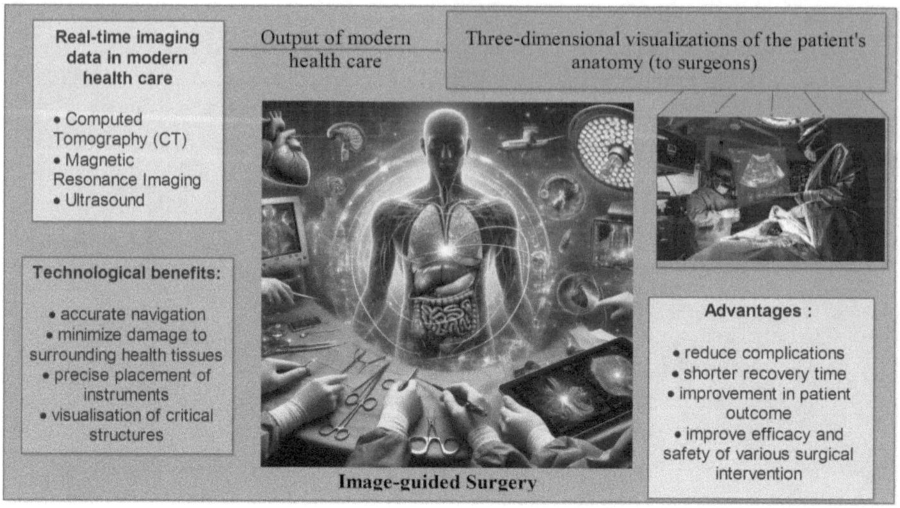

FIGURE 7.1 Overview of image-guided surgery.

7.1.2 Introduction to the Integration of ML and IoT in Surgical Procedures

The integration of ML and the IoT in surgical procedures represents a ground-breaking frontier in healthcare technology. This synergy heralds a new era of intelligent, data-driven decision-making and real-time connectivity within the surgical environment. ML, a subset of artificial intelligence (AI), empowers surgical systems to analyze vast amounts of patient data, aiding in diagnostics, preoperative planning, and personalized treatment strategies [5]. Concurrently, the IoT introduces interconnected devices and sensors into the surgical ecosystem, fostering seamless communication and data exchange [6]. This integration allows for continuous monitoring, enhances surgical navigation, and facilitates adaptive responses during procedures. The collective impact of ML and IoT in surgery is poised to revolutionize not only the precision and efficiency of medical interventions but also the overall patient experience. This introduction invites exploration into a transformative landscape where the amalgamation of advanced technologies reshapes the traditional boundaries of surgical capabilities, promising enhanced outcomes and a paradigm shift in healthcare practices.

Specifically, the chapter highlights the following key contributions:

1. Integration of cutting-edge technologies like ML and IoT into surgical environments. ML is for medical imaging analysis and real-time decision support, while IoT facilitates connectivity and data exchange within the surgical ecosystem.
2. It emphasizes the role of ML-powered smart surgical navigation systems in enhancing surgical precision and efficiency. By using ML algorithms for real-time data analysis and decision-making, these systems enable surgeons to navigate complex procedures with greater accuracy.

3. This chapter also presents real-world case studies that demonstrate the tangible benefits of ML and IoT in improving surgical outcomes.
4. Acknowledging the complexities inherent in deploying ML and IoT technologies in surgical settings, the chapter discusses challenges such as data security and ethical considerations. Raising awareness of these issues encourages a proactive approach to justifying risks and ensuring responsible deployment.
5. Emphasizing the collaborative efforts required to shape this evolving field by highlighting the potential for continued innovation and advancement, it inspires readers to contribute to the ongoing evolution of surgical precision through the dynamic integration of ML and IoT technologies.

This chapter unfolds systematically, commencing with an introduction to image-guided surgery's significance in modern healthcare (Section 7.1). It then proceeds to the foundations of ML in surgery (Section 7.2), elucidating ML algorithms and their role in analyzing medical imaging data. The subsequent section (Section 7.3) explores IoT-enabled surgical environments, discussing devices, sensors, and their role in data collection and connectivity. Section 7.4 delves into smart surgical navigation systems, providing a detailed examination and presenting case studies. Section 7.5 addresses critical considerations related to data security and privacy in the context of ML and IoT. Section 7.6 identifies current challenges and outlines potential future directions. Section 7.7 features in-depth case studies and success stories. The ethical implications of using ML and IoT in surgery are explored in Section 7.8. The chapter concludes in Section 7.9 with a summarization of key findings and a call to action for continued research and adoption of smart surgery technologies.

7.2 FOUNDATIONS OF ML IN SURGERY

The foundations of ML in surgery constitute a pivotal cornerstone in advancing the precision and efficacy of medical interventions. ML algorithms, driven by the analysis of vast datasets, have become instrumental in deciphering complex patterns within medical imaging, patient records, and genomic information [7]. In the context of surgery, ML plays a crucial role in preoperative planning, aiding surgeons in decision-making processes based on predictive analytics as shown in Figure 7.2. It enables the identification of subtle anomalies, assists in risk assessment, and optimizes personalized treatment strategies. The integration of ML in surgical workflows empowers healthcare professionals with intelligent tools that continuously learn and adapt, contributing to enhanced diagnostic accuracy and procedural outcomes. As the foundations of ML in surgery continue to evolve, the potential for ground-breaking advancements in precision medicine and tailored patient care emerges, promising a paradigm shift in how surgical interventions are conceptualized and executed in the modern healthcare landscape.

7.2.1 Explanation of ML Algorithms and Their Role in Analyzing Medical Imaging Data

In the realm of surgery, ML algorithms serve as sophisticated analytical tools that play a pivotal role in decoding intricate patterns within medical imaging data [8, 9].

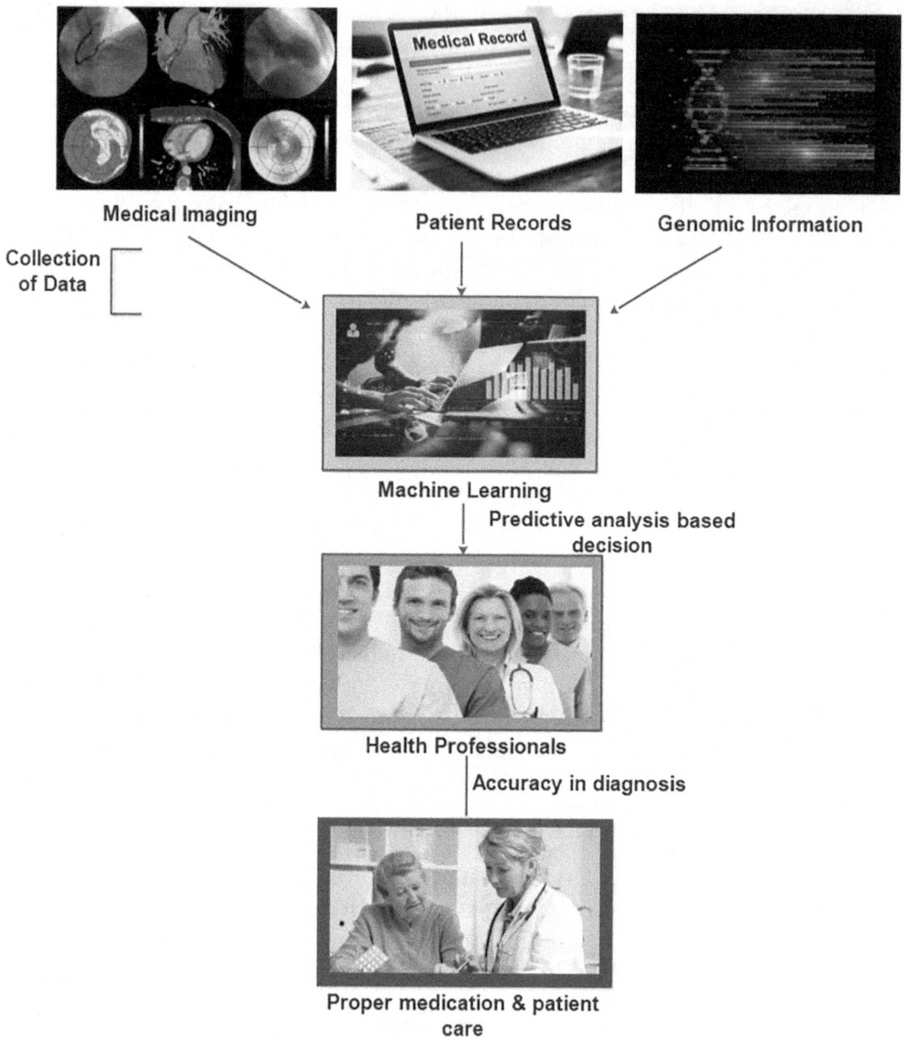

FIGURE 7.2 Utilization steps of ML in surgery.

These algorithms, ranging from traditional methods to deep learning approaches, are designed to autonomously learn and recognize subtle features in images generated by modalities such as CT, MRI, and X-rays. The chapter delves into the technical nuances of various ML algorithms, elucidating how they can efficiently process large datasets to identify anomalies, localize structures, and provide valuable insights to healthcare professionals. By unraveling the complexities inherent in medical images, ML algorithms enhance the precision and reliability of diagnostics, facilitating a more comprehensive understanding of anatomical structures and pathological conditions.

7.2.2 Showcase of ML's Ability to Assist in Preoperative Planning and Real-Time Decision Support

This section unveils the transformative impact of ML in the critical phases of preoperative planning and real-time decision support. ML algorithms excel in predicting potential complications, optimizing surgical pathways, and offering personalized insights based on patient-specific data. The chapter showcases instances where ML contributes to the creation of detailed surgical plans, taking into account individual patient profiles and optimizing procedural approaches. Furthermore, the narrative unfolds the dynamic role of ML in real-time decision support during surgeries. By processing and analyzing incoming data streams, ML algorithms assist surgeons with timely and data-driven recommendations, fostering a more adaptive and responsive surgical environment [10]. Through compelling case studies and practical applications, the chapter illustrates how ML's prowess enhances surgical precision and elevates decision-making processes, ultimately influencing positive outcomes for patients undergoing various surgical interventions.

7.3 IoT-ENABLED SURGICAL ENVIRONMENTS

The integration of the IoT into surgical environments signifies a revolutionary shift in healthcare infrastructure, creating interconnected ecosystems that enhance patient care and surgical processes [11]. IoT-enabled surgical environments leverage smart devices, sensors, and network connectivity to create a seamless flow of real-time data. This section of the chapter explores the multifaceted role of IoT in surgery, from the moment a patient enters the healthcare system to postoperative care.

IoT devices, strategically placed in operating rooms and medical facilities, facilitate continuous monitoring of vital signs, equipment status, and environmental conditions. This real-time data stream empowers surgical teams with valuable insights, contributing to proactive decision-making and early intervention in case of unexpected events. The chapter also delves into the utilization of IoT in tracking and managing medical equipment, ensuring their availability and functionality during surgical procedures.

Beyond the operating room, IoT extends its influence to patient monitoring, recovery, and postoperative care. Wearable devices and remote monitoring systems enable healthcare professionals to track patients' progress, vital signs, and adherence to postoperative care plans. This interconnected approach not only improves the overall efficiency of surgical workflows but also enhances patient outcomes by providing personalized, data-driven care throughout the entire surgical journey.

As the chapter unfolds, readers gain a comprehensive understanding of how IoT transforms surgical environments into intelligent, responsive ecosystems, fostering a new era of precision and connectivity in healthcare practices.

7.3.1 Exploration of IoT Devices and Sensors in the Surgical Ecosystem

The exploration of IoT devices and sensors within the surgical ecosystem reveals a transformative integration of intelligent technologies that revolutionize patient care and surgical processes [12]. IoT devices, ranging from smart sensors to connected instruments, are strategically embedded throughout the surgical environment, creating a networked ecosystem that enhances precision and efficiency.

Within operating rooms, IoT sensors monitor a spectrum of parameters, including temperature, humidity, and equipment status, in real time [13]. These sensors provide immediate feedback to surgical teams, enabling proactive adjustments to optimize the surgical environment. The chapter delves into specific instances where IoT devices contribute to surgical precision, such as smart instruments that provide real-time feedback on tissue characteristics, blood flow, and other vital metrics. This not only assists surgeons during procedures but also opens avenues for data-driven decision-making.

Furthermore, the exploration extends beyond the immediate surgical setting to include IoT applications in instrument sterilization, inventory management, and overall operational efficiency. By incorporating smart tags and RFID technology, hospitals can track the location and usage history of surgical instruments, ensuring compliance with sterilization protocols and minimizing the risk of errors.

In postoperative care, IoT devices continue to play a crucial role. Wearable sensors and remote monitoring devices facilitate continuous patient monitoring, allowing healthcare providers to track vital signs and recovery progress even after the surgical procedure has concluded.

Through this exploration, the chapter unravels the intricate web of IoT devices and sensors, showcasing their diverse applications within the surgical ecosystem. The integration of these technologies not only enhances the accuracy and safety of surgical procedures but also contributes to the broader goal of creating interconnected, intelligent healthcare systems.

7.3.2 Discussion on How IoT Contributes to Data Collection, Connectivity, and Monitoring during Surgeries

The exploration of IoT devices and sensors within the surgical ecosystem unveils a paradigm shift in healthcare, where interconnected technologies redefine the landscape of surgical procedures. In the operating room, IoT devices and sensors are strategically deployed to enhance real-time data acquisition, enabling a dynamic and responsive surgical environment [14]. These devices play a crucial role in monitoring vital signs, environmental conditions, and the status of medical equipment, providing surgeons and healthcare professionals with immediate insights for informed decision-making during procedures.

The chapter delves into specific applications, such as smart surgical instruments equipped with sensors that offer real-time feedback on tissue characteristics and procedural nuances. This level of precision not only enhances surgical outcomes but also exemplifies the potential of IoT to transform traditional instruments into intelligent, data-driven tools. Additionally, the exploration extends to IoT's role in optimizing the surgical workflow, from instrument sterilization processes monitored by smart sensors to inventory management systems that ensure the availability of necessary tools.

Beyond the operating room, the chapter navigates through the postoperative phase, highlighting the integration of wearable IoT devices for continuous patient monitoring. These devices enable healthcare providers to remotely track patients' vital signs, recovery progress, and adherence to postoperative care plans, fostering a more personalized and responsive approach to post-surgical care.

Ultimately, the exploration underscores how IoT devices and sensors converge to create a connected surgical ecosystem, where real-time data, enhanced precision, and streamlined processes contribute to improved surgical outcomes and patient experiences. This interconnected approach paves the way for a future where technology seamlessly integrates with healthcare practices, optimizing the entire surgical journey.

7.4 SMART SURGICAL NAVIGATION SYSTEMS

Smart surgical navigation systems [15] represent a transformative leap in the field of surgery, integrating advanced technologies to augment precision and decision-making during medical procedures. This section of the chapter delves into the intricacies of these navigation systems, elucidating their key components and profound impact on surgical interventions.

At the heart of these systems lie ML algorithms that process intricate medical data, enabling real-time analysis of patient anatomy. The chapter explores how these algorithms facilitate surgical planning by offering detailed, three-dimensional visualizations, aiding surgeons in understanding complex anatomical structures with unprecedented clarity. It also delves into the integration of navigation systems with preoperative imaging data, showcasing their ability to enhance accuracy in guiding surgical instruments and minimizing invasiveness.

The narrative unfolds with a detailed examination of the hardware components, such as augmented reality (AR) displays and robotic-assisted platforms that constitute smart surgical navigation systems [16]. By seamlessly overlaying critical information onto a surgeon's field of view, these systems enable precise instrument guidance, reducing the margin of error and optimizing surgical outcomes. The chapter delves into specific case studies and success stories, illustrating instances where smart navigation systems have significantly impacted procedures across various medical specialties.

As the chapter progresses, it explores the adaptability of these systems to different surgical contexts, emphasizing their potential in minimally invasive surgeries and complex interventions. The discussion also touches upon the ongoing advancements in smart surgical navigation, offering insights into the future trajectory of these systems and their potential to redefine the standards of surgical precision. In essence, the exploration of smart surgical navigation systems within this chapter unveils a transformative force that is reshaping the landscape of modern surgery, heralding a new era of accuracy and efficacy in medical interventions.

7.4.1 Detailed Examination of ML-Driven Navigation Systems for Precision-Guided Surgeries

The detailed examination of ML-driven navigation systems for precision-guided surgeries unveils a sophisticated integration of advanced technologies poised to redefine the landscape of surgical procedures [17]. This section meticulously dissects the components and functionalities of ML-driven navigation systems, elucidating their role in achieving unparalleled precision during surgeries. The chapter navigates through the intricate algorithms that power these systems, emphasizing their capacity to process and analyze vast datasets derived from various imaging modalities.

An in-depth exploration of ML's contribution to surgical precision unfolds, detailing how these algorithms create dynamic, real-time maps of the surgical field. The section delves into the seamless integration of ML with robotic platforms, showcasing how these systems collaborate to provide surgeons with enhanced guidance and decision-making capabilities. It further addresses the adaptability of ML algorithms to intraoperative changes, ensuring continuous, responsive navigation throughout the surgical process.

The examination extends to the user interface and display elements, exploring how AR and intuitive interfaces contribute to the surgeon's situational awareness and spatial understanding. This section aims to provide readers with a comprehensive understanding of the technological architecture underpinning ML-driven navigation systems, highlighting their capacity to optimize surgical workflows, reduce invasiveness, and ultimately elevate the precision of various medical interventions.

By scrutinizing the intricate details of ML-driven navigation systems, this chapter aims to not only demystify their technological foundations but also underscore their transformative potential in advancing the field of precision-guided surgeries, paving the way for more effective and personalized healthcare interventions.

7.4.2 Case Studies Demonstrating Successful Implementations and Improved Outcomes

This crucial section of the chapter unfolds a compelling tapestry of real-world applications, presenting a series of case studies that vividly illustrate the tangible successes resulting from the implementation of ML-driven navigation systems in surgical contexts [18]. These case studies span diverse medical specialties, providing a panoramic view of the transformative impact of ML on surgical precision and patient outcomes.

In neurosurgery, for instance, the chapter delves into cases where ML-driven navigation systems have enabled surgeons to navigate intricate brain structures with unprecedented accuracy, leading to reduced surgical times and minimized risks. Similarly, in orthopedic procedures, the implementation of such systems showcases improved implant placements and enhanced postoperative recovery.

The exploration extends to minimally invasive procedures, where ML-driven navigation has demonstrated its efficacy in guiding surgeons through complex anatomical landscapes with precision, resulting in reduced complications and shorter recovery times. Case studies emphasize instances where the technology has played a pivotal role in adapting to unforeseen challenges intraoperatively, showcasing the flexibility and responsiveness of ML-driven navigation systems.

Each case study dissects specific challenges addressed, innovative solutions implemented, and the subsequent positive impact on procedural efficacy. By weaving together these narratives, the chapter not only validates the theoretical promises of ML in surgery but also emphasizes its practical and transformative significance in diverse clinical settings. These real-world examples serve as beacons of success, inspiring confidence in the potential of ML-driven navigation systems to shape the future of precision-guided surgeries and contribute to improved patient outcomes.

7.5 DATA SECURITY AND PRIVACY CONSIDERATIONS

The section on data security and privacy considerations within the context of ML and IoT in surgical procedures critically examines the paramount importance of safeguarding sensitive medical information in an era of advanced healthcare technologies. This segment navigates through the complexities of managing patient data within interconnected systems, emphasizing the need for robust security protocols and ethical considerations [19].

The chapter explores the challenges associated with ensuring data security in the context of ML algorithms and IoT devices. It delves into encryption methods, access controls, and authentication mechanisms designed to protect patient records, surgical plans, and other confidential information from unauthorized access or cyber threats. The discussion extends to the secure transmission of data between devices, addressing potential vulnerabilities in the communication channels of interconnected systems.

Moreover, the narrative encompasses the privacy implications of utilizing ML algorithms and IoT devices in surgical settings. It scrutinizes how patient consent, data anonymization, and compliance with healthcare regulations contribute to maintaining the privacy and confidentiality of sensitive medical information. The section also considers the ethical dimensions of data usage, discussing the balance between leveraging patient data for improved healthcare outcomes and respecting individuals' rights to privacy.

By scrutinizing the intricate interplay between technological advancements, data security, and privacy concerns, this chapter seeks to provide a comprehensive understanding of the measures necessary to uphold the confidentiality and integrity of patient information in the age of ML and IoT in surgical procedures. This critical exploration aims to equip healthcare professionals, researchers, and policymakers with the insights needed to navigate the ethical and security challenges inherent in the adoption of these transformative technologies.

7.5.1 Discussion on the Importance of Securing Sensitive Medical Data in the Context of ML and IoT

This section delves into the imperative of securing sensitive medical data within the dynamic landscape of ML and the IoT in surgical procedures. Recognizing the pivotal role these technologies play in optimizing healthcare, the discussion emphasizes the critical need to fortify security measures to protect patient confidentiality and data integrity.

The chapter scrutinizes the unique challenges posed by ML algorithms and IoT devices in handling vast amounts of sensitive medical information. ML, with its ability to analyze intricate patterns and make data-driven decisions, requires robust safeguards to prevent unauthorized access or potential misuse. Similarly, the interconnected nature of IoT devices introduces new vulnerabilities that necessitate advanced security protocols to protect the entire data ecosystem [20].

The narrative unfolds with an exploration of encryption methods, access controls, and authentication mechanisms tailored to the intricacies of medical data. It delves into the significance of securing data both at rest and in transit, underscoring the importance of mitigating risks associated with potential breaches or cyber threats. The discussion extends to the role of healthcare institutions and technology providers in implementing and continually updating security measures to stay ahead of evolving threats.

Furthermore, the discourse underscores the ethical responsibility of stakeholders to prioritize patient privacy. It explores the delicate balance between leveraging medical data for advancements in ML-driven diagnostics and treatment while upholding the trust and confidentiality patients place in the healthcare system. As the chapter unfolds, it aims to provide a comprehensive understanding of the multifaceted challenges in securing sensitive medical data, offering insights to guide healthcare professionals, policymakers, and technologists in fortifying the ethical and secure implementation of ML and IoT in surgical contexts.

7.5.2 Overview of Strategies and Technologies to Ensure Patient Privacy and Compliance with Regulations

This crucial section provides a comprehensive overview of strategies and technologies essential for safeguarding patient privacy and ensuring compliance with stringent healthcare regulations in the context of ML and IoT applications within surgical procedures [21].

The chapter explores encryption as a fundamental strategy, shedding light on its role in securing sensitive medical data during storage and transmission. It delves into encryption algorithms, emphasizing their efficacy in protecting patient records, surgical plans, and other confidential information from unauthorized access. The discussion extends to technologies that enable secure data transmission, ensuring the privacy of patient information as it traverses interconnected devices and networks.

Access controls and authentication mechanisms are scrutinized as pivotal components of a robust privacy strategy. The chapter elucidates how implementing stringent access controls ensures that only authorized personnel can access sensitive medical data. Authentication technologies, such as biometrics or multi-factor authentication, are explored for their role in verifying the identity of users and preventing unauthorized entry into healthcare systems.

Moreover, the section navigates through technologies that facilitate data anonymization, allowing healthcare practitioners and researchers to glean valuable insights from medical data without compromising individual privacy. It also addresses the importance of consent management systems, empowering patients to control how their data is utilized while adhering to regulatory frameworks.

As the chapter unfolds, it emphasizes the significance of staying abreast of evolving healthcare regulations and industry standards. This involves adopting technologies that facilitate compliance monitoring, audit trails, and timely updates to security protocols. By providing a detailed overview of these strategies and technologies, this section aims to equip stakeholders in the healthcare ecosystem with the knowledge necessary to establish and maintain robust privacy measures amid the transformative integration of ML and IoT in surgical contexts.

7.6 CHALLENGES AND FUTURE DIRECTIONS

This pivotal section of the chapter navigates through the complex landscape of challenges inherent in the integration of ML and the IoT in surgical procedures, while concurrently illuminating potential future directions that promise to reshape the trajectory of healthcare technology [22].

The discussion begins by addressing current challenges, such as interoperability issues among diverse IoT devices and the need for standardized communication protocols to ensure seamless connectivity. It explores the computational demands and resource-intensive nature of ML algorithms, presenting hurdles in real-time decision support. The ethical conundrums surrounding data privacy and security, as well as the potential biases embedded in ML algorithms, are dissected with a critical lens.

Simultaneously, the chapter looks forward to future directions that could mitigate these challenges. It explores the potential of edge computing to alleviate computational burdens, making ML applications more agile and responsive in surgical settings. The discourse extends to the development of standardized frameworks for data interoperability among IoT devices, fostering a more cohesive and integrated healthcare ecosystem.

The narrative also contemplates the evolution of explainable AI, emphasizing the importance of transparency in ML algorithms to build trust among healthcare professionals and patients. Furthermore, the discussion touches on advancements in federated learning, allowing ML models to be trained across decentralized devices without compromising data privacy.

In charting the future directions, the chapter envisions the integration of AI-driven robotics, AR, and advanced sensors, amplifying the capabilities of ML and IoT in surgical environments. The potential of continuous learning algorithms is explored, adapting and improving over time based on accumulated experience and feedback.

By critically examining existing challenges and envisioning future trajectories, this section aims to provide a roadmap for stakeholders in healthcare and technology, fostering a proactive approach to overcoming obstacles and harnessing the full potential of ML and IoT for the advancement of precision-guided surgeries.

7.6.1 Identification of Current Challenges in Smart Surgery Implementation

This critical subsection delves into a comprehensive examination of the prevailing challenges that impede the seamless implementation of smart surgery, particularly in the integration of ML and the IoT. It brings to light the multifaceted obstacles that healthcare practitioners, technologists, and policymakers grapple with in their pursuit of elevating surgical precision through advanced technologies [23]. Some identified challenges are listed in Table 7.1.

By meticulously identifying these challenges, this section provides a foundation for understanding the intricacies and obstacles within the current landscape of smart surgery implementation. It sets the stage for the subsequent exploration of potential solutions and future directions, guiding stakeholders toward a more informed and strategic approach to overcoming these impediments.

TABLE 7.1
Overview of Current Challenges in Smart Surgery Implementation

Challenges	Overview	Solution
Interoperability conundrum	The interconnected tools and sensors, operating on diverse platforms, pose obstacles to seamless communication and data exchange within surgical settings.	This part emphasizes the necessity for standardized protocols to synchronize the functionality of these devices, ensuring a cohesive and interoperable ecosystem.
Computational demands of ML algorithms	With real-time decision support being crucial in surgical procedures, the intensive computational load on systems presents challenges.	The chapter navigates the complexities of balancing computational efficiency with the imperative for swift and accurate analyses, suggesting potential solutions like edge computing to tackle this obstacle.
Ethical considerations in data privacy and security	It explores the need to safeguard sensitive medical information and comply with privacy regulations.	The discourse extends to potential biases within ML algorithms, emphasizing the importance of mitigating algorithmic biases for equitable and unbiased healthcare outcomes.

7.6.2 Exploration of Potential Advancements and Future Directions for Research and Development

This forward-looking subsection embarks on an exploration of the exciting potential advancements and future directions in the realm of smart surgery, driven by the integration of ML and the IoT [24]. It envisions a roadmap for research and development that holds promise for overcoming current challenges and reshaping the landscape of precision-guided surgical interventions.

The discussion is initiated by delving into the burgeoning field of edge computing, foreseeing its transformative role in mitigating computational challenges. By bringing processing closer to the source of data, edge computing has the potential to enhance the agility and responsiveness of ML algorithms, paving the way for real-time decision support in surgical settings [25].

The chapter contemplates the evolution of standardized frameworks for data interoperability among IoT devices. The envisioned future sees the development of seamless communication protocols, fostering a more integrated and cohesive healthcare ecosystem. This exploration extends to the potential of blockchain technology, offering secure and transparent solutions for managing and sharing medical data across interconnected devices.

Explainable AI emerges as a crucial focal point in future research directions. The chapter envisions advancements in developing ML models that provide transparent insights into their decision-making processes, ensuring that healthcare professionals and patients can comprehend and trust the outcomes derived from these intelligent systems.

The narrative extends to the evolution of federated learning, anticipating a future where ML models can be trained across decentralized devices without compromising individual data privacy. This approach holds the potential to facilitate collaborative learning while respecting the sensitive nature of patient information.

The chapter concludes by envisioning the integration of AI-driven robotics, AR, and advanced sensors into smart surgical environments. These advancements are poised to amplify the capabilities of ML and IoT, providing surgeons with unprecedented precision and decision support during complex procedures.

By exploring these potential advancements and future directions, this subsection offers a glimpse into the transformative possibilities that lie ahead in the field of smart surgery. It serves as an inspiration for researchers, practitioners, and innovators, guiding them toward pioneering solutions that could redefine the landscape of surgical precision and patient care.

7.7 CASE STUDIES AND SUCCESS STORIES

This pivotal section of the chapter unfolds a rich tapestry of real-world applications, featuring case studies and success stories that illuminate the transformative impact of ML and the IoT in the domain of smart surgery [26, 27]. These narratives serve as compelling examples, showcasing how these advanced technologies have been instrumental in revolutionizing surgical precision and patient outcomes across diverse medical specialties.

The exploration begins with case studies in neurosurgery, where ML-driven navigation systems have empowered surgeons to navigate intricate brain structures with unprecedented accuracy. These cases delve into instances where precise guidance and decision support have led to reduced surgical times and minimized risks, illustrating the tangible benefits for both surgeons and patients.

Orthopedic procedures emerge as another focal point, demonstrating how ML algorithms have optimized implant placements and postoperative recovery. Success stories highlight the enhanced precision achieved through real-time feedback on tissue characteristics, leading to improved long-term outcomes and patient satisfaction.

In the realm of minimally invasive procedures, case studies illustrate how ML-driven navigation has guided surgeons through complex anatomical landscapes with unparalleled accuracy. These success stories underscore reduced complications and shorter recovery times, marking a paradigm shift in the field of minimally invasive surgery.

The section continues to unfold narratives that traverse various medical specialties, including cardiovascular surgery, oncology, and robotic-assisted procedures. Each case study is meticulously crafted to showcase the unique challenges addressed, innovative solutions implemented, and the subsequent positive impact on procedural efficacy.

By weaving together these real-world examples, the chapter not only validates the theoretical promises of ML and IoT in surgery but also emphasizes their practical and transformative significance in clinical settings. These case studies stand as beacons of success, inspiring confidence in the potential of smart surgery technologies to redefine standards and contribute to improved patient outcomes across the spectrum of surgical interventions.

7.7.1 In-depth Analysis of Notable Cases Where ML and IoT Have Significantly Impacted Surgical Outcomes

1. **Neurosurgery Precision Enhancement:** In a notable neurosurgery case, ML-driven navigation systems played a pivotal role in enhancing precision during a complex brain tumor resection. By analyzing preoperative imaging data in real time, the system provided the surgical team with high-resolution, three-dimensional maps of the patient's brain [28]. This allowed surgeons to navigate intricate structures with unprecedented accuracy, minimizing the risk of damage to surrounding healthy tissue. The integration of IoT sensors monitored the patient's vital signs and environmental conditions in real time, contributing to a responsive and adaptable surgical environment.
2. **Orthopedic Implant Optimization:** In an orthopedic case study, ML algorithms were employed to optimize implant placements during joint replacement surgery. The system analyzed patient-specific data, including bone density and joint biomechanics, to recommend optimal implant sizes and positions. IoT-enabled smart instruments provided real-time feedback on tissue characteristics and ensured precise implant placement [29]. This approach significantly improved the accuracy of the procedure, leading to enhanced postoperative recovery and reduced instances of implant-related complications.
3. **Minimally Invasive Precision in Cardiovascular Surgery:** A case in cardiovascular surgery highlighted the impact of ML-driven navigation in minimally invasive procedures. ML algorithms processed intricate cardiac imaging data, aiding surgeons in navigating complex coronary anatomy with exceptional precision [30]. Additionally, IoT devices continuously monitor the patient's hemodynamic parameters, ensuring real-time adjustments during the procedure. This integration of ML and IoT significantly contributed to reduced procedural risks, shorter recovery times, and improved overall outcomes in cardiovascular interventions.
4. **Oncological Surgery Decision Support:** In the field of oncology, ML-driven decision support systems demonstrated their efficacy in tailoring surgical approaches. By analyzing patient-specific tumor characteristics and integrating data from molecular profiling, the system provided surgeons with personalized recommendations for resection margins and lymph node dissection. IoT sensors tracked intraoperative variables, facilitating dynamic adjustments [31]. This comprehensive approach in oncological surgery showcased improved precision, reduced recurrence rates, and enhanced patient-specific treatment strategies.
5. **Robotic-Assisted Surgical Success:** A case in robotic-assisted surgery highlighted the synergy between ML algorithms and robotic platforms. ML-driven navigation systems, integrated with robotic instruments, facilitated real-time adjustments based on intraoperative data [32]. This collaborative approach enhanced the surgeon's dexterity and precision, leading to successful outcomes in procedures such as prostatectomy and gynecological surgeries. The incorporation of IoT devices ensured continuous monitoring and feedback, contributing to the overall success of robotic-assisted surgeries.

These in-depth analyses underscore the tangible impact of ML and IoT on surgical outcomes across diverse specialties. By leveraging advanced technologies for precision, decision support, and real-time adaptability, these cases exemplify the transformative potential of smart surgery in improving patient care and reshaping the landscape of modern surgical interventions.

7.7.2 Lessons Learned and Best Practices for Implementing Smart Surgery Solutions

The following categories mentioned in Figure 7.2 filter valuable lessons learned and best practices from the implementation of smart surgery solutions, drawing insights from successful cases and experiences. Table 7.2 shows lessons learned and best practices of different categories for implementing smart surgery solutions.

By embracing these lessons learned and adhering to best practices, healthcare institutions can navigate the complexities of implementing smart surgery solutions, ultimately enhancing patient care, surgical precision, and overall healthcare outcomes.

7.8 ETHICAL IMPLICATIONS

This section of the chapter delves into the ethical considerations surrounding the integration of ML and the IoT in smart surgery [33], highlighting the profound impact these technologies have on patient care, privacy, and the ethical responsibilities of healthcare professionals and technologists.

1. **Informed Consent and Autonomy:**
   - Ethical Consideration: The use of ML and IoT in surgery necessitates transparent communication with patients to ensure informed consent.
   - Implication: Surgeons and healthcare professionals must actively engage patients in discussions about the use of smart surgery technologies, providing comprehensive information about potential risks, benefits, and alternatives.

2. **Data Privacy and Security:**
   - Ethical Consideration: Protecting patient data is paramount to uphold privacy and trust.
   - Implication: Stringent measures must be in place to safeguard sensitive medical information, including robust encryption, access controls, and compliance with data protection regulations.

3. **Algorithmic Bias and Fairness:**
   - Ethical Consideration: ML algorithms may inherit biases, leading to disparities in healthcare outcomes.
   - Implication: Developers and healthcare professionals must actively work to identify and mitigate biases in algorithms, ensuring fair and equitable treatment for all patient demographics.

TABLE 7.2
Lessons Learned and Best Practices of Different Categories for Implementing Smart Surgery Solutions

Categories	Lesson Learned	Best Practice
Interdisciplinary Collaboration	Successful implementation requires interdisciplinary collaboration among surgeons, data scientists, engineers, and healthcare administrators.	Foster collaborative teams that facilitate open communication and shared understanding of clinical needs and technological capabilities.
Robust Data Governance	Data quality and governance are foundational to the success of ML-driven solutions.	Implement robust data governance frameworks, ensuring standardized data formats, accurate annotations, and adherence to privacy regulations.
Continuous Training and Education	The dynamic nature of smart surgery technologies necessitates ongoing training for healthcare professionals.	Establish continuous education programs to keep surgical teams updated on the latest advancements, ensuring proficiency in utilizing ML and IoT tools effectively.
Patient-Centric Approach	Patient outcomes are paramount, and solutions should be designed with a patient-centric focus.	Involve patients in the decision-making process, ensuring their understanding, consent, and comfort with the integration of smart surgery technologies.
Ethical Considerations and Bias Mitigation	Ethical considerations, including bias in algorithms, demand careful attention.	Best Practice: Prioritize fairness, transparency, and bias mitigation strategies in the development and deployment of ML algorithms, ensuring equitable outcomes for diverse patient populations.
Scalability and Interoperability	Scalability and interoperability are critical for widespread adoption.	Design solutions that can scale across different surgical specialties and seamlessly integrate with existing healthcare infrastructure, fostering interoperability among diverse devices and systems.
Security and Privacy Protocols	Robust security measures are imperative to protect sensitive medical data.	Implement end-to-end encryption, access controls, and regular security audits to safeguard patient information and comply with privacy regulations.
Iterative Development and Feedback Loops	Continuous refinement is essential for optimizing smart surgery solutions.	Establish iterative development cycles, incorporating feedback from surgeons, healthcare professionals, and patients to enhance the usability, accuracy, and overall efficacy of the technology.
Regulatory Compliance	Adherence to regulatory frameworks is crucial for deployment and acceptance.	Stay abreast of evolving healthcare regulations and standards, ensuring compliance throughout the development, testing, and deployment phases.
Robust Training and Support Infrastructure	Adequate training and support infrastructure are essential for successful implementation.	Provide comprehensive training programs, user manuals, and a responsive support system to assist surgical teams during the adoption and integration of smart surgery solutions.

4. **Accountability and Transparency:**
   - Ethical Consideration: Clear accountability for decisions made by ML algorithms is crucial for trust and ethical practice.
   - Implication: Healthcare professionals should have a deep understanding of how algorithms function, and transparent reporting mechanisms should be in place to trace decision-making processes.

5. **Impact on Healthcare Disparities:**
   - Ethical Consideration: The introduction of new technologies can inadvertently exacerbate existing healthcare disparities.
   - Implication: There is an ethical obligation to ensure that smart surgery solutions are accessible and beneficial across diverse populations, avoiding the perpetuation of disparities.

6. **Human Oversight and Decision-Making:**
   - Ethical Consideration: Balancing the autonomy of ML algorithms with human oversight is an ethical imperative.
   - Implication: Surgeons should retain ultimate responsibility for clinical decisions, with ML serving as a supportive tool rather than a replacement for human judgment.

7. **Patient Trust and Education:**
   - Ethical Consideration: Building and maintaining patient trust is essential for successful implementation.
   - Implication: Transparent communication and patient education initiatives are vital to instill confidence in the use of ML and IoT in smart surgery.

8. **Data Ownership and Consent Management:**
   - Ethical Consideration: Patients should have control over their medical data and how it is utilized.
   - Implication: Implementing systems for explicit consent management and clearly defining data ownership empower patients to make informed decisions about the use of their health information.

9. **Healthcare Professional Training:**
   - Ethical Consideration: Adequate training is essential to ensure the competent and ethical use of smart surgery technologies.
   - Implication: Continuous education programs must be established to equip healthcare professionals with the knowledge and skills required for ethical deployment and utilization of ML and IoT tools.

10. **Equitable Access to Technology:**
    - Ethical Consideration: Ensuring fair access to smart surgery technologies is an ethical imperative.
    - Implication: Efforts should be made to address socioeconomic disparities, providing equitable access to the benefits of ML and IoT in surgical interventions.

By addressing these ethical considerations, the healthcare community can navigate the implementation of ML and IoT in smart surgery with a commitment to patient welfare, fairness, and responsible innovation. This ethical framework lays the groundwork for a future where advanced technologies enhance healthcare outcomes while upholding the values of transparency, privacy, and equity.

7.8.1 Examination of Ethical Considerations in the Use of ML and IoT in Surgery

The integration of ML and the IoT in surgery brings forth a myriad of ethical considerations that demand careful examination. This section scrutinizes key ethical dimensions inherent in the utilization of these technologies [34]:

1. **Informed Consent and Patient Autonomy:**
   - **Ethical Concern:** The complexity of ML algorithms and IoT devices necessitates robust efforts to ensure patients comprehend the implications of their use.
   - **Examination:** Healthcare practitioners must prioritize clear communication, ensuring patients fully understand the involvement of smart technologies in their surgical care and obtain informed consent accordingly.

2. **Data Privacy and Security:**
   - **Ethical Concern:** The vast amount of sensitive medical data collected by IoT devices and utilized by ML algorithms raises concerns about patient privacy.
   - **Examination:** Stringent data protection measures, including encryption and access controls, must be in place to safeguard patient confidentiality, and healthcare providers must adhere to privacy regulations.

3. **Algorithmic Bias and Fairness:**
   - **Ethical Concern:** ML algorithms may inadvertently perpetuate biases, leading to disparities in healthcare outcomes.
   - **Examination:** Continuous scrutiny of algorithms is essential to identify and rectify biases. Developers must prioritize fairness, transparency, and regular audits to ensure equitable treatment for all patient demographics.

4. **Transparency and Explainability:**
   - **Ethical Concern:** The inherent complexity of ML algorithms poses challenges in explaining their decisions to both healthcare professionals and patients.
   - **Examination:** Ensuring transparency in algorithmic decision-making is crucial. Developers should strive to create explainable models, providing insights into how decisions are reached.

5. **Human Oversight and Accountability:**
   - **Ethical Concern:** Striking the right balance between the autonomy of ML algorithms and human oversight is an ethical imperative.

- **Examination:** Surgeons should maintain ultimate responsibility for clinical decisions, with ML serving as a supportive tool. Clear accountability structures must be in place to address any discrepancies or errors.

6. **Patient Trust and Education:**
   - **Ethical Concern:** Building and maintaining trust in smart surgery technologies is essential for successful implementation.
   - **Examination:** Transparent communication, patient education initiatives, and establishing a culture of openness regarding the use of ML and IoT contribute to fostering trust among patients.

7. **Data Ownership and Consent Management:**
   - **Ethical Concern:** Patients should have control over their medical data and its utilization in ML algorithms.
   - **Examination:** Implementing robust systems for explicit consent management ensures that patients are aware of and comfortable with how their health information is being utilized, respecting their autonomy.

8. **Equitable Access to Technology:**
   - **Ethical Concern:** Unequal access to smart surgery technologies may exacerbate existing healthcare disparities.
   - **Examination:** Efforts should be made to address socioeconomic disparities, ensuring that the benefits of ML and IoT in surgery are accessible to all patient populations.

9. **Healthcare Professional Training:**
   - **Ethical Concern:** Inadequate training can compromise the ethical use of smart surgery technologies by healthcare professionals.
   - **Examination:** Continuous education programs should be established to equip healthcare professionals with the necessary skills and knowledge for the ethical deployment and utilization of ML and IoT tools.

10. **Safety and Risk Mitigation:**
    - **Ethical Concern:** ML algorithms and IoT devices introduce new risks that must be actively managed.
    - **Examination:** Healthcare providers must prioritize patient safety, conduct thorough risk assessments, and implement mitigation strategies to minimize potential harm associated with the use of these technologies.

By comprehensively examining these ethical considerations, stakeholders in the healthcare ecosystem can navigate the integration of ML and IoT in surgery with a heightened awareness of their ethical responsibilities. This scrutiny lays the groundwork for ethically sound practices that prioritize patient welfare, fairness, and responsible innovation in the dynamic landscape of smart surgery.

7.8.2 Discussion on Maintaining the Balance between Technological Innovation and Ethical Responsibility

The integration of technological innovation, particularly ML and the IoT, into surgery, necessitates a delicate balance between pushing the boundaries of medical advancement and upholding ethical responsibility [35]. This discussion explores key considerations in maintaining this equilibrium:

1. **Ethical Frameworks and Guidelines:**
   - **Innovation:** Technological advancements should align with established ethical frameworks and guidelines that prioritize patient welfare, privacy, and fairness.
   - **Responsibility:** Striking a balance involves proactively incorporating ethical considerations into the development, deployment, and use of ML and IoT in surgery. Adherence to ethical guidelines ensures that innovation aligns with broader societal values and healthcare norms.

2. **Transparency and Explainability:**
   - **Innovation:** ML algorithms often operate as black boxes, making it challenging to understand their decision-making processes fully.
   - **Responsibility:** Ensuring transparency and explainability in algorithms is crucial. Innovations should prioritize the development of interpretable models, allowing healthcare professionals and patients to comprehend and trust the technology.

3. **Informed Consent and Patient Autonomy:**
   - **Innovation:** The complexity of ML and IoT may pose challenges in obtaining fully informed consent from patients.
   - **Responsibility:** Ethical responsibility demands transparent communication with patients, explaining the role of technology in their care. Innovations should include mechanisms for obtaining informed consent that respects patient autonomy.

4. **Algorithmic Bias and Fairness:**
   - **Innovation:** ML algorithms may inadvertently perpetuate biases in healthcare decision-making.
   - **Responsibility:** Innovators must actively address biases, employing techniques to identify, mitigate, and prevent unfair treatment. Regular audits and ongoing efforts to eliminate bias are essential to uphold ethical standards.

5. **Human Oversight and Accountability:**
   - **Innovation:** Autonomous decision-making by ML algorithms may raise questions about accountability and human oversight.
   - **Responsibility:** While embracing innovation, healthcare professionals must retain ultimate responsibility for clinical decisions. Clearly defined

lines of accountability ensure that ethical and legal considerations are addressed when technologies are integrated into patient care.

6. **Patient Trust and Education:**
   - **Innovation:** Rapid technological changes may lead to apprehension and mistrust among patients.
   - **Responsibility:** Upholding patient trust requires ongoing communication and education. Healthcare providers should actively engage patients, explaining the benefits and risks of innovative technologies, and fostering a culture of transparency and trust.

7. **Data Ownership and Consent Management:**
   - **Innovation:** The extensive use of patient data in ML and IoT introduces questions about ownership and consent.
   - **Responsibility:** Innovators must establish clear frameworks for data ownership and implement robust consent management systems. This ensures that patients have control over how their data is utilized, aligning with ethical principles.

8. **Equitable Access and Healthcare Disparities:**
   - **Innovation:** Technological innovations may inadvertently widen existing healthcare disparities if not implemented equitably.
   - **Responsibility:** Innovators bear the responsibility of actively working to bridge disparities. This involves considering socioeconomic factors, accessibility, and inclusivity in the design and deployment of technologies to ensure equitable access and benefits.

9. **Healthcare Professional Training:**
   - **Innovation:** The rapid pace of technological innovation requires healthcare professionals to continually update their skills.
   - **Responsibility:** Innovators and healthcare institutions must provide ongoing training programs to equip professionals with the knowledge and skills needed to navigate and ethically implement new technologies.

10. **Safety and Risk Mitigation:**
    - **Innovation:** Innovations may introduce new risks and uncertainties in patient care.
    - **Responsibility:** Ethical responsibility demands a proactive approach to risk mitigation. Innovators and healthcare providers should conduct thorough risk assessments, implement safeguards, and continuously monitor and address emerging risks.

Balancing technological innovation with ethical responsibility requires a collaborative effort from healthcare professionals, technologists, policymakers, and patients. Striking this balance ensures that advancements in ML and IoT contribute positively to patient care while upholding the core principles of ethics and responsible innovation in the ever-evolving landscape of modern healthcare.

7.9 CONCLUSION

In the dynamic intersection of ML and the IoT with surgery, the journey into image-guided precision and smart surgical interventions unfolds with transformative potential. This chapter has traversed the realms of technological innovation, ethical considerations, and real-world applications, shedding light on the intricacies of implementing ML and IoT in surgery.

From the foundations of ML algorithms analyzing medical imaging data to the exploration of IoT-enabled surgical environments, the integration of these technologies promises unprecedented precision, real-time decision support, and enhanced patient outcomes. The examined case studies and success stories have underscored the tangible impact of ML and IoT across diverse surgical specialties, from neurosurgery to orthopedics, cardiovascular surgery, and beyond.

Ethical considerations have been at the forefront of this exploration, acknowledging the delicate balance required between technological innovation and ethical responsibility. The discussions on informed consent, data privacy, algorithmic bias, and transparency underscore the importance of upholding ethical standards in the pursuit of medical advancements.

Lessons learned and best practices for implementing smart surgery solutions have been distilled from successful cases, emphasizing interdisciplinary collaboration, continuous training, and patient-centric approaches. The challenges and future directions discussed have provided a roadmap for navigating the complexities of ML and IoT integration in surgical settings.

As the chapter concludes, it becomes evident that the transformative potential of ML and IoT in surgery is accompanied by a profound responsibility. The ethical implications underscore the need for conscientious decision-making, transparency, and ongoing commitment to patient welfare. Striking the delicate balance between innovation and responsibility is imperative for shaping a future where technology augments the capabilities of healthcare professionals while prioritizing the well-being, autonomy, and trust of patients.

In essence, the journey into image-guided precision surgery through ML and IoT is not merely a technological evolution but a profound societal and ethical transition. As stakeholders in healthcare continue to navigate this transformative landscape, the overarching goal remains the same: to harness the power of innovation responsibly, ensuring that every advancement contributes to a future where healthcare is not just technologically advanced but, more importantly, humanely advanced.

7.9.1 Summarization of Key Findings and Insights

The exploration of image-guided precision surgery through the integration of ML and the IoT has yielded key findings and insights:

1. **Technological Advancements:**
   - ML algorithms, driven by vast datasets, have showcased their prowess in analyzing complex medical imaging data, providing surgeons with unprecedented insights for precision-guided surgeries.

- IoT-enabled surgical environments have introduced real-time data streams, facilitating dynamic decision support and creating interconnected ecosystems for enhanced surgical capabilities.

2. **Real-World Impact:**
   - Case studies across neurosurgery, orthopedics, cardiovascular surgery, and other specialties have demonstrated tangible improvements in surgical precision, reduced complications, and enhanced patient outcomes.
   - Smart surgery technologies, guided by ML and IoT, have become invaluable tools for surgeons, optimizing preoperative planning, intraoperative decision-making, and postoperative care.

3. **Ethical Considerations:**
   - Maintaining a delicate balance between technological innovation and ethical responsibility is imperative. Transparency, explainability, and addressing algorithmic biases are crucial for upholding ethical standards.
   - Patient-centric approaches, informed consent, and robust data privacy measures underscore the ethical imperative of ensuring patient autonomy, trust, and well-being in the adoption of smart surgery technologies.

4. **Best Practices:**
   - Interdisciplinary collaboration among surgeons, data scientists, and engineers is fundamental for successful implementation.
   - Continuous training programs for healthcare professionals, transparent communication with patients, and proactive efforts to mitigate algorithmic biases are essential best practices.

5. **Challenges and Future Directions:**
   - Challenges include interoperability issues, computational demands, and regulatory considerations. Future directions involve advancements in edge computing, standardized frameworks, and the evolution of explainable AI.
   - The integration of ML-driven navigation systems, IoT devices, and robotics is poised to redefine surgical precision and decision support.

6. **Security and Privacy:**
   - The importance of securing sensitive medical data in the context of ML and IoT has been emphasized. Robust encryption, access controls, and ethical responsibility are paramount for protecting patient information.

7. **Lessons Learned:**
   - Continuous refinement, iterative development, and patient trust-building efforts are critical lessons learned from successful implementations.
   - Ethical frameworks and guidelines must be integral to the development and deployment of smart surgery solutions.

8. **Conclusion:**
   - The journey into image-guided precision surgery through ML and IoT is marked by a transformative potential that comes with a profound responsibility.

- The chapter concludes with a call for responsible innovation, where technological advancements are aligned with ethical principles, patient welfare is prioritized, and the delicate balance between innovation and responsibility is maintained.

In summary, the exploration of ML and IoT in surgery signifies not just a technological evolution but a paradigm shift in healthcare, where innovation is deeply entwined with ethical considerations, patient-centric care, and a commitment to shaping a future where technology advances not only medical capabilities but also the fundamental principles of compassionate and responsible healthcare.

7.9.2 Call to Action for Continued Research and Adoption of Smart Surgery Technologies

The exploration of image-guided precision surgery through ML and the IoT has uncovered immense potential, but it is crucial to propel this transformative journey forward. A call to action is warranted for continued research and adoption of smart surgery technologies:

1. **Advanced Interdisciplinary Research:**
   - Encourage collaborative research involving surgeons, data scientists, engineers, ethicists, and policymakers to address evolving challenges and opportunities in smart surgery technologies.

2. **Invest in Education and Training Programs:**
   - Allocate resources to develop comprehensive educational programs for healthcare professionals, ensuring they are well-versed in the integration, utilization, and ethical considerations of ML and IoT in surgical settings.

3. **Foster Industry-Academia Collaboration:**
   - Facilitate collaboration between academic institutions and industry partners to bridge the gap between cutting-edge research and practical, scalable solutions that can be seamlessly integrated into healthcare systems.

4. **Promote Ethical Standards and Guidelines:**
   - Actively contribute to the development and refinement of ethical standards, guidelines, and regulatory frameworks that govern the implementation of ML and IoT in surgery, ensuring responsible and patient-centric practices.

5. **Encourage Real-world Implementations:**
   - Support initiatives that facilitate the real-world implementation of smart surgery technologies across diverse healthcare settings, fostering a deeper understanding of their impact on patient outcomes and healthcare workflows.

6. **Facilitate Data Sharing and Collaboration:**
    - Promote initiatives that encourage responsible data sharing and collaboration among healthcare institutions and researchers, facilitating the creation of larger datasets for training robust ML algorithms.

7. **Support Startups and Innovators:**
    - Provide support and resources for startups and innovators working on novel solutions in the smart surgery domain, fostering a culture of innovation and entrepreneurship in healthcare.

8. **Address Interoperability Challenges:**
    - Prioritize research efforts to address interoperability challenges, ensuring seamless communication and integration among various ML algorithms, IoT devices, and existing healthcare infrastructure.

9. **Explore Patient-Centric Design:**
    - Prioritize research on patient-centric design principles for smart surgery technologies, incorporating patient feedback and preferences into the development process to enhance usability and acceptance.

10. **Engage with Regulatory Bodies:**
    - Collaborate with regulatory bodies to ensure that frameworks and guidelines for smart surgery technologies are adaptive, accommodating technological advancements while safeguarding patient safety, privacy, and ethical standards.

11. **Encourage Global Collaboration:**
    - Foster international collaboration and knowledge exchange to leverage diverse perspectives, experiences, and expertise in advancing smart surgery technologies on a global scale.

12. **Promote Public Awareness and Trust:**
    - Engage in public awareness campaigns to demystify smart surgery technologies, address misconceptions, and foster trust among patients, healthcare professionals, and the wider public.

By embracing this call to action, the healthcare community can collectively contribute to the ongoing evolution of smart surgery technologies, ensuring that innovations are ethically sound, technologically robust, and, most importantly, dedicated to improving patient care and outcomes. Through continued research, collaboration, and responsible adoption, the future of smart surgery holds the promise of reshaping the landscape of healthcare delivery and advancing the frontiers of surgical precision.

REFERENCES

1. J. Bajwa, U. Munir, A. Nori, B. Williams, "Artificial intelligence in healthcare: Transforming the practice of medicine", *Future Healthcare Journal*, vol. 8, no. 2, pp. 188–194, 2021.

2. Z. N. Aghdam, A. M. Rahmani, M. Hosseinzadeh, "The role of the internet of things in healthcare: Future trends and challenges", *Computer Methods and Programs in Biomedicine*, vol. 199, no. 2, 2020.
3. D. G. Barone, T. A. Lawrie, M. G. Hart, "Image guided surgery for the resection of brain tumours", *Cochrane Database Systematic Review*, vol. 2014, no. 1, 2014.
4. Z. Lin, C. Lei, L. Yang, "Modern image-guided surgery: A narrative review of medical image processing and visualization", *Sensors*, vol. 23, no. 24, pp. 1–25, 2023.
5. M. Javaid, A. Haleem, R. P. Singh, R. Suman, S. Rab, "Significance of machine learning in healthcare: Features, pillars and applications", *International Journal of Intelligent Networks*, vol. 3, pp. 58–73, 2022.
6. F. Mulita, G. Verras, C. Anagnostopoulos, K. Kotis, "A smarter health through the internet of surgical things", *Sensors*, vol. 22, no. 12, 2022.
7. P. Satapathy, et al., "Application of machine learning in surgery research: Current uses and future directions", *International Journal of Surgery*, pp. 1550–2023.
8. K. Lam, et al., "Machine learning for technical skill assessment in surgery: A systematic review", *NPJ Digital Medicine*, vol. 5, no. 24, 2022.
9. N. Rashidian, M. A. Hilal, "Applications of machine learning in surgery: Ethical considerations", *Artificial Intelligence Surgery*, vol. 2, pp. 18–23, 2022.
10. R. H. Mithany, et al., "Advancements and Challenges in the application of artificial intelligence in surgical arena: A literature review", *Cureus*, vol. 15, no. 10, 2023.
11. A. Rejeb, et al., "The Internet of Things (IoT) in healthcare: Taking stock and moving forward", *Internet of things*, vol. 22, 2023.
12. B. Pradhan, S. Bhattacharyya, K. Pal, "IoT-based applications in healthcare devices", *Journal of Healthcare Engineering*, vol. 11, p. 266, 2021.
13. A. O. Affia, et al., "IoT health devices: Exploring security risks in the connected landscape", *IoT*, vol. 4, no. 2, pp. 150–182, 2023.
14. C. Li, J. Wang, S. Wang, Y. Zhang, "A review of IoT applications in healthcare", *Neurocomputing*, vol. 565, pp. 1–24, 2024.
15. S. Hwang, S. Lee, S. Kim, "Surgical navigation system for pedicle screw placement based on mixed reality", *International Journal of Control, Automation and Systems*, vol. 21, pp. 3983–3993, 2023.
16. S. Chiou, et al., "Augmented reality surgical navigation system integrated with deep learning", *Bioengineering*, vol. 10, no. 5, 2023.
17. M. Egert, J. E. Steward, C. P. Sundaram, "Machine learning and artificial intelligence in surgical fields", *Indian Journal of Surgical Oncology*, vol. 11, no. 4, pp. 573–577, 2020.
18. A. Mehta, S. Vijayakumar, "Unveiling the tapestry of machine learning: From basics to advanced applications", *International Journal of New Media Studies (IJNMS)*, vol. 5, no. 1, 2023.
19. W. Sun, Z. Cai, Y. Li, F. Liu, S. Fang, G. Wang, "Security and privacy in the medical internet of things: A review", *Security and Communication Networks*, pp. 1–9, 2018.
20. C. Butpheng, K. Yeh, H. Xiong, "Security and privacy in IoT-cloud-based e-health systems—a comprehensive review", *Symmetry*, vol. 12, no. 7, 2020.
21. V. Gugueoth, S. Safavat, S. Shetty, "Security of Internet of Things (IoT) using federated learning and deep learning—Recent advancements, issues and prospects", *ICT Express*, vol. 9, no. 5, pp. 941–960, 2023.
22. J. T. Kelly, K. L. Campbell, E. Gong, P. Scuffham, "The internet of things: Impact and implications for health care delivery", *Journal of Medical Internet Research*, vol. 22, no. 11, 2020.
23. S. Renukappa, P. Mudiyi, S. Suresh, W. Abdalla, C. Subbarao, "Evaluation of challenges for adoption of smart healthcare strategies", *Smart Health*, vol. 26, 2022.
24. D. F. Sittig, A. Wright, H. Singh, et al., "Current challenges in health information technology–related patient safety", *Health Informatics Journal*, vol. 26, no.1, pp. 181–189, 2020.

25. M. Z. Iqbal, E. Mangina, A. G. Campbell, "Current challenges and future research directions in augmented reality for education", *Multimodal Technologies and Interaction*, vol. 6, no. 9, 2022.
26. M. Elahi, S. O. Afolaranmi, J. L. M. Lastra, J. A. P. Garcia, "A comprehensive literature review of the applications of AI techniques through the lifecycle of industrial equipment", *Discover Artificial Intelligence*, vol. 3, no. 43, 2023.
27. S. Ahmad, F. Mehmood, A. Mehmood, D. Kim, "Design and implementation of decoupled IoT application store: A novel prototype for virtual objects sharing and discovery", *Electronics*, vol. 8, no. 3, 2019.
28. D. Patel, A. Nguyen, C. Fleeting, A. B. Patel, M. Mumtaz, B. Lucke-Wold, "Precision medicine in neurosurgery: The evolving role of theranostics", *INNOSC Theranostics and Pharmacological Sciences*, vol. 6, no. 2, 2023.
29. N. Kozic, S. Weber, P. Buchler, et al, "Optimisation of orthopaedic implant design using statistical shape space analysis based on level sets", *Medical Image Analysis*, vol. 10, no. 3, pp. 265–275, 2010.
30. R. B. Karsan, R. Allen, A. Powell, G. W. Beattie, "Minimally-invasive cardiac surgery: A bibliometric analysis of impact and force to identify key and facilitating advanced training", *Journal of Cardiothoracic Surgery*, vol. 17, no. 236, 2022.
31. S. Walsh, et al., "Decision support systems in oncology", *JCO Clinical Cancer Informatics*, vol. 3, no. 3, 2019.
32. S. Bramhe, S. S. Pathak, "Robotic surgery: A narrative review", *Cureus*, vol. 14, no. 9, 2022.
33. Z. Amiri, A. Heidari, et al., "The personal health applications of machine learning techniques in the internet of behaviors", *Sustainability*, vol. 15, no. 16, 2023.
34. K. Rasheed, et al., "Explainable, trustworthy, and ethical machine learning for healthcare: A survey", *Computers in Biology and Medicine*, vol. 149, pp. 1–23, 2022.
35. D. D. Farhud, S. Zokaei, "Ethical issues of artificial intelligence in medicine and healthcare", *Iran Journal of Public Health*, vol. 50, no. 11, 2021.

8 Classification and Detection of Brain Tumors in MRI Images Using Machine Learning Techniques

Ganesh Khekare, Gaurav Kumar Ameta, Rahul Sharma, Anil Turukmane, Pooja Sharma, Urvashi Khekare, and Rahul Agrawal

CONTENTS

8.1 INTRODUCTION

The use of machine learning techniques in medical imaging has shown great promise in improving diagnostic accuracy and facilitating early detection of diseases, particularly in the context of tumor detection. MRI is a frequently used medical imaging procedure known for its ability to provide detailed anatomical information. However, the interpretation of MRI images can be challenging and time-consuming for medical professionals, especially when identifying subtle tumor structures [1].

The main contribution of this research work is to explore and implement different machine learning algorithms and approaches to develop an efficient and accurate tumor detection system for MRI images. This research aimed to address the following objectives:

- **Literature Review:** Conducting an in-depth review of existing research papers, publications, and state-of-the-art techniques in the field of machine learning for medical image analysis and tumor detection in MRI.

DOI: 10.1201/9781003476207-8

- **Data Preparation:** Acquiring and preprocessing MRI datasets containing labeled tumor images and normal tissues, ensuring data quality and consistency for training and evaluation.
- **Architecture Selection:** Evaluating different Deep Learning architectures, such as ResNet, DenseNet, VGG19, VGG16, and custom-designed convolutional neural network (CNN) layers, to determine the most suitable models for tumor detection tasks.
- **Feature Extraction:** Investigating various feature extraction methods to represent MRI images effectively, capturing relevant information for tumor identification [2].
- **Model Training:** Training the selected machine learning models using the preprocessed MRI dataset to learn patterns and correlations between tumor regions and normal tissues.
- **Performance Evaluation:** Assessing the performance of the trained models using metrics such as accuracy.
- **Interpretability and Visualization:** Exploring techniques for model interpretability and visualizing the decision-making process to gain insights into the learned features and enhance the trustworthiness of the system [3].

The successful development of an accurate and reliable tumor detection system can significantly assist medical professionals in diagnosing and treating patients more effectively [4]. The field of medical imaging faces the critical challenge of timely and accurate identification of brain tumors using MRI pictures. The interpretation of these images is complex and time-consuming, often leading to delays in diagnosis and treatment planning. Conventional manual analysis by medical professionals may also result in subjective assessments and potential errors [5]. To address these issues, this research project aimed to harness the power of machine learning techniques to develop an efficient and reliable brain tumor detection and classification system. The primary problem at hand is to design and implement machine learning models capable of accurately distinguishing between normal brain images and those containing tumors. Furthermore, the research aimed to extend this capability to differentiate various types of brain tumors, enhancing the diagnostic process by providing insights into tumor characteristics. The complex nature of MRI images, coupled with the diversity of tumor shapes, sizes, and locations, presents a multifaceted problem. Developing models capable of capturing these intricate patterns and enabling rapid, non-invasive diagnosis requires a comprehensive exploration of various machine learning algorithms, advanced preprocessing techniques, and the integration of domain-specific knowledge [6].

The goal of this research work was to contribute to the improvement of medical diagnosis and patient care by creating a robust and interpretable brain tumor detection and classification system. Through the implementation of advanced artificial intelligence (AI) methodologies, the project sought to address the limitations of manual analysis and offer medical professionals a tool that can aid in early detection, accurate classification, and informed decision-making. By aligning the project with this problem definition, the research aimed to bridge the gap between cutting-edge machine learning techniques and the pressing need for efficient brain tumor analysis, potentially revolutionizing medical imaging practices and patient outcomes. The rest of the chapter is bifurcated as Section 8.2 provides a literature review, Section 8.3 describes the methodology used, Section 8.4 describes the implementation and result discussion, and Section 8.5 is the conclusion followed by references used. The chapter concludes by discussing future avenues for enhancing the project's outcomes, including more advanced preprocessing techniques, ensembling methods, and exploration of rare tumor types.

8.2 LITERATURE REVIEW

The paper by Ankit Ghosh and Alok Kole presents [7, 8] a comprehensive empirical analysis of machine learning algorithms for brain tumor identification. The authors explore the application of nine different machine learning algorithms, including Support Vector Machine (SVM) [9, 10], Random Forest, Logistic Regression, Gradient, Naïve Bayes, K means, Decision Tree, LSTM, XGBoost, etc. on data consisting of MRI brain pictures [11, 12]. The study evaluates the performance of these algorithms based on various parameters, like accuracy, recollect, exactitude, F1-Score, AUC-ROC slopes, and AUC-PR slopes. After rigorous iterations, the results indicate that Gradient Boosting provides better results of classification as compared to other machine learning classifiers tested [13, 14]. Additionally, the authors performed multi-class classification on various datasets consisting of brain MRI pictures of glioma, meningioma, pituitary, and non-tumor using SVM, Random Forest, K Nearest Neighbor, and XG Boost classifiers [15, 16]. The XGBoost classifier demonstrated superior performance, outperforming the other classifiers in accuracy, recall, precision, F1-score, and AUC-ROC score [17, 18]. Brain tumor detection in the early stage is still the biggest challenge faced by doctors.

In summary, the research paper "A Comparative Study of Enhanced Machine Learning Algorithms for Brain Tumor Detection and Classification" explores the use of machine learning classification techniques for brain tumor identification and classification from MRI pictures [19, 20]. The authors propose a hybrid method integrating CNNs and SVM to achieve high accuracy in classification [21, 22]. The results demonstrate that the hybrid CNN–SVM model outperforms individual SVM and CNN models in terms of accuracy. As a result of this study, the focus has shifted toward using deep learning methods [23, 24], particularly CNN–SVM hybrid models, due to their superior performance in achieving higher accuracy metrics in brain tumor classification [25].

The chapter presents a hybrid approach using CNN and SVM for tumor analysis of MRI brain images. The proposed system outperforms traditional machine learning methods [26] and shows significant improvements in accuracy [27]. The combination of CNN [28] and SVM [29] allows for better feature reuse and gradient flow, leading to enhanced model compactness and performance. The study emphasizes the importance of non-invasive, computer-aided diagnosis tools in handling brain tumors and improving diagnostic accuracy within seconds. Though lots of techniques are already available the system which predicts accurately is still missing. A strong robust system is needed which predicts the brain tumor promptly.

8.3 METHODOLOGY

This research focused on the analysis of brain MRI image datasets using AI methods, specifically for tumor detection and classification. Two datasets were utilized in the study. The first dataset involved binary classification to distinguish between healthy brain images and those with tumors. The second dataset comprised multi-class classification to analyze various types of brain tumors. Throughout the research, a series of well-defined stages are executed, including dataset preparation, model construction, training and evaluation, performance comparison, and result analysis. Initial efforts involved the development of a custom three-layer CNN that demonstrated impressive accuracy in binary classification. Subsequently, pre-trained models such as DenseNet, ResNet, VGG16, and VGG19 are employed for tumor-type classification.

The primary tasks in this research include:

1. **Dataset Preparation**: The brain MRI image datasets were collected from online sources, specifically from Kaggle. The datasets were preprocessed to ensure uniformity and eliminate any inconsistencies in the images. The preprocessing steps involved resizing, normalization, and noise reduction.
2. **Model Construction**: Several machine learning and deep learning models were developed for the tasks of tumor detection and classification. Commonly used models such as SVM, CNN, and others were considered.
3. **Training and Evaluation**: The prepared datasets were bifurcated into training and testing datasets. The systems were trained on the training dataset using appropriate optimization techniques. The trained models were then evaluated on the testing data to assess their performance.
4. **Performance Comparison**: The models' performances were compared based on various evaluation metrics, with accuracy being the primary metric of interest. The model with the highest accuracy was identified as the best-performing model.
5. **Result Analysis**: The final step involved analyzing the results of the models and interpreting their predictions. The insights gained from the analysis were used to conclude the effectiveness of different AI algorithms in brain tumor detection and classification tasks.

Throughout the project, the focus was on leveraging advanced AI techniques to handle medical image datasets, particularly MRI brain images. The aim was to develop accurate and efficient models that can aid in the quick identification and classification of brain tumors, contributing to improved medical diagnosis and treatment planning.

8.4 IMPLEMENTATION AND RESULT DISCUSSION

Work Stages:

- **Literature Review and Methodology Exploration:** Conducted a comprehensive review of relevant research papers and methodologies used in brain tumor detection and classification. Explored online courses, documentation of applied libraries, and machine learning methods.

- **Dataset Identification and Preparation:**
  Identified suitable brain MRI image datasets for the project's objectives. Prepared the datasets by ensuring uniformity and preprocessing steps like resizing normalization, and noise reduction, as output these kinds of pictures with labels as shown in Figures 7.1 and 7.2.
- **Initial Model Building and Training:** Started building preliminary models for binary classification (healthy vs. tumor) using the prepared dataset as shown in Figure 8.3. Trained these models and analyzed their performance.

The network consists of two main parts: a convolutional section (cnn_model) and a fully connected section (fc_model).

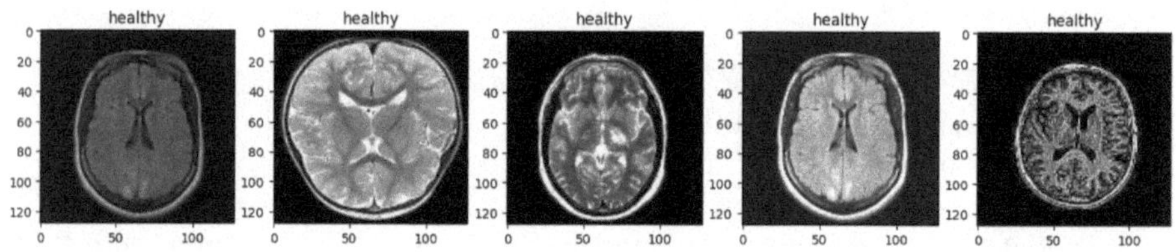

FIGURE 8.1 Pictures with no tumor.

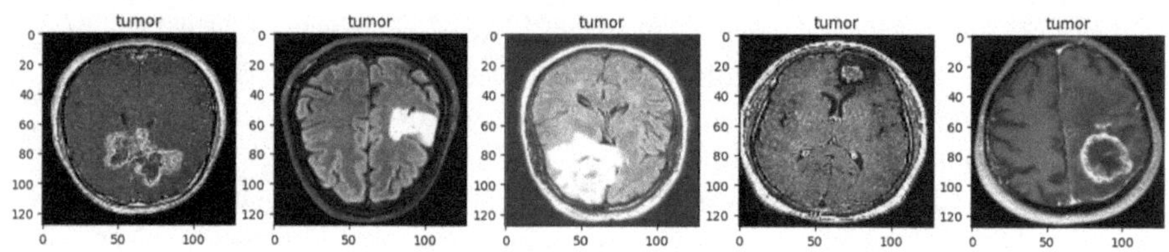

FIGURE 8.2 Pictures with a tumor.

```
CNN(
  (cnn_model): Sequential(
    (0): Conv2d(3, 6, kernel_size=(5, 5), stride=(1, 1))
    (1): Tanh()
    (2): AvgPool2d(kernel_size=2, stride=5, padding=0)
    (3): Conv2d(6, 16, kernel_size=(5, 5), stride=(1, 1))
    (4): Tanh()
    (5): AvgPool2d(kernel_size=2, stride=5, padding=0)
  )
  (fc_model): Sequential(
    (0): Linear(in_features=256, out_features=120, bias=True)
    (1): Tanh()
    (2): Linear(in_features=120, out_features=84, bias=True)
    (3): Tanh()
    (4): Linear(in_features=84, out_features=1, bias=True)
  )
)
```

FIGURE 8.3 Architecture of the constructed neural network.

The convolutional section (cnn_model) includes:

- **Convolutional Layer (Conv2d):** Applies a 5 × 5 convolutional kernel to the input image, generating six feature maps that represent different learned features.
- **Tanh Activation (Tanh):** Apply the hyperbolic tangent activation function to introduce non-linearity after each convolutional layer.
- **Average Pooling Layer (AvgPool2d):** Performs average pooling over 2 × 2 windows with a stride of 5, reducing dimensionality while retaining important features.
- **Repeats 2 and 3 for the Next Convolutional Layer:** Similar to the first convolutional layer, another convolution, activation, and pooling are applied.

The fully connected section (fc_model) includes:

- **Fully Connected Layer (Linear):** Transforms the data from the last convolutional layer into a vector and passes it through a fully connected layer. It has 256 input features and 120 output features.
- **Tanh Activation:** Applies the hyperbolic tangent activation function again.
- **Fully Connected Layer:** Takes the 120 input features and compresses them into 84 output features.
- **Tanh Activation:** Applies the hyperbolic tangent activation function once more.
- **Fully Connected Layer:** The final layer of the fully connected section has 1 output feature, which could indicate a binary classification or regression decision.

This CNN architecture extracts features from input images and makes decisions based on the specific task it's designed for. For MRI images in our case.

Let's consider one image as shown in Figure 8.4.

As it goes through the network—certain features stand out to send it to a fully connected layer

And that is sent to the fully connected layer (Figure 8.5). After training, the results are:

Test Accuracy: 0.940000 Through this graph it can be mentioned that the model has learned training samples on the 150th epoch as shown in Figure 8.6.

- **Dataset Selection for Multi-Class Classification:** Selecting a dataset for the categorization of different types of brain tumors.
- **Data Preparation for Multi-Class Classification:** Prepared the data for multi-class classification, ensuring it meets the requirements of the chosen models.
- **Pre-trained Model Exploration and Training:** Explored pre-trained models suitable for image analysis and utilized them for transfer learning. Trained these models on the selected dataset for brain tumor classification. Multiple training sessions were conducted due to the time-intensive nature of training each model.

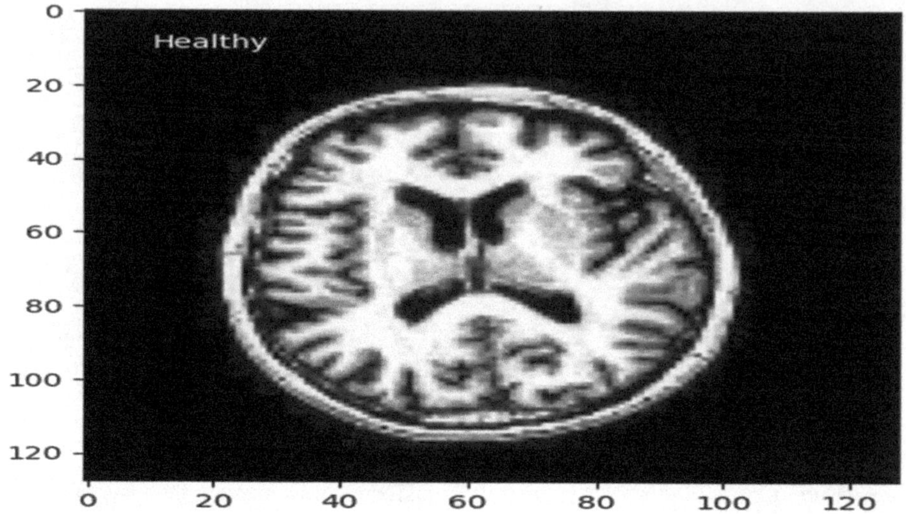

FIGURE 8.4 Random image from the dataset.

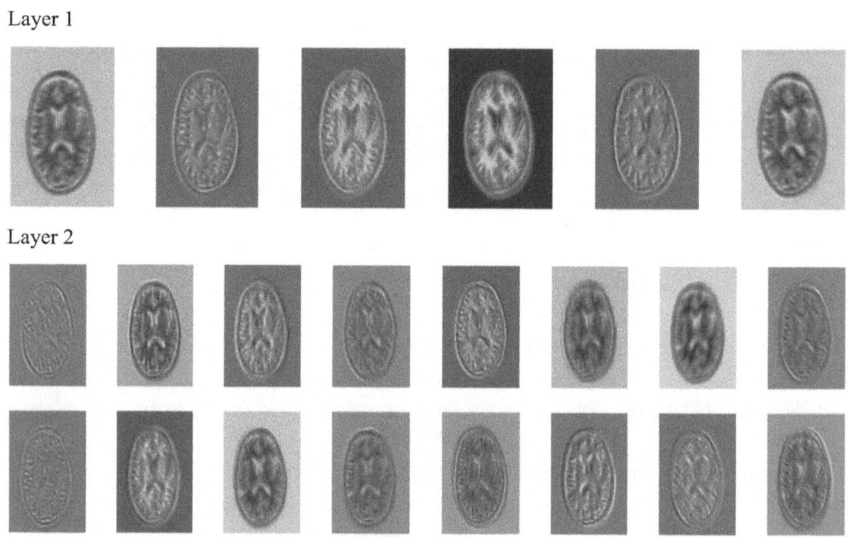

FIGURE 8.5 Fully connected layer.

- **Results Comparison and Analysis:** Compare the results of different models and evaluate their performance based on various metrics like accuracy.

Several graphs for accuracy on different models are shown in Figure 8.7.

Each model was trained for more than two hours. Throughout this research work, a significant portion of my time was dedicated to understanding the practical aspects

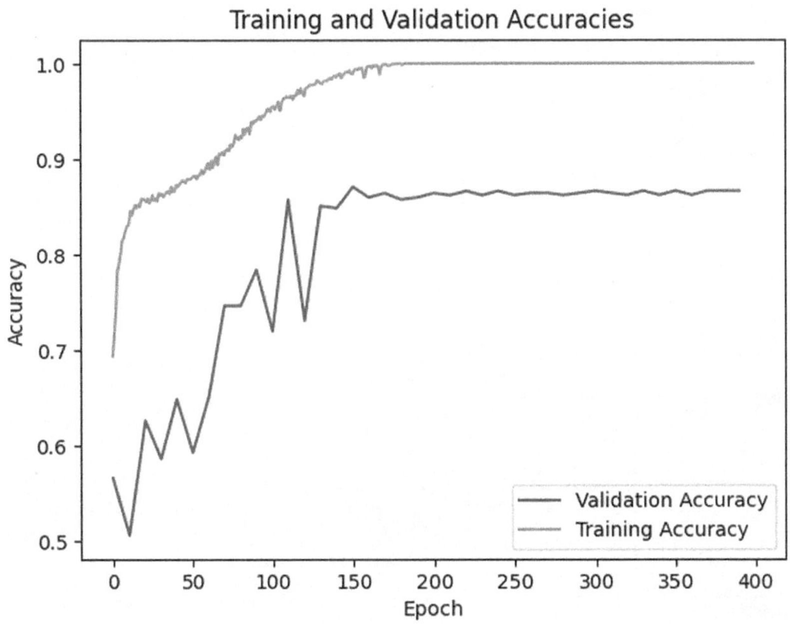

FIGURE 8.6 Validation and training accuracy.

of using existing tools and libraries for creating and training models. Learning how to work with pre-trained models and fine-tuning them for specific tasks was particularly time-consuming. This work allowed for a comprehensive exploration of brain tumor identification using AI techniques and provided valuable insights into medical image analysis applications.

The initial custom-built three-layer CNN with a simple architecture and fully connected layers demonstrated a remarkable test accuracy of 0.94 for the binary classification task, effectively distinguishing between healthy brain images and those with tumors. Subsequently, they employed pre-trained models, namely, DenseNet, ResNet, VGG16, and VGG19, to tackle the binary classification task. While these models exhibited only slight improvements in accuracy compared to the custom CNN, they showcased their true potential when confronted with the more challenging task of tumor-type classification.

For the tumor-type classification task, DenseNet achieved an accuracy of 0.8889, ResNet achieved an accuracy of 0.8720, VGG16 achieved an accuracy of 0.8575, and VGG19 achieved an accuracy of 0.8442. These models outperformed the custom CNN and showcased their ability to accurately classify brain tumor types into three categories: glioma, meningioma, and pituitary. The confusion matrixes revealed the models' capability to distinguish between the different tumor types, effectively contributing to medical diagnosis and treatment planning. Overall, the results highlight the superiority of pre-trained models for complex classification tasks involving brain tumor imaging datasets. The use of these models provides valuable insights into tumor classification, thereby enhancing the efficiency and accuracy of medical image analysis and diagnosis. This research work significantly contributed to the development and implementation of

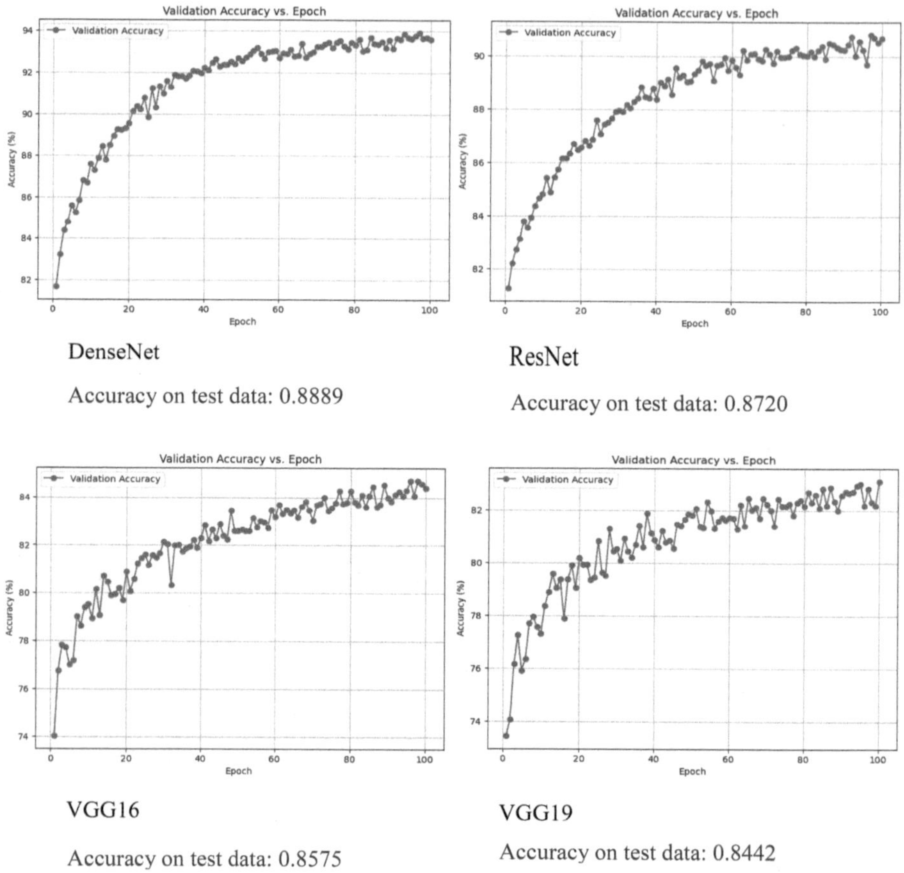

FIGURE 8.7 Comparative evaluation of model accuracy.

powerful machine learning models for brain tumor classification using MRI images. The achieved results demonstrate the potential of AI-based approaches in assisting medical professionals in accurate diagnosis and improved treatment decisions for brain tumor patients. The experience of exploring and utilizing pre-trained models, such as DenseNet, ResNet, VGG16, and VGG19, not only expanded knowledge but also demonstrated the versatility and power of transfer learning in medical image analysis. This research work has deepened my appreciation for the importance of domain-specific knowledge, data preprocessing, and the interpretability of model results in the medical domain. Moreover, extending the classification to include rarer tumor types and exploring the potential for transfer learning from other medical imaging domains could yield valuable insights and contribute to the advancement of medical research.

8.5 CONCLUSION

During this research work, significant progress was achieved in the field of brain tumor classification using MRI datasets. Initially, a custom-built three-layer CNN was developed, which demonstrated high accuracy in binary classification, effectively distinguishing between healthy brain images and those with tumors. The work was carried out via the Python language and the Pytorch libraries for working with deep learning. Further exploration involved the utilization of pre-trained models, including DenseNet, ResNet, VGG16, and VGG19, for the more challenging task of tumor-type classification. The pre-trained models exhibited improved performance compared to the custom CNN, accurately classifying brain tumor types into three categories: glioma, meningioma, and pituitary. The successful implementation of these models enables effective medical diagnosis and treatment planning by providing valuable insights into tumor classification based on MRI images. The results obtained are promising and underscore the potential for using advanced machine learning techniques in the medical imaging domain. While substantial progress was made during this research work, there are still areas for further improvement and exploration. One aspect that could be explored is the incorporation of more advanced preprocessing techniques to enhance the quality of input data. Additionally, the application of ensembling methods and other deep learning architectures might lead to further performance improvements.

Additionally, this research work provided an invaluable opportunity to immerse one in the world of machine learning, necessitating a significant amount of time devoted to learning and understanding the practical application of various methods. Working on the project allowed people to gain hands-on experience handling real-world datasets, preprocessing image data, selecting appropriate models, and tuning hyperparameters for optimal performance. The process of implementing and training different models, as well as analyzing their results, enhanced the understanding of the intricacies and challenges involved in applying machine learning techniques to medical imaging tasks.

REFERENCES

1. M. Rasool, N. A. Ismail, W. Boulila, A. Ammar, H. Samma, W. M. S. Yafooz, A. M. Emara, "A hybrid deep learning model for brain tumour classification," *Entropy (Basel)*. 2022 Jun 8;24(6):799. doi: 10.3390/e24060799. PMID: 35741521; PMCID: PMC9222774.
2. M. O. Khairandish, M. Sharma, V. Jain, J. M. Chatterjee, N. Z. Jhanjhi, "A hybrid CNN-SVM threshold segmentation approach for tumor detection and classification of MRI brain images," *IRBM*. 2021;42(5):307–316.
3. G. Huang, Z. Liu, L. Van Der Maaten, K. Q. Weinberger, "Densely connected convolutional networks," *Proceedings of the IEEE Conference on Computer Vision and Pattern Recognition (CVPR)*, Springer, Singapore, 2017, pp. 4700–4708.
4. A. Ghosh, A. Kole, "A comparative study of enhanced machine learning algorithms for brain tumor detection and classification", Institute of Electrical and Electronics Engineers (IEEE), 2021.
5. Khekare, G., Verma, P. (2021). Prophetic Probe of Accidents in Indian Smart Cities Using Machine Learning. In: Bhateja, V., Satapathy, S.C., Travieso-González, C.M., Aradhya, V.N.M. (eds) Data Engineering and Intelligent Computing. Advances in Intelligent Systems and Computing, vol 1407. Springer, Singapore. https://doi.org/10.1007/978-981-16-0171-2_18
6. J. S. Suri, Y. Chitre, "Multiclass magnetic resonance imaging brain tumor classification using artificial intelligence paradigm," *Computers in Biology and Medicine*. 2020;122:103804.

7. Z. Jia, D. Chen, "Brain tumor identification and classification of MRI images using deep learning techniques," *IEEE Access*. 10:230, doi: 10.1109/ACCESS.2020.3016319.
8. G. Khekare, K. Solanki, "Real time object detection with speech recognition using tensorflow lite," *Environment, Development and Sustainability*. 2021;24:10584–10594.
9. B. Deepa, M. Murugappan, M. G. Sumithra, M. Mahmud, M. S. Al-Rakhami, "Pattern descriptors orientation and MAP firefly algorithm based brain pathology classification using hybridized machine learning algorithm," *IEEE Access*. 2022;10:3848–3863, doi: 10.1109/ACCESS.2021.3100549.
10. Y. Ma *et al.*, "Multi-scale dynamic graph learning for brain disorder detection with functional MRI," *IEEE Transactions on Neural Systems and Rehabilitation Engineering*. 2023;31:3501–3512, doi: 10.1109/TNSRE.2023.3309847.
11. A. K. Budati, R. B. Katta, "An automated brain tumor detection and classification from MRI images using machine learning techniques with IoT," *Environment, Development and Sustainability*. 2022;24:10570–10584, doi: 10.1007/s10668-021-01861-8
12. N. Saeed, M. Ridzuan, H. Alasmawi, I. Sobirov, M. Yaqub, "MGMT promoter methylation status prediction using MRI scans? An extensive experimental evaluation of deep learning models," *Medical Image Analysis*. 2023;102989, ISSN: 1361-8415, doi: 10.1016/j.media.2023.102989.
13. Y. Ma *et al.*, "Multi-scale dynamic graph learning for brain disorder detection with functional MRI," *IEEE Transactions on Neural Systems and Rehabilitation Engineering*. 2023;31:3501–3512, doi: 10.1109/TNSRE.2023.3309847.
14. T. A. Soomro *et al.*, "Image segmentation for MR brain tumor detection using machine learning: A review," *IEEE Reviews in Biomedical Engineering*. 2023;16:70–90, doi: 10.1109/RBME.2022.3185292.
15. Z. Atha, J. Chaki, "SSBTCNet: Semi-supervised brain tumor classification network," *IEEE Access*. 2023;11:141485–141499, doi: 10.1109/ACCESS.2023.3343126.
16. B. Mallampati, A. Ishaq, F. Rustam, V. Kuthala, S. Alfarhood, I. Ashraf, "Brain tumor detection using 3D-UNet segmentation features and hybrid machine learning model," *IEEE Access*. 2023;11:135020–135034, doi: 10.1109/ACCESS.2023.3337363.
17. D. S. Vinod, S. P. S. Prakash, H. AlSalman, A. Y. Muaad, M. B. B. Heyat, "Ensemble technique for brain tumor patient survival prediction," *IEEE Access*. 2024;12:19285–19298, doi: 10.1109/ACCESS.2024.3360086.
18. B. Sandhiya, S. Kanaga Suba Raja, "Deep learning and optimized learning machine for brain tumor classification," *Biomedical Signal Processing and Control*. 2024;89:105778, ISSN: 1746-8094, doi: 10.1016/j.bspc.2023.105778.
19. S. Anantharajan, S. Gunasekaran, T. Subramanian, R. Venkatesh, "MRI brain tumor detection using deep learning and machine learning approaches," *Measurement: Sensors*. 2024;31:101026, ISSN: 2665-9174, doi: 10.1016/j.measen.2024.101026.
20. H. Hwang, S. E. Kim, H.-J. Lee, D. A. Lee, K. M. Park, "Identification of amnestic mild cognitive impairment by structural and functional MRI using a machine-learning approach," *Clinical Neurology and Neurosurgery*. 2024;108177, ISSN: 0303-8467, doi: 10.1016/j.clineuro.2024.108177.
21. G. Khekare, P. Verma, S. Raut, "The smart accident predictor system using internet of things," in *Cloud IoT*, pp. 163–175. Chapman and Hall/CRC, 2022.
22. G. Khekare, *et al.*, "Optimizing network security and performance through the integration of hybrid GAN-RNN models in SDN-based access control and traffic engineering," *International Journal of Advanced Computer Science and Applications (IJACSA)*. 2023;14(12), doi: 10.14569/IJACSA.2023.0141262.
23. G. Khekare, Midhunchakkravarthy, "Smart image recognition system for the visually impaired people," *2023 International Conference on Energy, Materials and Communication Engineering (ICEMCE)*, Madurai, India, 2023, pp. 1–6, doi: 10.1109/ICEMCE57940.2023.10434130.

24. A. V. N. Reddy, P. K. Mallick, B. Srinivasa Rao, P. Kanakamedala, "An efficient brain tumor classification using MRI images with hybrid deep intelligence model," *The Imaging Science Journal*, 2023;11, 110, doi: 10.1080/13682199.2023.2207892.
25. S. Aluri, S. S. Imambi, "Brain tumour classification using MRI images based on Lenet with golden teacher learning optimization," *Network: Computation in Neural Systems*. 2024;35:1, 27–54, doi: 10.1080/0954898X.2023.2275720.
26. M. Kordemir, K. K. Cevik, A. Bozkurt, "A mask R-CNN approach for detection and classification of brain tumours from MR images," *Computer Methods in Biomechanics and Biomedical Engineering: Imaging & Visualization*. 2024;85, 455, doi: 10.1080/21681163.2023.2301391.
27. S. Raju, V. R. P. Veera, "Classification of brain tumours from MRI images using deep learning-enabled hybrid optimization algorithm," *Network: Computation in Neural Systems*. 2023;34:4, 408–437, doi: 10.1080/0954898X.2023.2275045.
28. M. Ahmadi, A. Sharifi, M. J. Fard, N. Soleimani, "Detection of brain lesion location in MRI images using convolutional neural network and robust PCA," *International Journal of Neuroscience*. 2023;133:1, 55–66, doi: 10.1080/00207454.2021.1883602.
29. R. D. Chougala, R. H. Havaldar, Systematic assessment and review of techniques based on tumour detection in brain using MRI," *Computer Methods in Biomechanics and Biomedical Engineering: Imaging & Visualization*. 2023;11(5):1708–1716, doi: 10.1080/21681163.2023.2181020.

9 Advanced Deep Learning for Early Alzheimer's Detection

A Comparative Analysis

J. Deepika Roselind, G. Logeswari, and G. Sudhakaran

CONTENTS

9.1 INTRODUCTION

Alzheimer's disease (AD) stands as a formidable challenge in the realm of global public health, characterized by its progressive neurodegenerative nature and its far-reaching impact on cognitive functions. With an aging population and a surge in the incidence of neurodegenerative disorders, the need for effective early diagnosis and intervention in AD has become increasingly critical [1]. Conventional diagnostic approaches frequently depend on clinical evaluations and cognitive tests, which might lack the sensitivity to identify subtle early indicators. This imperative has fueled research into innovative approaches, with advanced deep learning (DL) models emerging as promising tools for the timely prediction of Alzheimer's.

The ascent of DL in the healthcare domain marks a significant technological advancement. Nested within machine learning, DL has demonstrated remarkable proficiency in diverse tasks [2]. Its integration into healthcare practices has gained momentum, showcasing notable achievements in areas like medical imaging analysis, disease prediction, and drug discovery. The unique capability of DL models,

DOI: 10.1201/9781003476207-9

particularly convolutional neural networks (CNN), to discern intricate patterns and representations from complex datasets positions them as formidable tools for tasks demanding nuanced analysis, such as the interpretation of medical images [3]. This research endeavors to address the gap in understanding the comparative performance of various DL models in predicting Alzheimer's.

This chapter holds immense significance in shedding light on the application of DL models for AD prediction. Through a systematic comparison of diverse CNN architectures, the research strives to offer valuable insights that can guide researchers and healthcare practitioners in selecting optimal models for early detection. The findings of this research may play a pivotal role in advancing the development of more accurate and efficient diagnostic tools. Ultimately, this has the potential to enhance patient outcomes and contribute to the evolution of personalized medicine approaches in the realm of neurodegenerative disorders. As the global healthcare landscape continues to evolve, the integration of advanced technologies holds immense promise for addressing complex challenges. This research contributes to the ongoing dialogue on leveraging DL for improved AD prediction, fostering interdisciplinary collaboration between the fields of computer science and healthcare.

The chapter aims to conduct an extensive comparative analysis of state-of-the-art DL models specifically designed for predicting AD, recognizing the significant global health impact of this condition on cognitive function and daily life. By utilizing advanced CNN architectures such as VGG19, VGG16, ResNet50, ResNet101, Xception, MobileNet, MobileNetV2, DenseNet169, DenseNet121, and InceptionV3, the study seeks to evaluate their effectiveness in early detection using medical imaging data. Through a thorough examination of model structures, training methodologies, and predictive capabilities, the research endeavors to provide insights into the unique strengths and limitations of each model. Furthermore, the chapter aims to validate its findings through rigorous evaluation of benchmark datasets, ultimately contributing to the evolving understanding of leveraging sophisticated machine learning techniques for the timely diagnosis of neurodegenerative conditions, particularly AD. The remaining sections of this chapter are structured as follows: Section 2 presents the literature survey, Section 3 outlines the methodology, Section 4 covers results and discussion, and Section 5 provides the conclusion.

9.2 LITERATURE REVIEW

Tanveer et al. [4] systematically explore various machine learning methods for AD diagnosis. It emphasizes the urgency for accurate diagnostic tools given the rising global prevalence of Alzheimer's. The study addresses challenges in classifying AD and mild cognitive impairment (MCI), highlighting the importance of predicting Mild Cognitive Impaired (MCI-to-AD) conversion. Utilizing open-source databases and tools like AD neuroimaging initiative (ADNI), the paper discusses the stability of Support Vector Machines (SVM), local optimization in artificial neural networks (ANN), and feature extraction integration in DL. The conclusion outlines subsequent sections exploring the practical applications of SVM, ANN, and DL in AD diagnosis.

Trambaiolli et al. [5] address the pressing need for early AD characterization, acknowledging current diagnostic challenges relying on autopsy or biopsy. It explores machine learning techniques as innovative approaches for more accurate AD diagnosis, considering the limitations of current neuropsychological screenings. The study proposes quantitative electroencephalography, a non-invasive method, particularly focusing on spectral analysis (SpecA) and coherence (Coh), as a potential screening tool. Emphasizing alpha rhythms as diagnostic markers, the research aims to develop SVM models to classify digital electroencephalograph (EEG) signal patterns, offering a promising avenue for earlier AD diagnosis.

Asim et al. [6] address the critical need for improved early detection of AD through a multi-modal, multi-atlas-based machine learning approach. Focused on the amnestic impairment stage, a precursor to AD, the research reviews structural magnetic resonance imaging (MRI), functional MRI, and fludeoxyglucose-18—positron emission tomography (FDG-PET) imaging modalities. Emphasizing structural MRI and atlas-based methods, the study proposes combining features from different atlases to enhance classification accuracy, aiming for a more nuanced understanding of brain features. The paper outlines the methodology, including feature extraction and classification, and presents experimental results, contributing to the advancement of AD diagnosis with an innovative approach for enhanced accuracy in early detection.

The paper [7] addresses the critical need for accurate AD staging to optimize treatment strategies, highlighting the urgency of early diagnosis given the increasing prevalence of AD. Recognizing the progressive nature of AD and patient response variability, the paper advocates categorizing patients into distinct subgroups based on disease stages to enhance treatment effectiveness and overall quality of life. Acknowledging the challenge of unstructured data in electronic health records (EHRs), the paper proposes the use of machine learning and data mining tools to extract valuable patterns from EHRs, specifically focusing on the application of these techniques to the (ADNI) dataset. The primary objective is to classify different AD stages, provide a nuanced approach to treatment planning, and identify distinguishing attributes within the ADNI dataset, aligning with the broader trend of leveraging data mining for efficient disease prognosis and classification in healthcare research.

The research [8] underscores the urgent need for early AD detection, emphasizing its impact on treatment decisions and complications prevention. Distinguishing Alzheimer's from other dementias, it highlights the absence of a cure and focuses on research to slow symptoms. Acknowledging treatment limitations, the paper suggests machine learning (ML) and DL algorithms for early AD detection, proposing a novel approach. The subsequent sections cover the state-of-the-art in Alzheimer's detection, the methodology, experimental results, and discussions, emphasizing ML and DL techniques' potential for more effective early interventions and improved outcomes.

Escudero et al. [9] explore recent technological advancements and ML's potential in clinical decision-making, addressing a gap in personalized diagnostic approaches. Unlike standardized methods, the study proposes an innovative approach tailored to individual patients, incorporating feature selection, classifiers, and measures of similarity for continuous variables. Leveraging data from the ADNI database, the research focuses on variables like gender, age, education, body mass index, and various biomarkers from MRI, PET, and blood samples.

The study in [10] introduces a novel DL architecture, using stacked auto-encoders and a softmax output layer, for accurate AD and MCI diagnosis. It addresses shortcomings in prior research on computer-aided design of AD, offering the ability to analyze multiple classes simultaneously with fewer labeled training samples. The study [11] utilizes the voice-based AD dataset, collected from 23 elderly individuals using a wearable Internet of Things device continuously recording voice data. An algorithm extracts spectrogram features from the collected speech data, training a ML model for Alzheimer's identification.

The study [12] introduces an innovative method for early AD identification using first-order statistical features extracted from 3D brain MRI. Emphasizing the importance of early detection for optimal disease control, the approach targets grey and white matter regions affected by AD. Through voxel-based feature extraction and ML algorithms, the process involves computing first-order statistical features, with Principal component analysis (PCA) applied for feature vector identification. Diverse classifiers use these features to predict AD or healthy control (HC) class, achieving an impressive accuracy rate of 90.9%, surpassing alternative techniques.

In summary, the existing literature offers various approaches to AD detection, incorporating ML and innovative methods like IoT devices and speech analysis. However, a noticeable gap exists in the detailed exploration and comparison of DL models specifically designed for AD diagnosis. This gap is addressed in the upcoming chapter, which undertakes a thorough investigation of ten distinct DL models. The chapter aims to provide a comprehensive comparative analysis, revealing the individual strengths and weaknesses of these models in the context of AD detection. This exploration is crucial for guiding practitioners and researchers in selecting the most effective DL architecture for personalized and accurate early-stage diagnosis of AD.

9.3 METHODOLOGY

In this chapter, an extensive comparative analysis of various DL models is undertaken with the main objective of predicting AD. The evaluated models encompass VGG16, ResNet50, ResNet101, Xception, MobileNet, MobileNetV2, DenseNet169, DenseNet121, and InceptionV3.

9.3.1 Data Preprocessing

The dataset utilized for this study comprises 3D brain MRI scans. The initial processing step involves segmenting the white and grey matter images from the 3D structural brain MRI data. After segmentation, the dataset undergoes a partitioning process to establish separate training and validation sets [13, 14].

9.3.2 Model Architecture

When implementing each DL model, the base architecture is initialized with pre-trained weights derived from the ImageNet dataset. Following this, modifications are applied to the top layers of the model to customize it for the particular task of predicting AD. This transfer learning strategy leverages the insights acquired from ImageNet to improve the model's capacity to identify pertinent features in the context of AD prediction. A typical adjustment involves freezing the layers of the pre-trained models to preserve learned features and mitigate overfitting on the constrained AD dataset. The ultimate dense layer is adjusted to generate probabilities for the AD classes.

First-order statistical features are derived from 2D slices obtained in the coronal, sagittal, and axial orientations of the preprocessed images. This process is crucial for capturing pertinent information about the structural attributes of the brain. To handle the dimensionality of the feature vectors, PCA is employed. PCA identifies and preserves the most meaningful features, enabling a more concise and targeted analysis in the subsequent phases of the study.

9.3.3 Implementation

The implementation of all models utilizes TensorFlow and Keras. TensorFlow's data pipeline is employed for the efficient loading and processing of the dataset into the models. The code is organized to enhance reproducibility, and the essential dependencies are explicitly outlined for clarity. During this phase, an interpretability analysis is executed to uncover the decision-making mechanisms of each DL model. Methods such as layer-wise relevance propagation and gradient-weighted class activation mapping are utilized to emphasize areas in the brain MRIs that play a substantial role in the prediction. The objective of this step is to improve the transparency of model predictions, offering valuable insights into the features influencing AD classification.

9.3.4 Model Training and Evaluation

During the training phase, the preprocessed and feature-extracted data are inputted into each model for 50 epochs. The training advancement is observed on the validation set, and the optimal weights are stored. Performance metrics, such as accuracy and AUC, are assessed on the validation set to gauge the predictive effectiveness of each model in identifying AD. The models are built using the Adam optimizer and Categorical Cross-entropy loss function. Metrics like AUC and accuracy are tracked throughout the training process. To mitigate overfitting, an early stopping callback is incorporated, set with patience of 8 epochs to revert to the best weights when the validation loss reaches a plateau [15, 16]. To evaluate the models' robustness, two forms of cross-validation are executed. Leave-one-out cross-validation is utilized to systematically assess model performance by excluding one subject for testing in each iteration. Furthermore, three-fold cross-validation is carried out to confirm the predictive capability of the selected features across various subsets of the dataset.

Each model is tailored to address specific architectural nuances and characteristics. VGG16 and VGG19 emphasize simplicity and uniformity in layer structure. ResNet models utilize residual connections to address vanishing gradient issues, while InceptionV3 incorporates parallel convolutions to enhance feature extraction. MobileNet and MobileNetV2 are tailored for efficiency in mobile and edge devices, whereas DenseNet optimizes feature reuse through dense connections between

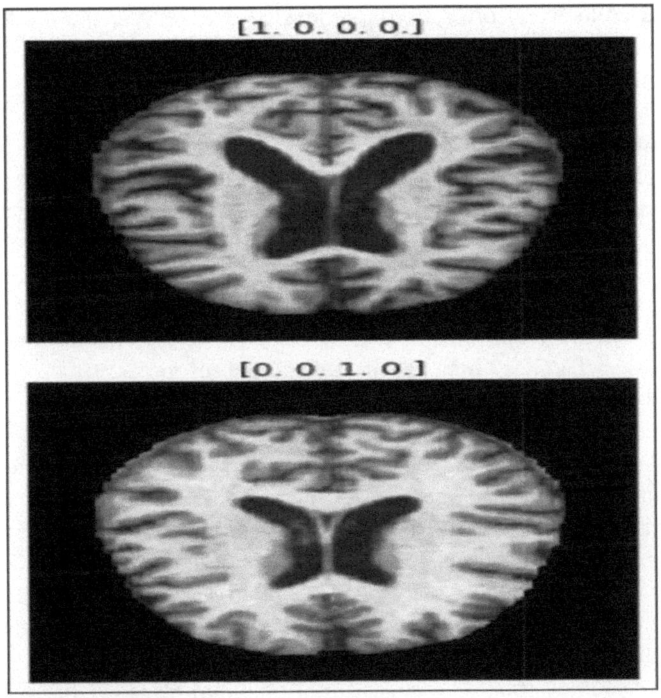

FIGURE 9.1 Sample images from the training dataset.

layers. To further improve predictive accuracy, an ensemble learning approach is implemented. This ensemble leverages the diversity of individual models, potentially mitigating biases and enhancing overall performance. The ensembled models undergo additional training, and their collective predictions are evaluated to assess the potential for increased accuracy in AD prediction. Figure 9.1 shows the sample image of the training dataset.

9.3.5 Ethical Considerations

In medical imaging studies, privacy and ethical considerations take precedence. The dataset employed adheres strictly to ethical guidelines, guaranteeing the anonymity and confidentiality of patient information. The study centers on evaluating model performance and generalization, with no intention of compromising patient privacy. This methodology is designed to offer a systematic and comparative analysis of DL models for AD prediction. It aims to illuminate the strengths and weaknesses of these models in dealing with datasets related to neurodegenerative diseases.

9.4 RESULT AND ANALYSIS

After concluding the training of each DL model, a thorough review of the epoch results yields valuable insights into their performance. The mean accuracy, loss, and

AUC metrics collectively offer a comprehensive overview of the model's learning dynamics and discriminative capabilities. In the following sections, a detailed analysis of each model is presented, elucidating their convergence patterns and effectiveness in discerning between AD and HC. Table 9.1 shows the performance analysis of various existing models in terms of loss, AUC, and accuracy. The performance analysis is pictorially presented in Figures 9.2, 9.3, and 9.4.

In this comparison of DL models for predicting AD, each architecture unveils unique strengths and considerations, providing insights into their nuanced performances. VGG19 stands out as a strong candidate, demonstrating a well-balanced combination of high accuracy (70.13%) and excellent discrimination capabilities (AUC: 0.911). Despite its promising attributes for Alzheimer's detection, the computational intensity of VGG19 may require substantial resources.

VGG16 closely trails behind, sustaining competitive discrimination capabilities and an admirable AUC of 0.907. Despite a slightly elevated loss (0.7391), the model attains a robust accuracy of 67.47%. These findings underscore the effectiveness of VGG16 in categorizing Alzheimer's cases, though there are minor opportunities for optimization. ResNet50 distinguishes itself with an impressive accuracy of 84.29%, showcasing expertise in precise classification. The model's accuracy and loss metrics suggest effective discrimination. However, the relatively elevated loss (1.0272) raises considerations regarding potential overfitting or optimization requirements.

ResNet101 displays competitive discrimination (AUC: 0.858) but struggles to achieve high accuracy (60.2%), suggesting a potential trade-off between discrimination capabilities and overall predictive accuracy. Further investigation into model refinement is warranted. Xception exhibits moderate discrimination (AUC: 0.8246) with a balanced accuracy (58.24%) and loss (1.7824). Despite the higher loss, Xception remains a viable option with the potential for optimization. MobileNet demonstrates a balanced architecture, with an accuracy of 68.49% and an AUC of 0.8495. While effective in discriminating between classes, further improvements could enhance overall performance. MobileNetV2 maintains effective discrimination (AUC: 0.8196)

TABLE 9.1
Comparison of Various Models

Model	Loss	AUC	Accuracy
VGG19	0.70285	0.91103	0.70132
VGG16	0.73917	0.90706	0.6747
ResNet50	1.02722	0.82253	0.84299
ResNet101	1.06966	0.85804	0.60203
Xception	1.78240	0.82461	0.58248
MobileNet	2.43283	0.84957	0.68491
MobileNetV2	2.38945	0.81963	0.61376
DenseNet169	2.47222	0.82823	0.63017
DenseNet121	1.59514	0.84106	0.58717
InceptionV3	2.90277	0.75880	0.51837

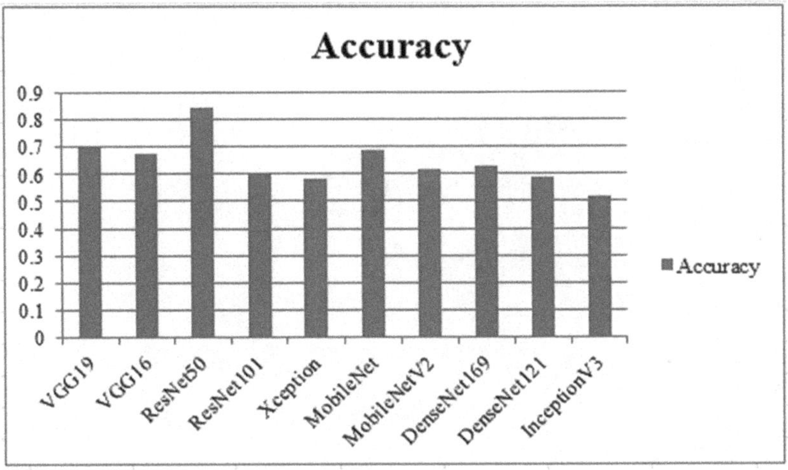

FIGURE 9.2 Accuracy for different models.

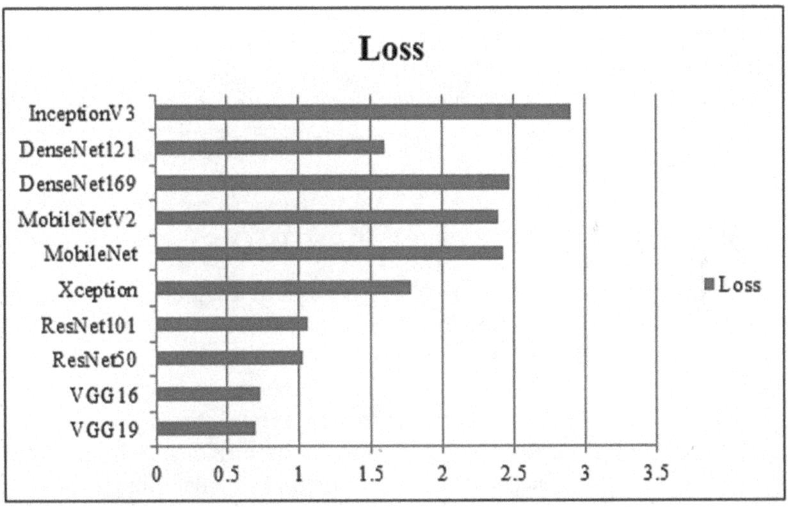

FIGURE 9.3 Loss for different models.

and a balance between accuracy (61.37%) and loss (2.3894). Optimization opportunities exist, suggesting avenues for refining its predictive capabilities.

DenseNet169 exhibits effective discrimination (AUC: 0.8282) and balanced metrics, with an accuracy of 63.01% and a loss of 2.4722, presenting a viable option with potential for further enhancements. DenseNet121 demonstrates moderate discrimination (AUC: 0.841) but faces challenges in achieving higher accuracy (58.71%), suggesting potential areas for improvement and optimization. InceptionV3 encounters challenges with lower accuracy (51.83%) and a higher loss (2.9027), indicating

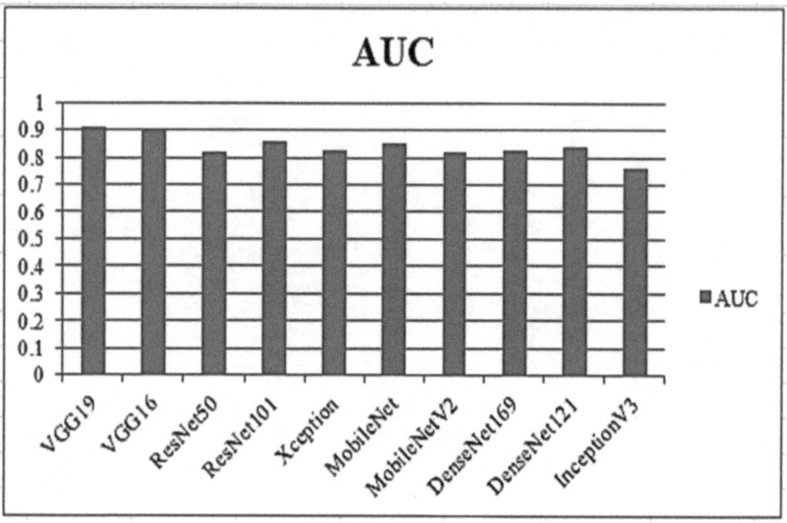

FIGURE 9.4 AUC for different models.

potential limitations in its suitability for this specific prediction task. These findings underscore the importance of considering various factors, including discrimination capabilities, accuracy, and computational complexity, in selecting an appropriate model for AD prediction in 3D brain MR images.

9.5 CONCLUSION AND FUTURE DIRECTIONS

The study delved into the application of DL models in the prediction of D) by analyzing 3D brain MR images, providing valuable insights into various architectural approaches. Notably, significant performances were observed in models such as VGG19, VGG16, and ResNet50, showcasing their potential in AD prediction. Among these, VGG19 emerged as particularly promising, demonstrating an accuracy rate of 70.13% and an AUC value of 0.911, indicating its proficiency in distinguishing between AD and non-AD cases. However, challenges were identified in other models like ResNet101 and DenseNet121, which may indicate limitations in their ability to effectively capture the intricate patterns present in the MR images related to AD diagnosis. The comprehensive comparative analysis conducted in the study elucidated nuanced distinctions among these models, underscoring the importance of balancing discrimination capability with overall accuracy. Looking ahead, the study suggests several promising avenues for future research. This includes focusing on refining model optimization techniques to enhance predictive performance further. Hyper-parameter tuning represents another crucial area for exploration, as fine-tuning model parameters can significantly influence predictive accuracy. Moreover, strategies for mitigating overfitting, a common challenge in DL, warrant attention to ensure the generalizability of models across diverse datasets. Furthermore, exploring ensemble methods, which combine predictions from multiple models, could lead to the development of more robust and reliable predictive systems. By leveraging the complementary strengths of different architectures, ensemble methods have the potential to enhance prediction accuracy and resilience to variations in input data. In essence, this study not only sheds light on the efficacy of DL models in AD prediction but also sets the stage for future research aimed at refining these models and advancing our understanding of neurodegenerative disorders.

REFERENCES

1. Venugopalan, J., Tong, L., Hassanzadeh, H. R., & Wang, M. D. (2021). Multimodal deep learning models for early detection of Alzheimer's disease stage. *Scientific Reports*, 11(1), 3254.
2. Altinkaya, E. Trambaiolli, & Barakli, B. (2020). Detection of Alzheimer's disease and dementia states based on deep learning from MRI images: A comprehensive review. *Journal of the Institute of Electronics and Computer*, 1(1), 39–53.
3. Ramzan, F., Khan, M. U. G., Rehmat, A., Iqbal, S., Saba, T., Rehman, A., & Mehmood, Z. (2020). A deep learning approach for automated diagnosis and multi-class classification of Alzheimer's disease stages using resting-state fMRI and residual neural networks. *Journal of Medical Systems*, 44, 1–16.
4. Tanveer, M., Richhariya, B., Khan, R. U., Rashid, A. H., Khanna, P., Prasad, M., & Lin, C. T. (2020). Machine learning techniques for the diagnosis of Alzheimer's disease: A review. *ACM Transactions on Multimedia Computing, Communications, and Applications (TOMM)*, 16(1s), 1–35.
5. Trambaiolli, L. R., Lorena, A. C., Fraga, F. J., Kanda, P. A., Anghinah, R., & Nitrini, R. (2011). Improving Alzheimer's disease diagnosis with machine learning techniques. *Clinical EEG and Neuroscience*, 42(3), 160–165.
6. Asim, Y., Raza, B., Malik, A. K., Rathore, S., Hussain, L., & Iftikhar, M. A. (2018). A multi-modal, multi-atlas-based approach for Alzheimer detection via machine learning. *International Journal of Imaging Systems and Technology*, 28(2), 113–123.
7. Shahbaz, M., Ali, S., Guergachi, A., Niazi, A., & Umer, A. (2019, July). Classification of Alzheimer's disease using machine learning techniques. In *Data* (pp. 296–303). Springer.
8. Dashtipour, K., Taylor, W., Ansari, S., Zahid, A., Gogate, M., Ahmad, J.,. . . Abbasi, Q. (2021, December). Detecting Alzheimer's disease using machine learning methods. In *EAI International Conference on Body Area Networks* (pp. 89–100). Springer International Publishing.
9. Escudero, J., Ifeachor, E., Zajicek, J. P., Green, C., Shearer, J., & Pearson, S. (2012). Machine learning-based method for personalized and cost-effective detection of Alzheimer's disease. *IEEE Transactions on Biomedical Engineering*, 60(1), 164–168.
10. Liu, S., Liu, S., Cai, W., Pujol, S., Kikinis, R., & Feng, D. (2014, April). Early diagnosis of Alzheimer's disease with deep learning. In *2014 IEEE 11th International Symposium on Biomedical Imaging (ISBI)* (pp. 1015–1018). IEEE.
11. Liu, L., Zhao, S., Chen, H., & Wang, A. (2020). A new machine learning method for identifying Alzheimer's disease. *Simulation Modelling Practice and Theory*, 99, 102023.
12. Aruchamy, S., Haridasan, A., Verma, A., Bhattacharjee, P., Nandy, S. N., & Vadali, S. R. K. (2020, February). Alzheimer's disease detection using machine learning techniques in 3D MR images. In *2020 National Conference on Emerging Trends on Sustainable Technology and Engineering Applications (NCETSTEA)* (pp. 1–4). IEEE.
13. Ghazal, T. M., Abbas, S., Munir, S., Khan, M. A., Ahmad, M., Issa, G. F., & Hasan, M. K. (2022). Alzheimer disease detection empowered with transfer learning. *Computers, Materials & Continua*, 70(3).

14. Li, S., Shi, F., Pu, F., Li, X., Jiang, T., Xie, S., & Wang, Y. (2007). Hippocampal shape analysis of Alzheimer disease based on machine learning methods. *American Journal of Neuroradiology*, 28(7), 1339–1345.
15. Sethi, M., Ahuja, S., Rani, S., Koundal, D., Zaguia, A., & Enbeyle, W. (2022). An exploration: Alzheimer's disease classification based on convolutional neural network. *BioMed Research International*, 2022;20, 233.
16. Pahuja, G., & Nagabhushan, T. N. (2021). A comparative study of existing machine learning approaches for Parkinson's disease detection. *IETE Journal of Research*, 67(1), 4–14.

10 Artificial Intelligence and Machine Learning in Biomedical Signal Processing

Aditya Kumar, Niharika Koch, Sk Imran, and Jainath Yadav

CONTENTS

10.1 INTRODUCTION

A signal can be defined as a function that conveys information about a physical phenomenon or a process. In the context of signal processing, a signal is a time-varying or spatially varying quantity that can be measured, recorded, and analyzed [1, 2]. Signals can take many forms, including electromagnetic waves, sound waves, and biological signals such as electroencephalograms (EEGs), electromyograms (EMGs), and electrocardiograms (ECGs). Retrieving meaningful information from these

DOI: 10.1201/9781003476207-10

signals is the aim of signal processing; this information can then be utilized for additional analysis, interpretation, or system control. Mathematically, a signal can be described as a function of one or more independent variables. For a continuous-time signal, the function is often specified over time (t), and it can be written as x(t). The function is defined over a discrete domain, which is often a sequence of integers (n), and can be denoted as x[n] in the case of a discrete-time signal. A continuous-time signal, x(t), can be described mathematically as:

$$x(t) = \int_{-\infty}^{\infty} X(\omega)e^{j\omega t}d\omega \tag{1}$$

where X(ω) is the Fourier transform of the signal. The discrete-time signal x[n] can be written as follows:

$$x[n] = \sum_{k=-\infty}^{\infty} X[k]e^{j2\pi kn/N} \tag{2}$$

where X[k] is the discrete-time Fourier transform of the signal and N is the length of the sequence. The analysis and processing of biological signals frequently makes use of these mathematical representations of signals.

10.1.1 Biomedical Signals and Their Types

Biomedical signals are electrical, chemical, or physical signals that are produced within the body and convey information related to physiological or pathological processes [3]. These signals can be recorded and analyzed to diagnose diseases, monitor the progress of treatment, and provide insights into the underlying mechanisms of various biological processes. These signals are measured using specialized instruments and equipment and require expertise in signal processing and analysis for accurate interpretation. Figure 10.1 illustrates the several kinds of biological signals, which include:

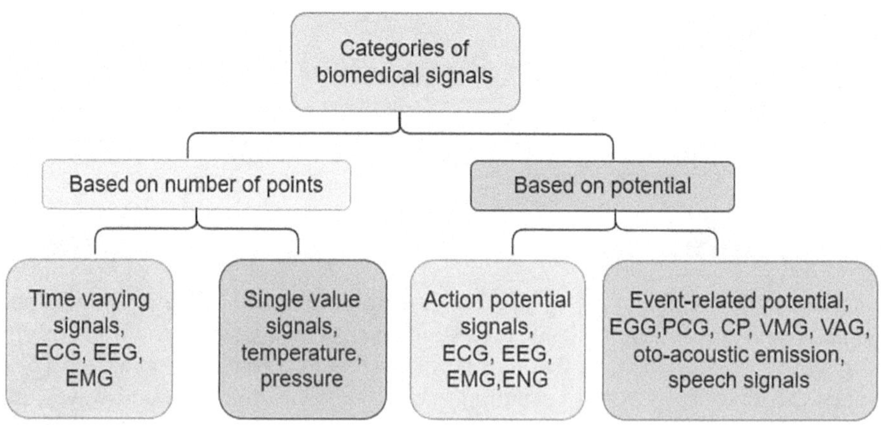

FIGURE 10.1 Categories of biomedical signals.

- **ECG or EKG:** This signal is used to identify a variety of cardiac problems and measures the heart's electrical activity.
- **EMG:** This signal is recorded in the skeletal muscles' electrical activity and used to diagnose diseases of the neuromuscular system.
- **EEG:** This signal is used to record brain electrical activity and diagnose neurological issues.
- **Blood pressure (BP):** This signal measures the pressure of blood flow through arteries and is used to diagnose hypertension and other cardiovascular conditions.
- **Respiration rate (RR):** This signal measures the rate and depth of breathing and is used to diagnose respiratory disorders.
- **Electrooculography (EOG):** This signal records eye movements and is used to diagnose sleep disorders and other conditions affecting eye movements.
- **Photoplethysmogram (PPG):** Because it monitors variations in blood volume in the tissue's microvascular bed, this signal is used to diagnose respiratory and circulatory disorders.
- **Galvanic skin response:** This signal measures changes in skin conductance and is used to diagnose various psychological and emotional conditions.

10.1.2 Biomedical Signal Processing

The study area known as "biomedical signal processing" is concerned with the evaluation, deciphering, and modification of biological signals. These signals, which can comprise ECG, EEG, EMG, EOG, and other signal types, are primarily collected from the human body. Biomedical signal processing is required to extract useful information from these signals for the purpose of diagnosing, monitoring, and treating a wide range of medical conditions. For this, sophisticated mathematical and computational methods for signal processing and analysis are required, in addition to an extensive knowledge of the physiological mechanisms behind the signals. Signal capture, preprocessing, feature extraction, and classification are the fundamental processes in biomedical signal processing.

1. **Signal Acquisition**: Signal acquisition is the process of recording biological signals from the human body using electrodes or sensors. For example, an ECG machine uses electrodes applied to the skin to record heart electrical activity, whereas EEG equipment uses electrodes applied to the scalp to capture brain electrical activity.
2. **Signal Preprocessing**: Once the signals are acquired, they must be preprocessed to remove noise, artifacts, and other unwanted components. This may involve filtering the signals to remove high-frequency noise, baseline drift, or other types of interference.
3. **Feature Extraction**: The next process is feature extraction, which entails finding and removing pertinent features from the signals. This may involve measuring the amplitude, frequency, or other properties of the signals, or extracting more complex features using methods like time-frequency analysis or wavelet transforms [4].

4. **Classification**: Finally, classification or diagnosis is performed using the retrieved features. To categorize the signals based on the collected features, may include using machine learning (ML) algorithms like neural networks or Support Vector Machines.

There are several uses for biomedical signal processing in the medical industry. For instance, it can be used to identify and keep tabs on a variety of illnesses, including heart disease, epilepsy, and sleep disorders. It can also be utilized to create novel medical devices that interface with the human body and depend on the interpretation of biological signals, including pacemakers and neuroprosthetics. In general, the subject of biomedical signal processing is expanding quickly and has the potential to completely change how different medical problems are diagnosed and treated. Researchers and physicians can learn new things about how the human body works and create novel, more effective treatments, and therapies that are tailored to the needs of specific patients by gleaning information from biological signals.

The chapter significantly contributes to the field of biomedical signal processing by:

- Introducing the types, characteristics, and applications of biomedical signals.
- Establishing the foundational understanding necessary for further exploration.
- Highlighting their crucial role in advancing medical diagnosis, monitoring, and treatment.

The chapter is structured to first introduce the importance of signal processing. It then explores various types of biomedical signals, such as action potentials, ECGs, EEGs, EMGs, and brain–computer interface (BCI) signals. Following this, it discusses the application of ML and deep learning (DL) techniques in processing these signals. Subsequent sections address the applications of biomedical signals in healthcare, the challenges they pose, and emerging trends in the field. Finally, the chapter concludes by summarizing key points and emphasizing the critical role of biomedical signal processing in advancing healthcare.

10.2 BIOELECTRIC SIGNALS

The human body is an intricate mechanism made up of several interrelated systems and subsystems that cooperate to carry out a wide range of physiological operations. These processes are influenced and controlled by a variety of stimuli and outputs, such as physical, biochemical, or informational nerve or hormonal inputs and outputs. It is crucial to analyze the signals generated by these physiological processes to study and comprehend how the human body functions since they can offer important insights into how the body's many systems operate. Bioelectric signals, which are electrical signals generated by the body's numerous physiological processes, are among the most significant kinds of signals in the human body. EEG, ECG, and EMG are just a few of the methods and tools that can be used to identify and measure these signals. Each of these methods is used to assess bioelectric signals coming from particular bodily organs like the heart, muscles, and brain, as shown in Figure 10.2.

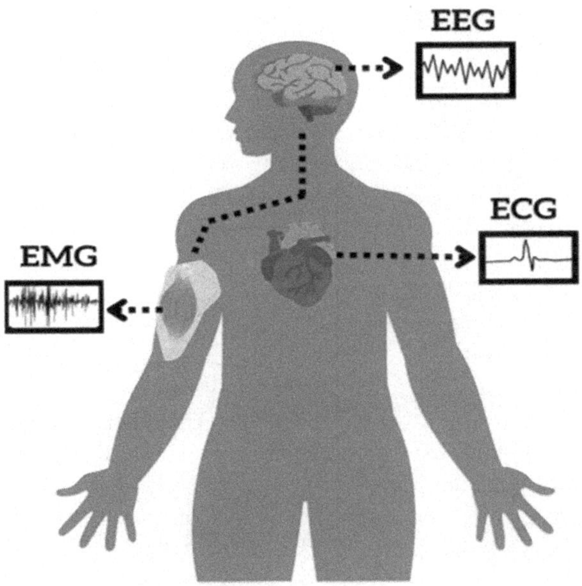

FIGURE 10.2 Bioelectric signals.

One of the most used methods for detecting bioelectric impulses in the human body is the ECG. It records the electrical activity of the heart, which can reveal important details about how the heart is beating, including its rhythm and pace. Diagnoses of illnesses like cardiac disease and arrhythmia can be made using this information. EEG, a method for assessing brain electrical activity, is a vital tool for measuring bioelectric impulses. EEG can be used to diagnose a variety of neurological conditions, such as epilepsy and sleep disorders, and can also be used in research to gather information about brain function and activity. EMG is another technique used to measure bioelectric signals in the body. EMG measures the electrical activity of muscles and can be used to diagnose conditions such as muscular dystrophy and carpal tunnel syndrome.

In addition to bioelectric signals, the human body produces a variety of other types of signals, including biochemical and physical signals. Hormones and neurotransmitters are examples of biochemical signals. These chemical messengers are produced by different glands and organs in the body and are engaged in a variety of physiological processes, including metabolism, growth, and reproduction. Physical signals, such as temperature and pressure, are also important in the human body. For example, the sense of touch is mediated by pressure receptors in the skin, while the sense of temperature is mediated by temperature receptors. Due to this, the study of physiological signals is an essential aspect of understanding the workings of the human body and diagnosing various medical conditions. Advances in technology have made it possible to measure and analyze these signals with increasing precision and accuracy, opening up new possibilities for research and diagnosis.

10.2.1 Action Potential

The action potential is a fundamental process that underlies the communication and functioning of cells in the human body, particularly nerve and muscle cells. It involves modifications in the electrical properties of the cell membrane, resulting in depolarization and subsequent repolarization. This phenomenon allows cells to transmit signals and carry out their specific functions [5]. In a resting state, cells are polarized, with a negative charge inside the cell compared to the outside. The specific passage of ions through specialized channels across the cell membrane maintains this resting potential. When a cell is stimulated by an electrochemical signal or an external stimulus, the cell membrane changes its permeability, allowing sodium ions (Na^+) to enter the cell. The influx of Na^+ ions constitutes an ionic current, reducing the membrane barrier for Na^+ ions and causing depolarization. As a result, the inside of the cell becomes positive relative to the outside. This change in electrical potential represents the beginning of the action potential, with a peak value of around +20 mV for most cells. During depolarization, the positive charge inside the cell can stimulate adjacent cells, propagating the action potential along nerve or muscle fibers. This transmission occurs through specialized structures called axons and synapses, which allow the impulse to pass from one cell to the next. After a certain period of time, the cell repolarizes, returning to its resting potential. Repolarization is facilitated by the movement of potassium ions (K^+) out of the cell. Voltage-dependent potassium channels change the membrane permeability, allowing K^+ ions to flow out of the cell. Since K^+ concentration is higher inside the cell, the net efflux of K^+ ions causes the inside of the cell to become more negative, leading to repolarization. The duration of the action potential varies depending on the type of cell. Nerve and muscle cells typically repolarize rapidly, with an action potential duration of about 1 ms. In contrast, heart muscle cells repolarize more slowly, with an action potential duration of 150–300 ms.

The human body needs to go through the depolarization and repolarization processes. It allows cells to transmit electrical signals, communicate with each other, and carry out essential physiological processes. Action potentials are vital for various functions, such as muscle contractions, nerve impulses, sensory perception, and coordination of bodily functions. Understanding the working of action potentials is essential for studying and diagnosing various medical conditions. For example, abnormalities in the action potential can lead to neurological disorders, cardiac arrhythmias, and other pathological conditions. Healthcare practitioners can learn more about the health and functioning of the human body by examining and interpreting the features of action potentials, which can help with disease diagnosis and therapy.

10.2.2 Electrocardiogram

A common diagnostic technique in medicine for determining the electrical activity of the heart is the ECG. A broad spectrum of cardiac disorders, including arrhythmias, myocardial infarction, and heart failure, can be identified using the non-invasive ECG test. By capturing the electrical potentials produced as the heart muscle contracts and relaxes, the ECG records the electrical activity of the heart. Electrodes positioned on the patient's skin can find these electrical potentials. The ECG signal, which varies in voltage over time, is routinely captured for anywhere between a few seconds and many minutes. A vector, which represents the total electrical activity of all the heart's separate cells, can be used to describe the electrical activity of the organ. By placing electrodes on the skin, this vector can be measured at the skin's surface. The electrical vector moves through these electrodes during the cardiac cycle, resulting in voltage changes at these electrodes, which are recorded to produce the ECG signal.

The ECG signal is typically composed of a series of waves and intervals that reflect the different phases of the cardiac cycle, as shown in Figure 10.2. The P wave is the first wave in the ECG signal and represents the depolarization of the atria. The QRS complex represents the depolarization of the ventricles, and the T wave represents their repolarization. The PR interval represents the time interval between the onset of the P wave and the onset of the QRS complex, and the QT interval represents the time interval between the onset of the QRS complex and the end of the T wave. The ECG signal can be mathematically represented as a time-varying voltage signal, V(t), that is measured across two electrodes that are placed on the skin of the patient. The ECG signal is typically recorded using a standard 12-lead configuration, which involves placing 10 electrodes on the patient's limbs and chest. The standard 12-lead ECG provides a comprehensive view of the electrical activity of the heart from different angles.

There are several approaches to analyze the ECG signal to diagnose different heart diseases. One kind of arrhythmia, such as atrial fibrillation, ventricular tachycardia, or heart block, might be indicated by abnormalities in the amplitude, duration, or shape of the waves and intervals in the ECG signal. Additionally, alterations in the ST segment of the ECG signal may be a symptom of cardiac muscle ischemia or damage. Performing a Fourier transform to transform the signal from the time domain to the frequency domain is a typical technique for analyzing the ECG signal. As a result, it is possible to identify particular frequency components in the signal that can be utilized to identify different kinds of arrhythmias. For example, the presence of a high-frequency component in the signal may indicate the presence of atrial fibrillation, while the absence of a low-frequency component may indicate the presence of heart block. Another common method for analyzing the ECG signal is to perform a wavelet transform, which allows for the identification of specific time-frequency patterns in the signal. This can be particularly useful for detecting changes in the ST segment, which can be indicative of ischemia or injury to the heart muscle. In addition to these methods, a number of other techniques have been developed for analyzing the ECG signal, including ML algorithms, which can be utilized to automatically detect and diagnose various cardiac conditions based on features extracted from the ECG signal [6, 7].

In general, the ECG signal is a vital instrument for identifying and keeping track of a number of heart problems. Clinicians can learn important information about the electrical activity of the heart and the operation of its various parts by examining the different waves and pauses in the ECG signal. This may aid in determining the best course of treatment and enhance patient results.

10.2.3 Electroencephalography

EEG is a non-invasive technique used to measure the electrical activity of the brain. The EEG signal is generated by the activity of the neurons in the brain, which communicate with each other through electrical impulses. These electrical impulses produce tiny electric currents that can be detected by electrodes placed on the scalp. EEG signals are used in clinical settings to diagnose and monitor a wide range of neurological conditions, including epilepsy, sleep disorders, and brain injuries. The EEG signal is a complex mixture of various components that arise from different sources in the brain. The EEG signal is generated by the synchronous activity of millions of neurons in the brain, which produce electrical fields that can be measured on the scalp, as shown in Figure 10.4. The amplitude of the EEG signal is in the range of microvolts and is therefore extremely small. To detect these signals, electrodes are placed on the scalp at different locations to record the electrical activity of the brain. Figure 10.3 shows capturing ECG signals.

The EEG signal can be divided into different frequency bands, which are associated with different states of consciousness and cognitive processes. The frequency bands of the EEG signal are usually classified as delta (0.5–4 Hz), theta (4–8 Hz), alpha (8–12 Hz), beta (12–30 Hz), and gamma (30–100 Hz). Each of these frequency bands has a distinct physiological and cognitive function. Delta waves are usually observed in deep sleep and are associated with restorative processes in the brain. Theta waves are observed during the early stages of sleep and are associated with the transition from wakefulness to sleep. Alpha waves are observed during wakeful relaxation and are associated with the inhibition of sensory processing. Beta waves are observed during active cognitive processing and are associated with alertness, attention, and motor activity. Gamma waves are observed during cognitive processing and are associated with higher-order cognitive functions such as perception, memory, and attention. The EEG signal is generated by the electrical activity of the brain, which is influenced by a variety of factors, including genetics, age, gender, and environmental factors. The EEG signal can be affected by a variety of neurological

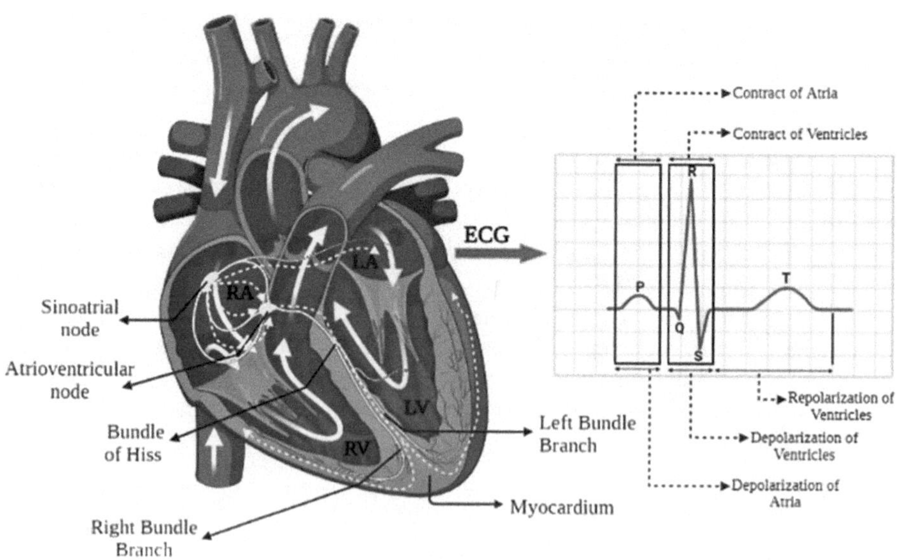

FIGURE 10.3 Capturing ECG signals.

conditions, such as epilepsy, stroke, and brain injuries. In these conditions, the electrical activity of the brain is altered, resulting in changes in the EEG signal. The EEG signal can be analyzed using various signal processing techniques, such as time-domain analysis, frequency-domain analysis, and time-frequency analysis. Time-domain analysis involves the analysis of the EEG signal in the time domain, which includes measuring the amplitude, duration, and frequency of the signal. The frequency-domain analysis involves the analysis of the EEG signal in the frequency domain, which includes measuring the power spectral density (PSD) of the signal. Time-frequency analysis involves the analysis of the EEG signal in both the time and frequency domains, which includes measuring the changes in the PSD over time. One of the most common uses of the EEG signal is in the diagnosis and monitoring of epilepsy. Epilepsy is a neurological disorder characterized by recurrent seizures, which are caused by abnormal electrical activity in the brain. EEG signals are used to diagnose and monitor epilepsy by detecting abnormal patterns of electrical activity in the brain. During an epileptic seizure, the EEG signal shows a characteristic pattern of high-amplitude, high-frequency activity, known as a spike or a sharp wave. The EEG signal is also used to localize the source of the seizure activity in the brain, which is important for surgical planning in patients with drug-resistant epilepsy. In addition to epilepsy, the EEG signal is used to diagnose and monitor other neurological conditions, such as sleep disorders and brain injuries. Sleep disorders, such as sleep apnea and insomnia, are characterized by disruptions in the normal sleep-wake cycle, which can be detected by changes in the EEG signal. Brain injuries, such as traumatic brain injury (TBI), can cause disruptions in the normal electrical activity of the brain, which can also be detected by changes in the EEG signal. For example,

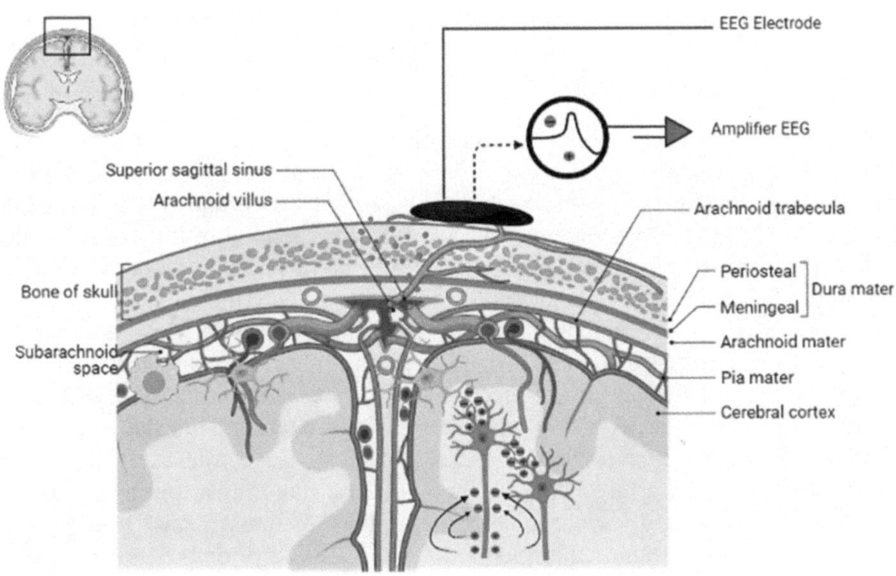

FIGURE 10.4 Capturing EEG signals.

after a TBI, there may be an increase in slow-wave activity and a decrease in alpha activity. The EEG signal can also be used to monitor the depth of anesthesia during surgery. Anesthesia affects the electrical activity of the brain, and monitoring the EEG can help ensure that the patient remains in a safe and appropriate level of anesthesia. EEG can also be used to monitor brain function during other medical procedures, such as deep brain stimulation for Parkinson's disease or epilepsy.

The analysis of EEG signals can provide insights into the underlying neural processes and can help to identify abnormalities in brain function. One common technique used to analyze EEG signals is spectral analysis, which involves decomposing the signal into its frequency components. This can reveal information about the power and distribution of different frequency bands in the EEG signal, which can be indicative of different brain states and functions. Another technique used to analyze EEG signals is event-related potential analysis, which involves averaging the EEG signal across many repetitions of a specific stimulus or task. This can reveal the time course and characteristics of neural processing related to that stimulus or task, such as the onset and duration of sensory processing, attentional modulation, and motor preparation. In recent years, there has been growing interest in using ML techniques to analyze EEG signals for clinical applications [8, 9]. ML algorithms can be trained to identify patterns in the EEG signal that are associated with specific neurological conditions, such as epilepsy or Alzheimer's disease. These algorithms can also be used to predict outcomes, such as the likelihood of seizure recurrence or cognitive decline [10, 11]. Overall, the EEG signal is a valuable tool for studying brain function and diagnosing neurological conditions. Its non-invasive nature, high temporal resolution, and sensitivity to changes in brain activity make it a versatile and widely used technique in neuroscience and clinical medicine. As technology continues to advance, it is likely that EEG will continue to play an important role in understanding the human brain and developing new treatments for neurological disorders.

10.2.4 Electromyography

EMG is a diagnostic technique used to assess the electrical activity of muscles and the nerves controlling them. It involves the measurement and recording of the electrical signals generated by muscle fibers during contraction and relaxation. EMG provides valuable information about muscle function, helping in the diagnosis and management of neuromuscular disorders, as well as in research and rehabilitation settings [12]. The electrical signals generated by muscle activity are known as action potentials. These action potentials propagate along the muscle fibers and can be detected and measured using specialized electrodes. There are two main types of electrodes used in EMG: surface electrodes and needle electrodes. Surface electrodes are placed on the skin overlying the muscle of interest. They detect the electrical activity from the superficial muscles and provide a non-invasive method of EMG measurement. Surface EMG is commonly used in clinical settings to assess muscle function, identify abnormalities, and guide treatment plans. Needle electrodes, also called intramuscular electrodes, are inserted directly into the muscle tissue. They allow for more precise and detailed measurements, particularly for deep muscles. Needle EMG is often used in specialized cases or research settings where a higher level of accuracy is required. During an EMG examination, the patient is typically asked to relax or contract specific muscles. The electrical signals generated by the muscle activity are picked up by the electrodes and amplified for analysis. The signals are then processed and displayed on a monitor or recorded for further evaluation. EMG recordings can provide valuable insights into muscle activation patterns, motor unit recruitment, muscle fatigue, and nerve conduction abnormalities. Abnormal EMG findings may indicate muscle or nerve dysfunction, such as muscle weakness, nerve compression, neuropathy, or neuromuscular disorders like muscular dystrophy or myasthenia gravis.

In addition to diagnostic purposes, EMG is used in research and rehabilitation settings. Researchers utilize EMG to study muscle physiology, motor control, and movement patterns. In rehabilitation, EMG biofeedback is sometimes used to help individuals regain control and strength in their muscles through visual or auditory feedback based on their EMG signals. In short, electromyography is a valuable diagnostic tool that measures the electrical activity of muscles and provides insights into neuromuscular function. It is widely used in clinical practice, research, and rehabilitation to assess and understand muscle and nerve abnormalities, guide treatment plans, and monitor progress. It involves the use of specialized electrodes to detect and amplify the electrical signals generated by muscle fibers. The detailed working of EMG can be explained in several steps:

1. **Electrode Placement**: To perform EMG, electrodes are placed on the skin overlying the muscle or inserted directly into the muscle tissue. Surface electrodes are commonly used, which consist of adhesive patches with conductive elements that pick up the electrical signals from the surface of the skin. Needle electrodes, on the other hand, are thin, fine wires that are inserted into the muscle tissue to measure the activity of deeper muscles.
2. **Signal Detection and Amplification**: Once the electrodes are in place, they detect the electrical activity of the muscles. The electrical signals generated by the muscle fibers are very small and require amplification for accurate measurement. The electrodes are connected to an EMG amplifier, which increases the strength of the signals and filters out unwanted noise.
3. **Signal Processing**: The amplified electrical signals are then processed using various techniques to extract useful information. Commonly used processing techniques include filtering, rectification, and smoothing. Filtering removes unwanted noise and interference from the signals, rectification converts the signals to a unidirectional form, and smoothing further refines the signals to provide a clearer representation of muscle activity.
4. **Display and Analysis**: The processed EMG signals are displayed on a monitor or recorded for further analysis. The EMG waveform shows the amplitude and frequency characteristics of the muscle activity over time. The shape and duration of the waveform can provide insights into the muscle's contraction and relaxation patterns, as well as the timing and coordination of muscle activation.
5. **Interpretation**: Trained professionals, such as neurologists or physiatrists, interpret the EMG data to assess muscle function and diagnose any

abnormalities. They analyze various parameters of the EMG signals, such as amplitude, duration, recruitment patterns, and motor unit action potentials, to identify any signs of muscle or nerve dysfunction. Abnormalities in the EMG patterns can indicate muscle weakness, nerve damage, neuromuscular disorders, or other pathologies.

6. **Clinical Applications**: EMG is widely used in clinical practice for diagnostic purposes. It helps in identifying and localizing the source of muscle weakness, assessing nerve conduction abnormalities, diagnosing neuromuscular disorders, and monitoring disease progression or treatment effectiveness. EMG findings are often correlated with other clinical information, such as patient history, physical examination, and imaging studies, to provide a comprehensive assessment.
7. **Research and Rehabilitation**: In addition to diagnostic applications, EMG is extensively used in research to study muscle physiology, motor control, and movement patterns. It provides insights into muscle activation patterns, muscle coordination, muscle fatigue, and other aspects of neuromuscular function. In rehabilitation settings, EMG biofeedback techniques may be employed to help individuals regain control and strength in their muscles by providing real-time feedback based on their EMG signals [13].

Overall, electromyography is a valuable tool that enables the assessment of muscle and nerve function through the measurement and analysis of electrical signals generated by muscles. It has broad applications in clinical practice, research, and rehabilitation, providing valuable insights into neuro-muscular function and aiding in the diagnosis, treatment, and monitoring of various conditions.

10.3 BRAIN–COMPUTER INTERFACE

A BCI is a type of technology that enables direct communication between the brain and an external device or computer system. It allows individuals to control and interact with computers or other devices using only their brain activity [14]. The technology has the potential to transform the lives of people with disabilities, including those with spinal cord injuries, ALS, and other conditions that limit movement, as shown in Figure 10.5. The concept of BCI has been around since the 1970s, but current developments in neuroscience, ML, and computer technology have led to significant progress in the field. There are different types of BCI systems, but they generally involve the use of sensors or electrodes to record and analyze brain activity, and then translate this activity into commands or signals that can be used to control a computer or other device. Two primary categories of BCI systems exist: invasive and non-invasive. Invasive BCI systems involve the use of electrodes that are implanted directly into the brain tissue, while non-invasive systems use external sensors that are placed on the scalp or other parts of the body. Invasive BCI systems have the advantage of providing more precise and reliable signals, but they also carry greater risks and require invasive surgery to implant the electrodes. Non-invasive BCI systems are safer and less invasive, but they tend to be less accurate and reliable due to the attenuation and distortion of the signals as they pass through the skull and other tissues.

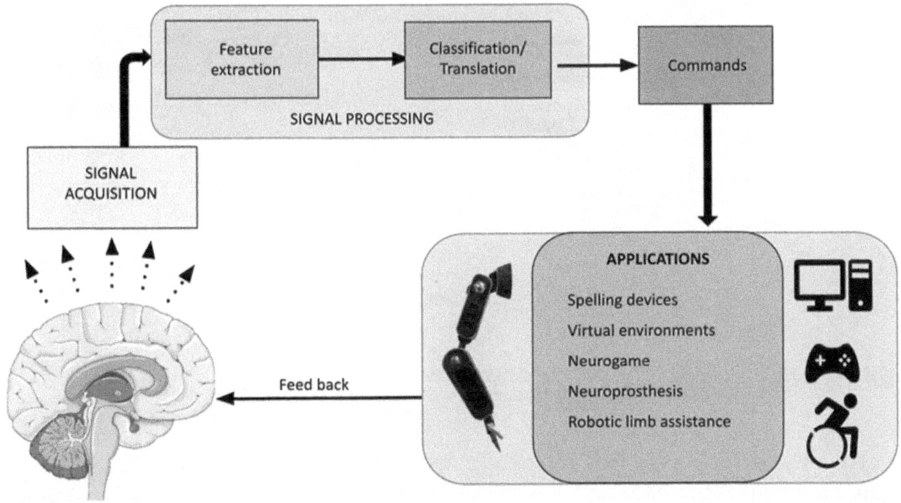

FIGURE 10.5 Brain–computer interface.

One of the key challenges in developing BCI systems is to extract meaningful signals from the complex and noisy activity of the brain [15]. This involves the use of advanced signal processing and ML algorithms to analyze and decode the brain activity, and to identify patterns or features that can be used to generate useful commands or signals. Several different types of brain signals can be utilized for BCI, including EEG, magnetoencephalography, functional magnetic resonance imaging, and single-unit recordings [16]. The selection of the signal relies on the particular application and specifications of the BCI system. Each type of signal has advantages and disadvantages of its own.

Signal capture, signal processing, feature extraction, classification, and feedback are some of the phases involved in creating commands or signals from brain activity. The brain signals are captured using sensors or electrodes during the signal acquisition step as shown in Figure 10.6, when they are then amplified and filtered to remove noise and artifacts. After processing the data, valuable features are extracted from them that can be used to categorize various brain states or activities. To do this, sophisticated signal processing methods like wavelet transformations, independent component analysis, and time-frequency analysis are used to find patterns and characteristics in the brain signals. ML algorithms like artificial neural networks, Support Vector Machines, and random forests are used to classify various brain states or activities after the features have been retrieved. Using labeled data, which comprises brain signals connected to certain commands or actions, classification algorithms are learned. The final stage of the BCI process is feedback, where the output of the classification algorithm is used to control a computer or other device. This involves mapping the brain signals to specific commands or actions, such as moving a cursor on a screen or controlling a robotic arm. BCI technology has the potential to revolutionize the way we interact with computers and other devices and

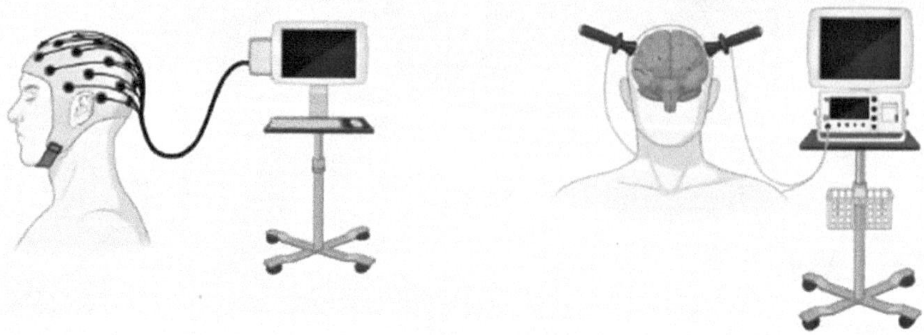

FIGURE 10.6 Different types of electrodes for capturing brain signals.

to provide new opportunities for people with disabilities. However, there are still many challenges that need to be addressed, including improving the accuracy and reliability of the BCI systems, reducing the invasiveness of the implantation procedures, and developing more robust and intuitive feedback mechanisms. Despite these challenges, BCI research is advancing rapidly, and there is growing interest and investment in the technology from both the academic and commercial sectors. As technology continues to evolve and improve, it has the potential to transform a wide range of fields, including medicine, education, entertainment, and even defense. One potential application of BCI technology is in the field of medicine. BCIs have the potential to provide new ways to diagnose, treat, and manage neurological disorders and conditions. For example, BCIs could be used to help restore movement and communication abilities in patients with spinal cord injuries, stroke, or other neurological disorders. Researchers are also exploring the use of BCIs for managing chronic pain, epilepsy, and other conditions. Another potential application of BCI technology is in the field of education. BCIs could be used to help individuals with learning disabilities or cognitive impairments to communicate and interact with their environment. For example, BCIs could be utilized to support individuals with autism to communicate more effectively or to help individuals with attention-deficit hyperactivity disorder to focus and concentrate. Additionally, BCIs have the power to completely transform the entertainment industry. They might be applied to develop fully immersive gaming environments where users can manipulate the game with their emotions or thoughts. Real-time virtual reality settings that react to a user's motions and ideas could also be made with BCIs. Finally, BCIs could also have important applications in defense and security. They could be used to operate other remote-controlled devices, such as unmanned aerial vehicles, solely with the operator's thoughts. BCIs could also be used to monitor the mental states of soldiers and other personnel, helping to identify and prevent stress-related conditions such as post-traumatic stress disorder (PTSD).

In a nutshell, brain–computer interfaces (BCIs) are a rapidly advancing field with many potential applications across a range of domains. Despite the challenges associated with developing effective and reliable BCIs, there is growing interest and investment in the technology from both the academic and commercial sectors. As

BCIs continue to evolve and improve, they have the potential to revolutionize fields such as medicine, education, entertainment, and defense, improving the lives of millions of people around the world.

10.4 ML AND DL TECHNIQUES FOR BIOMEDICAL SIGNAL PROCESSING

ML and DL techniques have revolutionized biomedical signal processing, playing a crucial role in analyzing complex biomedical data and extracting meaningful insights. Biomedical signal processing involves the acquisition, analysis, and interpretation of physiological signals, such as ECG, EEG, and medical images, to aid in the diagnosis, monitoring, and treatment of various medical conditions [17].

The design and development of statistical models and techniques that let computers learn from data and make judgments or predictions without explicit programming are known as ML. ML techniques are particularly well-suited for analyzing large volumes of biomedical data, which often exhibit complex patterns and relationships. By training ML models on labeled datasets, patterns can be identified, and predictions can be made on unseen data. DL is a subset of ML that focuses on training artificial neural networks with multiple layers to automatically learn hierarchical representations of data. DL models, such as convolutional neural networks (CNNs) and recurrent neural networks (RNNs), have shown remarkable success in various biomedical signal-processing tasks, surpassing traditional feature extraction methods [18, 19]. DL models excel at learning intricate features directly from raw data, eliminating the need for manual feature engineering [20].

One of the significant applications of ML and DL in biomedical signal processing is disease diagnosis and prediction. By leveraging large datasets of labeled biomedical signals, ML models can learn to classify signals into different disease categories, as shown in Figure 10.7. For example, in ECG analysis, ML algorithms can accurately detect abnormalities associated with cardiac arrhythmias, myocardial infarction, or heart failure. DL models can learn complex patterns in raw ECG signals and achieve state-of-the-art performance in detecting and classifying abnormal cardiac rhythms. ML and DL techniques also play a vital role in biomedical signal denoising and enhancement. Biomedical signals are often contaminated with noise, making it challenging to extract meaningful information. ML models can be trained to remove noise from signals, improving their quality and enabling more accurate analysis. For instance, ML algorithms can effectively denoise EEG signals, enhancing the detection of specific brain activity patterns associated with neurological disorders.

Furthermore, ML and DL methods have been successfully applied to medical image analysis. Medical imaging techniques, such as magnetic resonance imaging and computed tomography, generate vast amounts of image data that require sophisticated analysis for disease diagnosis and treatment planning. ML algorithms can be trained on labeled medical images to identify and localize abnormalities, aiding radiologists in the detection of tumors, lesions, or other pathologies. DL models, particularly CNNs, have shown exceptional performance in image classification, segmentation, and reconstruction tasks. ML and DL techniques also have applications in physiological signal monitoring and real-time analysis. Continuous monitoring of

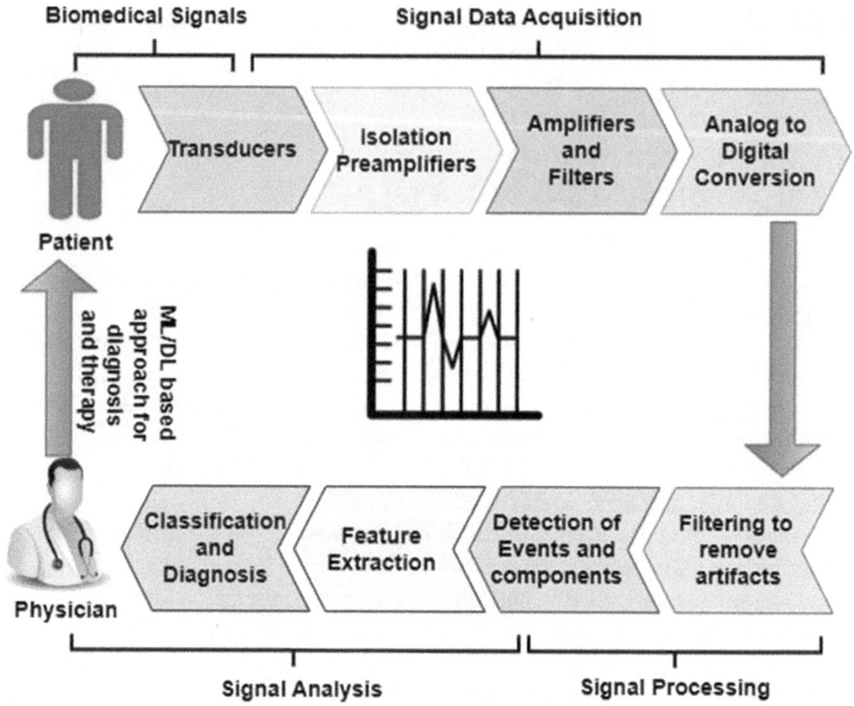

FIGURE 10.7 Illustrating ML/DL-based approach for diagnosis and therapy.

vital signs, such as heart rate, BP, and RR, is essential for patient care in critical care settings. ML algorithms can be employed to analyze real-time physiological signals and provide early warnings for deteriorating health conditions. DL models, with their ability to learn temporal dependencies, can capture dynamic patterns in time series data, enabling accurate prediction of future physiological states or events.

Despite the significant advancements and potential of ML and DL in biomedical signal processing, several challenges exist. First, the availability of high-quality labeled datasets for training ML models can be limited, particularly for rare diseases or conditions. The acquisition and annotation of biomedical signals require expert knowledge and resources. Therefore, efforts are being made to develop open-access datasets and encourage collaborations to address this challenge. Second, the interpretability of ML and DL models in biomedical signal processing is crucial for clinical acceptance and trust. Deep neural networks, with their complex architectures, often act as black boxes, making it challenging to understand the underlying mechanisms and reasoning behind their predictions. Interpretable ML and DL models that provide insights into decision-making are being actively researched to address this issue. Techniques such as attention mechanisms and saliency maps aim to highlight important features or regions in the input signals that contribute to the model's output. Another challenge is the generalizability of ML and DL models across different patient populations and clinical settings. Biomedical signals can exhibit significant inter-individual and inter-site variations, making it difficult to develop models that perform well in diverse scenarios. Transfer learning techniques, which leverage knowledge from pre-trained models on large datasets, can help mitigate this challenge by adapting models to specific target domains or populations with limited data. Data privacy and security also pose concerns in biomedical signal processing. Biomedical signals often contain sensitive information, and maintaining patient privacy is of utmost importance. Techniques such as federated learning, where models are trained collaboratively on distributed data without sharing raw data, are being explored to ensure privacy while still benefiting from collective knowledge. Furthermore, the integration of ML and DL models into clinical practice requires addressing regulatory and ethical considerations. Robust validation, standardization, and regulatory frameworks need to be established to ensure the safety and effectiveness of these techniques. Additionally, ethical aspects, such as transparency, fairness, and accountability, must be carefully addressed to avoid biases and ensure equitable healthcare outcomes.

In conclusion, ML and DL techniques have emerged as powerful tools in biomedical signal processing, enabling accurate diagnosis, denoising, monitoring, and analysis of various physiological signals. Their ability to learn complex patterns directly from raw data and make predictions has revolutionized the field, offering new insights and possibilities for improving healthcare outcomes. However, challenges such as data availability, interpretability, generalizability, privacy, and ethics need to be carefully addressed to unlock the full potential of these techniques in clinical practice. Continued research, collaborations, and advancements in these areas will further enhance the role of ML and DL in biomedical signal processing, ultimately leading to improved patient care and outcomes.

10.5 APPLICATIONS, CHALLENGES, AND EMERGING TRENDS IN BIOMEDICAL SIGNAL PROCESSING

Biomedical signal processing has diverse applications in healthcare, including ECG, EEG, EMG, and medical imaging, aiding in diagnosis, monitoring, and treatment. Challenges include handling large data volumes, addressing signal variability and artifacts, and ensuring data security and privacy. Emerging trends involve the integration of intelligent algorithms, ML, and artificial intelligence techniques for improved accuracy, automation, and personalized healthcare.

10.5.1 Applications of Biomedical Signals

Emerging trends in biomedical signals play a crucial role in healthcare, providing valuable information about the physiological state of individuals [21]. These signals are collected through various sensors and devices and can be utilized in several applications to aid in the diagnosis, monitoring, treatment, and overall healthcare management. Here are some key applications of biomedical signals in healthcare:

- **Disease Diagnosis:** Biomedical signals can be utilized to diagnose a wide range of diseases and conditions. For example, ECG signals are used to

detect abnormalities in heart rhythm and diagnose conditions such as heart failure, myocardial infarction, and arrhythmias. Similarly,
EEG signals are used in the diagnosis of epilepsy, sleep disorders, and neurological conditions. Other signals like EMG, BP, and respiratory signals are also used for disease diagnosis.

- **Patient Monitoring:** Biomedical signals are extensively used for monitoring patients in various healthcare settings. Vital indicators like oxygen saturation, respiratory rate, BP, and heart rate are frequently monitored because they give important clues about a patient's health. These signals can be collected in real time and analyzed to detect any abnormalities or changes that may require immediate medical attention. Remote patient monitoring systems utilize biomedical signals to monitor patients in non-hospital environments, allowing for early detection of complications and timely intervention.
- **Personalized Medicine:** Biomedical signals contribute to the development of personalized treatment plans for patients. By monitoring and analyzing signals such as genetic data, biomarkers, and physiological parameters, healthcare professionals can tailor treatment strategies to individual patients. With this strategy, treatments are optimized based on the unique requirements, characteristics, and responses of each patient, producing greater results and fewer negative effects.
- **Rehabilitation and Physical Therapy:** Biomedical signals are utilized in rehabilitation and physical therapy to assess the progress of patients and guide their treatment. For instance, motion capture systems use signals from sensors placed on the body to track and analyze movements during rehabilitation exercises. These signals provide objective feedback to therapists and patients, helping in the assessment of motor function and the effectiveness of therapeutic interventions.
- **Prosthetics and Assistive Devices:** Biomedical signals are instrumental in the development and control of prosthetic limbs and assistive devices. Signals such as EMG can be used to detect and interpret muscle activity, enabling individuals with limb loss to control prosthetic devices using their residual muscle signals. With the help of BCIs, people with severe motor difficulties can communicate and operate external devices by using neural signals like EEG.

• **Sleep Analysis:** Biomedical signals, such as EEG and respiratory signals, are used in sleep analysis to evaluate sleep patterns, detect sleep disorders, and assess the quality of sleep. These signals are tracked during sleep investigations that are carried out at sleep laboratories or at home to identify disorders such as sleep apnea, narcolepsy, insomnia, and restless legs syndrome. The analysis of these signals helps in understanding sleep-related problems and guides treatment interventions [22].

- **Mental Health Monitoring:** Biomedical signals are increasingly being explored for monitoring and assessing mental health conditions [23, 24]. EEG and heart rate variability signals can provide insights into mental states, stress levels, and emotional responses. Using these signals, objective diagnostic and monitoring tools are created for mental health illnesses such as anxiety, depressive disorders, and PTSD.

- **Health and Wellness Tracking:** Biomedical signals are employed in various wearable devices and smartphone applications to track health and wellness parameters. These devices collect signals like heart rate, activity level, sleep patterns, and stress levels to provide users with insights into their overall health and well-being. This information can motivate individuals to make positive lifestyle changes and enable them to take proactive steps toward maintaining a healthy lifestyle.
- **Drug Development and Clinical Trials:** Biomedical signals play a crucial role in drug development and clinical trials. ECG and EEG signals are used to evaluate the efficacy and safety of new medicines and medical interventions. These signals help researchers monitor the effects of treatments on the cardiovascular and neurological systems, providing valuable data for evaluating drug responses and identifying potential side effects.
- **Sports Performance Monitoring:** Biomedical signals are utilized in sports medicine to monitor athletes' performance, track their physiological responses, and prevent injuries. Signals such as BP, heart rate, oxygen saturation, and muscle activity can provide insights into an athlete's physical exertion, recovery, and overall fitness level. By monitoring these signals, coaches and sports scientists can optimize training programs, prevent overexertion, and enhance performance.
- **Telemedicine and Remote Healthcare:** Biomedical signals play a vital role in telemedicine and remote healthcare, enabling healthcare professionals to monitor patients remotely and provide timely interventions. With the help of wearable devices and wireless sensors, patients can transmit their biomedical signals to healthcare providers from the comfort of their homes. This approach facilitates regular monitoring and early detection of abnormalities and reduces the need for in-person visits, especially for patients in remote areas or with limited mobility.
- **Medical Research and Data Analysis:** Biomedical signals serve as valuable resources for medical research and data analysis. Large datasets of biomedical signals, collected from diverse populations, enable researchers to gain insights into disease patterns, treatment responses, and population health trends. ML and data mining techniques can be applied to these datasets to uncover hidden patterns, identify predictive markers, and develop advanced diagnostic and prognostic models.

In a nutshell, biomedical signals have numerous applications in healthcare, ranging from disease diagnosis and patient monitoring to personalized medicine, rehabilitation, and mental health assessment. These signals provide valuable insights into the physiological state of individuals, enabling healthcare professionals to make informed decisions and deliver personalized care. With advancements in technology, such as ML and DL, the analysis and interpretation of biomedical signals continue to evolve, promising further improvements in healthcare outcomes, early detection of diseases, and the development of innovative treatment approaches.

10.5.2 Challenges and Limitations of Using Biomedical Signals in Healthcare

While biomedical signals have great potential in healthcare, there are several challenges and limitations that need to be considered. Here are some of them:

- **Noise and Artifacts:** The quality and dependability of the measurements can be impacted by the ease with which noise and artifacts can contaminate biomedical signals. Various factors such as motion artifacts, electrode impedance, electrical interference, and environmental factors can introduce noise and distortions into the signals.
- **Interpretation Complexity:** Biomedical signals often require specialized knowledge and expertise to interpret correctly. The analysis and interpretation of signals like ECG, EEG, or medical imaging data can be complex and may require skilled professionals, which can limit accessibility in certain healthcare settings.
- **Individual Variations:** Biomedical signals can exhibit significant variations among individuals due to factors such as age, gender, physiological conditions, and disease states. These variations make it challenging to establish generalized and accurate reference ranges or models applicable to diverse populations.
- **Data Volume and Storage:** Biomedical signals, especially high-resolution signals, or continuous streaming data, can generate large volumes of data. Managing, storing, and processing these large datasets require robust infrastructure and efficient algorithms, which can pose challenges in terms of storage capacity, computational resources, and data management.
- **Ethical and Privacy Concerns:** Biomedical signals often contain sensitive and personal health information. Maintaining patient privacy, ensuring data security, and adhering to ethical considerations when collecting, storing, and sharing biomedical signal data present significant challenges in healthcare settings.
- **Validation and Standardization:** New strategies for processing and analyzing biomedical signals must be rigorously assessed and validated against industry-recognized best practices or clinical results. Standardization of data acquisition protocols, signal processing algorithms, and interpretation criteria is crucial to ensure consistent and reliable results across different healthcare settings.
- **Integration and Interoperability:** Integrating biomedical signal data from different sources or devices and interoperability among various healthcare systems can be challenging due to differences in data formats, protocols, and standards. Achieving seamless data exchange and integration for comprehensive patient care and research collaborations requires efforts in data standardization and interoperability frameworks.
- **Cost and Accessibility:** Access to advanced biomedical signal acquisition devices and analysis tools can be costly, limiting their widespread use and availability in certain healthcare settings, particularly in resource-constrained environments or developing countries.

Addressing these challenges and limitations requires collaboration among researchers, healthcare professionals, engineers, and policymakers to develop robust methodologies, improve data quality, enhance signal processing techniques, establish data sharing and privacy frameworks, and ensure the ethical and responsible use of biomedical signals in healthcare.

10.5.3 Emerging Trends and Future Directions in Biomedical Signal Processing

Biomedical signal processing is a rapidly evolving field with several emerging trends and future directions [25]. Here are some key areas that show promise for advancements in biomedical signal processing:

- **Deep Learning and Artificial Intelligence (AI):** CNNs and RNNs, two types of DL techniques, are increasingly being used for biomedical signal processing problems. AI-based methods can extract complex features from signals, improve classification and prediction accuracy, and enable automated analysis and decision-making in healthcare [26].
- **Wearable and Mobile Health Technologies:** The proliferation of wearable devices and mobile health applications has created new opportunities for continuous monitoring of biomedical signals in real-world settings. These devices can capture signals like electrocardiography (ECG), photoplethysmography (PPG), and accelerometry, enabling remote patient monitoring, early detection of abnormalities, and personalized healthcare [27].
- **Internet of Things (IoT) and Cloud Computing:** The integration of biomedical devices, sensor networks, and cloud computing platforms allows for efficient storage, processing, and analysis of large-scale biomedical signal data. IoT-based healthcare systems enable real-time monitoring, secure data transmission, and remote access to biomedical information, facilitating personalized and data-driven healthcare [28].
- **Multimodal Signal Fusion:** Combining information from multiple modalities, such as physiological signals, imaging data, and clinical records, can provide a more comprehensive understanding of a patient's health status. Fusion of multimodal signals can enhance diagnostic accuracy, improve treatment planning, and enable personalized healthcare interventions [29, 30].
- **Real-Time and Adaptive Signal Processing:** Real-time processing of biomedical signals is crucial for timely decision-making and intervention. Advancements in signal processing algorithms, hardware accelerators, and embedded systems enable efficient real-time analysis of signals, facilitating point-of-care diagnostics, continuous monitoring, and closed-loop therapeutic interventions [31].
- **Explainable and Interpretable Models:** As ML techniques become more prevalent in biomedical signal processing, there is a growing need for models that provide transparent and interpretable results. Explainable AI methods aim to enhance model interpretability, ensuring that the decision-making process of algorithms can be understood and trusted by healthcare professionals.

- **Big Data Analytics and Data-Driven Approaches:** The increasing availability of large-scale biomedical signal datasets provides opportunities for data-driven approaches and advanced analytics. Big data analytics, combined with signal processing techniques, can uncover hidden patterns, discover biomarkers, and enable precision medicine through personalized treatment strategies.
- **Ethical Considerations and Privacy Protection:** As biomedical signal processing technologies advance, ensuring patient privacy, data security, and ethical considerations become paramount. Striking a balance between data access for research and protecting individual privacy rights requires the development of robust data anonymization techniques, secure data sharing frameworks, and ethical guidelines.

Personalized medicine, better patient outcomes, and industrial transformation are all possible with these new developments and directions in biomedical signal processing. Effective implementation of these improvements requires collaboration among researchers, healthcare professionals, engineers, and policymakers to stimulate innovation and overcome obstacles.

10.6 CONCLUSIONS

As discussed, biomedical signals play a crucial role in healthcare and medical research, providing valuable insights into the functioning of the human body. The numerous biomedical signal types, including ECG, EEG, EMG, and several more, each offer particular insights into specific physiological processes. We gave an overview of the various categories of biomedical signals, along with their distinctive features and uses, in this chapter. We also discussed the challenges and limitations in acquiring and processing biomedical signals, such as noise, artifacts, and data variability. Future technological developments and ML methods offer hope for increasing the accuracy as well as efficiency of biomedical signal analysis. As data collection and processing methods continue to improve, the potential for early diagnosis and personalized treatment options will become more feasible. Additionally, the integration of biomedical signals with other sources of health data, such as genomics and imaging, will provide a more comprehensive understanding of health and disease.

REFERENCES

1. Alan V Oppenheim, Alan S Willsky, Syed Hamid Nawab, and Jian-Jiun Ding. *Signals and systems*, volume 2. Upper Saddle River, NJ: Prentice Hall, 1997.
2. Lawrence R Rabiner and Bernard Gold. *Theory and application of digital signal processing*. Englewood Cliffs: Prentice-Hall, 1975.
3. Rangaraj M Rangayyan. *Biomedical signal analysis*. Paris: John Wiley & Sons, 2015.
4. Beatriz Remeseiro and Veronica Bolon-Canedo. A review of feature selection methods in medical applications. *Computers in Biology and Medicine*, 112:103375, 2019.
5. Mark W Barnett and Philip M Larkman. The action potential. *Practical Neurology*, 7(3):192–197, 2007.
6. Monu Malik, Tanya Dua, and Snigdha. Biomedical signal processing: ECG signal analysis using machine learning in matlab. In *Recent advances in metrology: Select proceedings of AdMet 2021*, pages 121–127. Paris: Springer, 2022.

7. Mahsa Bahrami and Mohamad Forouzanfar. Sleep apnea detection from single-lead ecg: A comprehensive analysis of machine learning and deep learning algorithms. *IEEE Transactions on Instrumentation and Measurement*, 71:1–11, 2022.
8. Pavlos Christodoulides, Andreas Miltiadous, Katerina D Tzimourta, Dimitrios Peschos, Georgios Ntritsos, Victoria Zakopoulou, Nikolaos Giannakeas, Loukas G Astrakas, Markos G Tsipouras, Konstantinos I Tsamis, et al. Classification of EEG signals from young adults with dyslexia combining a brain computer interface device and an interactive linguistic software tool. *Biomedical Signal Processing and Control*, 76:103646, 2022.
9. Seyed Morteza Ghazali, Mousa Alizadeh, Jalil Mazloum, and Yasser Baleghi. Modified binary salp swarm algorithm in EEG signal classification for epilepsy seizure detection. *Biomedical Signal Processing and Control*, 78:103858, 2022.
10. Akshansh Gupta, Riyaj Uddin Khan, Vivek Kumar Singh, Muhammad Tanveer, Dhirendra Kumar, Anirban Chakraborti, and Ram Bilas Pachori. A novel approach for classification of mental tasks using multiview ensemble learning (MEL). *Neurocomputing*, 417:558–584, 2020.
11. Nalini Pusarla, Anurag Singh, and Shrivishal Tripathi. Learning densenet features from EEG based spectrograms for subject independent emotion recognition. *Biomedical Signal Processing and Control*, 74:103485, 2022.
12. Luzheng Bi, Cuntai Guan, et al. A review on EMG-based motor intention prediction of continuous human upper limb motion for human-robot collaboration. *Biomedical Signal Processing and Control*, 51:113–127, 2019.
13. Sami Briouza, Hass'ene Gritli, Nahla Khraief, Safya Belghith, and Dil-bag Singh. EMG signal classification for human hand rehabilitation via two machine learning techniques: KNN and SVM. In *2022 5th International Conference on Advanced Systems and Emergent Technologies (IC ASET)*, pages 412–417. Paris: IEEE, 2022.
14. Luis Fernando Nicolas-Alonso and Jaime Gomez-Gil. Brain computer interfaces, a review. *Sensors*, 12(2):1211–1279, 2012.
15. Ashwin Kamble, Pradnya Ghare, and Vinay Kumar. Machine-learning-enabled adaptive signal decomposition for a brain-computer interface using EEG. *Biomedical Signal Processing and Control*, 74:103526, 2022.
16. Reza Abiri, Soheil Borhani, Eric W Sellers, Yang Jiang, and Xiaopeng Zhao. A comprehensive review of EEG-based brain–computer interface paradigms. *Journal of Neural Engineering*, 16(1):011001, 2019.
17. Abdulhamit Subasi. *Practical guide for biomedical signals analysis using machine learning techniques: A MATLAB based approach*. Paris: Academic Press, 2019.
18. Haya Alaskar. Convolutional neural network application in biomedical signals. *Journal of Computer Science and Information Technology*, 6(2):45–59, 2018.
19. Lan Lan, Lei You, Zeyang Zhang, Zhiwei Fan, Weiling Zhao, Nianyin Zeng, Yidong Chen, and Xiaobo Zhou. Generative adversarial networks and its applications in biomedical informatics. *Frontiers in Public Health*, 8:164, 2020.
20. Ryad Zemouri, Noureddine Zerhouni, and Daniel Racoceanu. Deep learning in the biomedical applications: Recent and future status. *Applied Sciences*, 9(8):1526, 2019.
21. Walid A Zgallai. *Biomedical signal processing and artificial intelligence in healthcare*. Academic Press, 2020.
22. Rym Nihel Sekkal, Fethi Bereksi-Reguig, Daniel Ruiz-Fernandez, Nabil Dib, and Samira Sekkal. Automatic sleep stage classification: From classical machine learning methods to deep learning. *Biomedical Signal Processing and Control*, 77:103751, 2022.
23. K Mohanavelu, S Poonguzhali, A Janani, and S Vinutha. Machine learning-based approach for identifying mental workload of pilots. *Biomedical Signal Processing and Control*, 75:103623, 2022.
24. Lou Ancillon, Mohamed Elgendi, and Carlo Menon. Machine learning for anxiety detection using biosignals: A review. *Diagnostics*, 12(8):1794, 2022.

25. Luis Miguel Lopez-Ramos. Future perspectives on automated machine learning in biomedical signal processing. In *Intelligent Technologies and Applications: 4th International Conference, INTAP 2021,* Grimstad, Norway, October 11–13, 2021, Revised Selected Papers, pages 159–170. Paris: Springer, 2022.
26. Katarzyna J Blinowska and Jaroslaw Z˙ygierewicz. *Practical biomedical signal analysis using MATLAB®*. CRC Press, 2021.
27. Aishwarya Balakrishnan, Jeevan Medikonda, Pramod Kesavan Namboothiri, et al. Role of wearable sensors with machine learning approaches in gait analysis for Parkinson's disease assessment: A review. *Engineered Science*, 19:5–19, 2022.
28. Pantea Keikhosrokiani and Nor Saralyna Azwa Binti Kamaruddin. IoT-based in-hospital-in-home heart disease remote monitoring system with machine learning features for decision making. In *Connected e-Health: Integrated IoT and Cloud Computing*, pages 349–369. Paris: Springer, 2022.
29. Aditya Kumar, Vipin Kumar, and Sapna Kumari. A graph coloring based framework for views construction in multi-view ensemble learning. In *2021 2nd International Conference on Secure Cyber Computing and Communications (ICSCCC)*, pages 84–89. Paris: IEEE, 2021.
30. Md Tanveer Alam, Vipin Kumar, and Aditya Kumar. A multi-view convolutional neural network approach for image data classification. In *2021 International Conference on Communication information and Computing Technology (ICCICT)*, pages 1–6. Paris: IEEE, 2021.
31. Mingkan Shen, Peng Wen, Bo Song, and Yan Li. An EEG based real-time epilepsy seizure detection approach using discrete wavelet transform and machine learning methods. *Biomedical Signal Processing and Control*, 77:103820, 2022.

11 Machine Learning and Internet of Things Biomedical Technologies

Ruchin Kacker, Sanjay Kumar Singh, and Amit Arora

CONTENTS

DOI: 10.1201/9781003476207-11

11.1 INTRODUCTION

11.1.1 Brief Overview of the Evolution of ML and IoT in Biomedical Engineering

The confluence of machine learning (ML) and Internet of Things (IoT) has ushered in a revolutionary era in biomedical engineering, fundamentally transforming the landscape of healthcare delivery and patient outcomes. Over the past few decades, the relentless progress in ML algorithms and IoT technologies has given rise to a fundamental change in the method of collecting biomedical data, its processing, and utilization. ML, with its capacity to discern patterns and glean insights from vast datasets, has become an indispensable tool in deciphering the complexities of biomedical information. Simultaneously, the pervasive integration of IoT devices, ranging from wearables to sophisticated medical sensors, has enabled the seamless collection and transmission of real-time patient data. This section provides a chronological overview of the evolutionary trajectory of ML and IoT in biomedical engineering, highlighting key milestones and breakthroughs that have paved the way for their symbiotic integration. By exploring this historical context, we set the stage for a comprehensive understanding of the synergies and applications that characterize the intersection of ML and IoT in the biomedical domain.

11.1.2 Significance and Impact of Integrating ML and IoT in Healthcare and Biomedical Applications

The fusion of ML and IoT in healthcare and biomedical applications holds profound significance, ushering in transformative changes with far-reaching impacts [1]. Central to this integration is the capacity to utilize the power of data for enhanced decision-making, personalized treatments, and improved patient outcomes [2].

- **Data-Driven Precision:** The marriage of ML and IoT empowers healthcare professionals with unprecedented access to real-time, high-dimensional data. ML algorithms, trained on diverse datasets, excel in discerning intricate patterns within this information, allowing for precise diagnostics, prognostics, and treatment recommendations. This data-driven precision is particularly valuable in fields such as genomics, where individualized treatment plans can be tailored based on a patient's unique genetic makeup [3].
- **Remote Patient Monitoring:** IoT devices, seamlessly integrated into wearable technologies and medical sensors, enable continuous remote monitoring of patients. ML algorithms analyze the streaming data, facilitating the

early detection of anomalies or changes in health metrics. This proactive approach not only enhances patient care but also reduces the burden on healthcare systems by minimizing the need for frequent in-person visits.

- **Predictive Analytics:** ML algorithms excel in predicting outcomes based on historical data. In healthcare, this translates to the ability to anticipate disease progression, identify at-risk populations, and optimize resource allocation. Predictive analytics powered by ML and IoT contribute to preventive medicine strategies, reducing the incidence of diseases through early intervention and targeted interventions.
- **Personalized Medicine:** The integration of ML and IoT supports the realization of personalized medicine, where treatment plans are tailored to individual patient characteristics. This level of customization extends beyond genetics to include real-time physiological data, lifestyle factors, and environmental influences. As a result, healthcare interventions become not only more effective but also better aligned with the unique needs of each patient.

As we explore the significance and impact of this integration, it becomes evident that ML and IoT are not mere technological enhancements; they represent a paradigm shift toward data-driven, patient-centric healthcare practices with the potential to revolutionize the entire biomedical field

11.1.3 Objectives of the Chapter

The aims of this chapter are diverse, seeking to offer a thorough exploration of the symbiotic relationship between ML and the IoT in the realm of biomedical engineering [4]. The overarching goals include:

- **Comprehensive Overview:** Furnish a detailed understanding of the evolutionary trajectory of ML and IoT technologies in the context of biomedical engineering. By tracing their historical development, we aim to offer readers a nuanced perspective on the milestones and breakthroughs that have paved the way for their integration.
- **Foundational Concepts:** Elucidate fundamental ML concepts pertinent to biomedical applications. Delve into the algorithms driving data analytics, decision support systems, and predictive modeling in healthcare. Simultaneously, explore the basics of IoT, elucidating the interconnected devices that form the foundation of real-time patient data collection [5].
- **Intersection of ML and IoT:** Examine the intersection of ML and IoT in biomedical engineering, emphasizing how ML algorithms enhance the processing and interpretation of vast datasets acquired through IoT devices. Illustrate how this intersection contributes to more informed decision-making, personalized treatment plans, and advancements in disease prediction and diagnostics.

- **Case Studies:** Showcase real-world case studies that exemplify the successful synergy of ML and IoT in biomedical applications. Highlight instances where this integration has led to significant improvements in disease management, patient care, and healthcare resource optimization. These case studies serve to underscore the practical impact of ML and IoT technologies.
- **Challenges and Solutions:** Address the challenges associated with the amalgamation of ML and IoT in biomedical contexts. Explore issues such as privacy concerns, security risks, and ethical considerations. Provide insights into potential solutions and best practices for safeguarding sensitive health information and navigating regulatory frameworks.
- **Future Directions:** Outline emerging trends and future directions in ML and IoT biomedical technologies. Identify opportunities for advancements in remote patient monitoring, predictive healthcare analytics, and precision medicine. This section aims to stimulate discussion on the evolving landscape of biomedical engineering.

Through the achievement of these objectives, the chapter aspires to contribute a valuable resource that not only informs readers about the current state of ML and IoT in biomedical engineering but also inspires future research, innovation, and collaboration in this dynamic field.

11.2 FOUNDATIONS OF ML IN BIOMEDICAL ENGINEERING

11.2.1 Overview of ML Concepts Relevant to Biomedical Applications

ML plays a pivotal role in advancing biomedical engineering by providing robust tools for extracting meaningful insights from complex and diverse datasets. In this section, we offer a comprehensive overview of key ML concepts that are particularly pertinent to biomedical applications [4–6].

- **Supervised Learning:** In the context of biomedical engineering, supervised learning is a cornerstone. It involves training ML models on labeled datasets, where each data point is associated with a known outcome. This approach is extensively applied in tasks such as disease classification, prognosis, and treatment response prediction.
- **Unsupervised Learning:** Unsupervised learning techniques, such as clustering and dimensionality reduction, are crucial for uncovering patterns within unlabeled biomedical data. This is especially valuable in scenarios where the underlying structure of the data is not well-defined or where discovering inherent relationships is of paramount importance.
- **Feature Selection and Engineering:** Given the intricate nature of biomedical data, feature selection and engineering are vital. ML models benefit from a thoughtful curation of significant attributes that enhance the predictive accuracy and interpretability of the model. Feature engineering entails converting raw data into insightful representations, enhancing the model's ability to discern subtle patterns.

- **Deep Learning:** The advent of deep learning, a subfield of ML, has ushered in groundbreaking advancements in biomedical applications. Neural networks, notably convolutional neural networks (CNNs) and recurrent neural networks (RNNs), excel in tasks such as medical imaging analysis, sequence data processing, and natural language understanding. These architectures have demonstrated remarkable success in areas like image-based diagnostics, genomics, and electronic health record analysis.
- **Transfer Learning:** Leveraging insights obtained from pre-trained models on extensive datasets can be immensely valuable in biomedical settings where labeled data may be limited. Transfer learning allows the application of insights from one domain to another, facilitating effective model training with smaller, domain-specific datasets.
- **Explainability and Interpretability:** The interpretability of ML models is crucial in biomedical contexts where decisions impact patient well-being. Methods for model explainability, for example, SHAP (Shapley additive explanations) values and LIME (local interpretable model-agnostic explanations), represent essential for ensuring transparency and fostering confidence in the decision-making process.

This section sets the stage for a deeper exploration of how these ML concepts are specifically applied in the biomedical domain. By understanding these foundational principles, readers gain insight into the underpinnings of ML techniques that drive advancements in healthcare and biomedical engineering.

11.2.2 Examples of ML Algorithms Commonly Used in Healthcare Settings

ML algorithms have found widespread application in healthcare settings, transforming the landscape of medical diagnostics, treatment planning, and patient care. The following are prominent examples of ML algorithms [7, 8] that are frequently employed in various healthcare contexts:

- **Support Vector Machines (SVM):** SVM is a supervised learning algorithm utilized for classification and regression purposes. In healthcare, SVM is applied to tasks such as disease classification based on patient data, predicting treatment outcomes, and identifying potential risks.
- **Random Forests:** Random Forests are an ensemble learning technique that amalgamates numerous decision trees to enhance predictive accuracy. In healthcare, Random Forests are utilized for tasks like disease prediction, identifying influential factors in patient outcomes, and feature selection in large datasets.
- **Neural Networks:** Neural networks, particularly deep learning architectures like CNNs and RNNs, are instrumental in medical imaging analysis, natural language processing, and genomics. CNNs excel in tasks such as image-based diagnostics, while RNNs are applied to sequence data, such as patient records and genetic data.

- **K-Nearest Neighbors (KNN):** KNN is a straightforward yet potent algorithm for both classification and regression assignments. In healthcare, KNN is employed for tasks such as patient similarity analysis, disease clustering, and personalized medicine.
- **Decision Trees:** Decision Trees are widely used for their interpretability. In healthcare, decision trees aid in diagnostic reasoning, treatment planning, and risk assessment. They are particularly useful when transparency in decision-making is crucial.
- **Naive Bayes:** Naive Bayes is a probabilistic method frequently employed for classification purposes. In healthcare, Naive Bayes is applied to tasks like disease prediction, risk assessment, and identifying relevant factors influencing patient outcomes.
- **Linear Regression:** Linear regression serves as a foundational algorithm for forecasting numerical values. In healthcare, linear regression models are employed to predict variables such as patient recovery time, dosage optimization, and resource utilization.
- **Clustering Algorithms (e.g., K-Means):** Clustering algorithms are used for grouping similar data points. In healthcare, K-Means clustering can be applied to patient data for segmentation, identifying patient cohorts with similar characteristics, which is valuable for personalized treatment strategies.
- **Ensemble Learning (e.g., AdaBoost):** Ensemble learning methods combine multiple models to improve overall performance. In healthcare, AdaBoost and other ensemble methods enhance predictive accuracy in tasks like disease diagnosis, prognosis, and treatment response prediction.

Figure 11.1 provides an overview of commonly used ML algorithms in healthcare. Classifications include algorithms for disease prediction, diagnostics, and personalized treatment plans. Understanding these algorithms is fundamental to appreciating their role in transforming healthcare practices. Understanding the diverse applications of these ML algorithms in healthcare sets the stage for their integration with IoT technologies in the subsequent sections of this chapter.

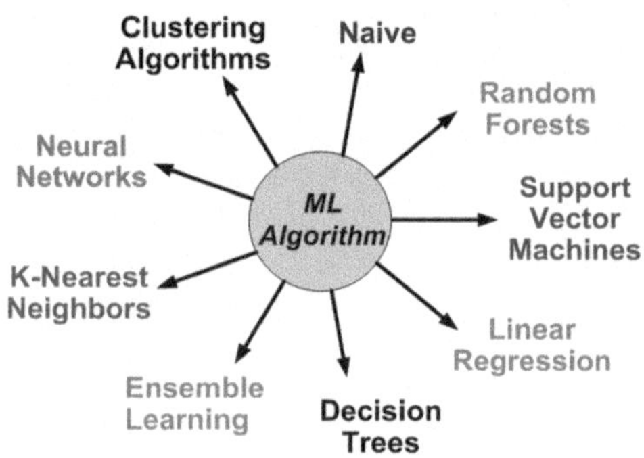

FIGURE 11.1 Examples of ML algorithms commonly used in healthcare settings [9].

11.2.3 Discussion on the Role of ML in Processing and Analyzing Biomedical Data

The integration of ML in biomedical engineering has revolutionized the way vast and complex datasets are processed, interpreted, and transformed into actionable insights [10]. This section explores the pivotal role of ML in handling biomedical data and its transformative impact on healthcare practices.

- **Pattern Recognition and Classification:** One of the primary contributions of ML in biomedical data processing is its ability to recognize intricate patterns within datasets. ML algorithms, particularly those in the realm of supervised learning, excel in classifying and categorizing biomedical data. Whether it's distinguishing between healthy and diseased states, identifying anomalies in medical images, or predicting patient outcomes, ML brings a level of precision and accuracy that traditional methods struggle to achieve [11].
- **Predictive Modeling and Prognostics:** ML models are adept at building predictive models based on historical data. In biomedical applications, this capability is harnessed for prognostics—predicting the likelihood of disease progression, treatment response, and patient outcomes. These predictive models inform clinicians, enabling them to make timely and informed decisions tailored to the individual patient.
- **Feature Extraction and Dimensionality Reduction:** Biomedical datasets are often high-dimensional, containing a multitude of variables. ML techniques, such as feature extraction and dimensionality reduction, play a pivotal role in distilling pertinent information. By identifying the most influential features, these techniques streamline the analysis process, improve model efficiency, and enhance the interpretability of results.
- **Personalized Medicine and Treatment Optimization:** ML contributes significantly to the realization of personalized medicine by tailoring treatments to the unique characteristics of individual patients. Through the analysis of patient-specific data, encompassing genetic information and lifestyle factors, and treatment histories, ML algorithms can recommend optimized treatment plans, minimizing adverse effects and maximizing therapeutic efficacy.
- **Image and Signal Processing:** In medical imaging and signal processing, ML algorithms have demonstrated remarkable success. CNNs, for instance, excel in image-based tasks such as tumor detection in radiological images. Signal processing techniques, enhanced by ML, enable the analysis of physiological signals, such as electrocardiograms and brainwave patterns, for diagnostic and monitoring purposes.
- **Real-Time Monitoring and Early Detection:** ML's capacity for real-time analysis is invaluable in scenarios that require continuous monitoring. In the context of biomedical data, this translates into early detection of abnormalities and timely intervention. For example, ML algorithms integrated with wearable devices can monitor vital signs and alert healthcare

professionals to deviations from normal patterns, facilitating proactive healthcare management.

- **Integration with Electronic Health Records (EHR):** ML plays a crucial role in extracting meaningful insights from EHR. Natural Language Processing algorithms enable the analysis of unstructured clinical narratives, contributing to a holistic understanding of patient histories and supporting clinical decision-making.

By processing and analyzing biomedical data, ML not only enhances the efficiency of healthcare processes but also opens avenues for novel discoveries and advancements in diagnostics and treatment strategies. As we explore the integration of ML with the IoT in the subsequent sections, it becomes evident that the synergistic interplay of these technologies propels biomedical engineering into a new era of data-driven, patient-centric healthcare.

11.3 FUNDAMENTALS OF IoT IN BIOMEDICAL ENGINEERING

11.3.1 Introduction to IoT and Its Applications in Healthcare

The IoT is a transformative paradigm that interconnects physical devices, sensors, and systems, enabling them to communicate and exchange data seamlessly [11]. In the context of biomedical engineering, IoT emerges as a powerful enabler, revolutionizing the way healthcare is delivered, monitored, and managed.

- **Connectivity and Sensor Integration:** At the core of IoT in healthcare is the seamless connectivity between a myriad of devices and sensors. Wearable devices, medical sensors, implantable technologies, and monitoring devices are integrated into a network, collectively forming an interconnected ecosystem. This connectivity facilitates the continuous collection of real-time data, providing a holistic view of patients' health and well-being.
- **Remote Patient Monitoring:** One of the hallmark applications of IoT in healthcare is remote patient monitoring. Wearable devices embedded with sensors track vital signs, physical activity, and other health parameters in real time. This continuous monitoring allows healthcare professionals to remotely assess patient health, detect anomalies, and intervene promptly, particularly valuable for managing chronic conditions and postoperative care.
- **Smart Medical Devices:** IoT technologies contribute to the development of smart medical devices that enhance diagnostics and treatment. From smart inhalers and insulin pumps to connected prosthetics, these devices offer personalized and adaptive healthcare solutions. They often leverage data analytics to optimize treatment plans based on individual patient needs.
- **Asset and Inventory Management:** IoT applications extend beyond patient care to streamline hospital operations. RFID tags and sensors enable the tracking of medical equipment, pharmaceuticals, and other assets in real time. This not only enhances efficiency in resource utilization but also aids in preventing loss or theft of critical assets.

- **Environmental Monitoring:** IoT plays a role in maintaining optimal healthcare environments. Sensors monitor factors such as temperature, humidity, and air quality in hospital settings. This ensures the well-being of both patients and healthcare practitioners, contributing to infection control and overall safety.
- **Data Integration with EHR:** The integration of IoT-generated data with EHR is integral to creating comprehensive and real-time patient profiles. This holistic approach enhances clinical decision-making by providing a more complete understanding of patients' health trajectories.
- **Emergency Response Systems:** IoT facilitates the implementation of advanced emergency response systems. Wearables and sensors can detect emergencies, such as falls or sudden changes in vital signs, triggering automated alerts to healthcare providers or emergency services. This rapid response is critical in situations where timely intervention is paramount.

As we delve deeper into the IoT landscape in subsequent sections, the focus will shift toward how ML complements these IoT fundamentals, creating a synergistic framework that propels biomedical engineering into an era of intelligent, data-driven healthcare.

11.3.2 Overview of IoT Devices Used in Biomedical Monitoring and Data Collection

The widespread adoption of IoT devices has heralded a new era of biomedical monitoring and data collection, transforming the way healthcare is delivered and monitored [12]. The following are key categories of IoT devices extensively employed in the biomedical domain:

- **Wearable Health Trackers:** Wearable devices, ranging from smartwatches to fitness trackers, have become ubiquitous in the realm of biomedical monitoring. Equipped with sensors such as accelerometers, heart rate monitors, and GPS, these wearables provide real-time data on physical activity, sleep patterns, and vital signs. Wearable health trackers are instrumental in promoting proactive health management and facilitating continuous monitoring of individuals.
- **Medical Sensors and Implants:** IoT-enabled medical sensors and implants have revolutionized patient care by providing continuous and personalized health data. Implants, such as pacemakers and insulin pumps, are equipped with IoT capabilities to transmit data to healthcare providers. Medical sensors, embedded in clothing or attached to the skin, monitor parameters like glucose levels, temperature, and hydration, offering a non-intrusive and real-time approach to health monitoring.
- **Remote Monitoring Devices:** IoT devices designed for remote patient monitoring extend beyond wearables to include specialized devices for monitoring specific health conditions. For instance, remote glucose monitors for diabetes management, blood pressure monitors, and respiratory

monitoring devices enable patients to manage chronic conditions remotely, offering healthcare professionals invaluable data for timely interventions.

- **Smart Inhalers and Medication Adherence Devices:** IoT technologies are integrated into inhalers and medication adherence devices to track and optimize medication usage. Smart inhalers, for example, record inhalation patterns and dosage adherence, providing insights into respiratory conditions. Medication adherence devices leverage sensors and connectivity to ensure patients adhere to prescribed medication regimens, enhancing treatment effectiveness.
- **Biometric and Biochemical Sensors:** Biometric and biochemical sensors offer a comprehensive approach to health monitoring by measuring specific physiological parameters. Biometric sensors, such as fingerprint or iris scanners, contribute to secure patient identification. Biochemical sensors, including those for measuring biomarkers in bodily fluids, provide valuable diagnostic information for conditions such as cardiovascular disease, cancer, and infectious diseases.
- **Smart Home Health Devices:** The integration of IoT extends to smart home health devices that contribute to holistic health monitoring. Smart scales, sleep monitoring devices, and environmental sensors within the home environment offer additional layers of data for a more complete understanding of an individual's well-being.
- **IoT-Enabled Medical Imaging Devices:** Medical imaging apparatuses, like X-ray machines, MRI scanners, and CT scanners, are increasingly equipped with IoT capabilities. These devices transmit imaging data securely, allowing for remote diagnostics, collaborative decision-making among healthcare professionals, and integration with patient records.
- **Assistive Technologies:** IoT devices play a crucial role in providing assistance to individuals with disabilities. Smart prosthetics, IoT-enabled wheelchairs, and sensory aids are designed to improve the quality of life for individuals with mobility impairments or sensory challenges.

Figure 11.2 depicts the diverse IoT device ecosystem employed in biomedical monitoring. It includes wearables, medical sensors, and other connected devices, showcasing their roles in collecting real-time patient data. Understanding this ecosystem is crucial for appreciating the breadth of data sources in modern healthcare. This diverse array of IoT devices forms the backbone of a connected healthcare ecosystem, contributing to personalized medicine, proactive health management, and the optimization of healthcare resources. As we delve further into the chapter, the convergence of ML with these IoT devices will be explored, uncovering synergies that redefine the landscape of biomedical engineering.

11.3.3 Discussion on the Integration of IoT with Existing Healthcare Infrastructure

The seamless integration of the IoT with existing healthcare infrastructure marks a transformative shift in how healthcare is delivered, monitored, and managed [14]. This section explores the key aspects and implications of this integration:

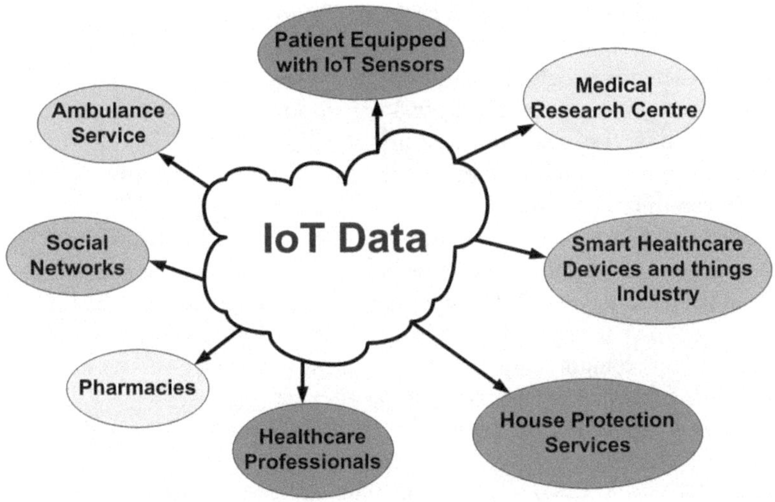

FIGURE 11.2 IoT device ecosystem in biomedical monitoring [13].

- **Enhanced Connectivity and Data Flow:** The integration of IoT introduces a new level of connectivity within healthcare systems. IoT devices, ranging from wearables to medical sensors, are integrated with existing networks, facilitating the continuous flow of real-time data. This enhanced connectivity ensures that healthcare providers have timely access to critical patient information, enabling informed decision-making.
- **Interoperability for Comprehensive Patient Profiles:** IoT integration promotes interoperability among diverse healthcare systems and devices. Data from wearables, medical sensors, and other IoT devices seamlessly integrate with EHR and other health information systems. This interoperability creates comprehensive patient profiles, providing a holistic view of a patient's health history, current conditions, and ongoing treatment plans.
- **Remote Patient Monitoring and Telehealth:** The integration of IoT supports the implementation of remote patient monitoring programs and telehealth services. Healthcare providers can remotely monitor patients with chronic conditions, ensuring continuity of care outside traditional clinical settings. Telehealth consultations leverage IoT devices to capture real-time data during virtual visits, enhancing the quality of remote diagnostics and patient engagement.
- **Efficient Resource Utilization:** IoT-enabled devices contribute to more efficient resource utilization within healthcare facilities. Smart inventory management systems, equipped with IoT sensors, automate the tracking of medical supplies, reducing waste and ensuring that essential resources are readily available. This efficiency extends to the scheduling and allocation of medical equipment, optimizing workflows, and minimizing downtime.

- **Security and Privacy Considerations:** The integration of IoT in healthcare necessitates a robust focus on security and privacy. As devices continuously transmit sensitive health data, it becomes paramount to implement stringent security measures to protect against unauthorized access and data breaches. Encryption, secure communication protocols, and compliance with healthcare data protection regulations are critical components of a secure IoT healthcare infrastructure.
- **Scalability for Future Growth:** IoT integration allows healthcare infrastructure to be scalable, accommodating future growth and technological advancements. As new IoT devices and technologies emerge, the infrastructure can evolve to support these innovations. Scalability ensures that healthcare systems remain adaptable and resilient in the face of evolving patient care needs and technological landscapes.
- **Real-time Analytics for Informed Decision-Making:** The influx of real-time data generated by IoT devices empowers healthcare providers with actionable insights. ML algorithms, when integrated with IoT data streams, facilitate real-time analytics. This enables predictive analytics, early detection of health issues, and informed decision-making, ultimately improving patient outcomes and the efficiency of healthcare delivery.

In conclusion, the integration of IoT with existing healthcare infrastructure lays the foundation for a connected, intelligent healthcare ecosystem. As we progress in this chapter, the intersection of ML with IoT in the biomedical domain will be explored, showcasing how these technologies synergize to redefine patient care, diagnostics, and healthcare management.

11.4 SYNERGIES BETWEEN ML AND IoT IN BIOMEDICAL APPLICATIONS

11.4.1 Exploration of How ML and IoT Technologies Complement Each Other in Healthcare

The intersection of ML and the IoT in healthcare creates a symbiotic relationship that extends the capabilities of both technologies, offering unprecedented opportunities for improved diagnostics, personalized medicine, and enhanced patient care [3].

- **Data Enrichment and Contextual Understanding:** IoT devices generate vast streams of data, capturing a myriad of patient parameters and environmental factors. ML algorithms excel at processing and analyzing this data, extracting valuable insights, and discerning patterns that may not be apparent through traditional methods. By integrating ML with IoT, healthcare providers gain a more nuanced and contextual understanding of patient health, leading to more accurate diagnostics and tailored interventions.
- **Predictive Analytics for Early Intervention:** ML algorithms, when applied to IoT-generated data, enable predictive analytics that go beyond retrospective analysis. These algorithms can forecast potential health issues,

complications, or changes in patient conditions. For example, predicting the likelihood of disease exacerbation or identifying patterns indicative of impending health challenges allows for timely and proactive interventions, potentially preventing adverse outcomes.

- **Personalized Treatment Plans:** The combination of ML and IoT facilitates the development of personalized treatment plans based on individual patient data. ML algorithms analyze diverse datasets, including genetic information, lifestyle choices, and real-time physiological data from IoT devices. This holistic approach allows healthcare providers to tailor treatment strategies to the unique characteristics and needs of each patient, optimizing therapeutic outcomes.
- **Continuous Monitoring and Real-Time Alerts:** IoT devices provide continuous monitoring of patient health parameters, generating a constant stream of data. ML algorithms can analyze this real-time data and generate alerts or notifications for healthcare professionals when deviations from normal patterns are detected. This capability is particularly valuable in critical care situations, where early detection of abnormalities is crucial for rapid response and intervention.
- **Enhanced Disease Diagnosis and Risk Stratification:** ML algorithms, trained on diverse datasets encompassing IoT-generated data, contribute to more accurate disease diagnosis and risk stratification. For example, in medical imaging analysis, ML can enhance the accuracy of identifying anomalies or early signs of diseases. Integrating IoT data with ML models enables a comprehensive approach to assessing risk factors, aiding in the identification of high-risk patient populations.
- **Optimized Resource Utilization:** ML algorithms applied to IoT data contribute to optimizing resource utilization in healthcare settings. By predicting patient admission rates, resource demands, and peak activity periods, healthcare providers can allocate resources efficiently. This proactive approach ensures that healthcare facilities are adequately prepared for fluctuations in demand, minimizing wait times and improving overall patient satisfaction.
- **Adaptive and Learning Systems:** The adaptive nature of ML allows systems to learn and evolve based on new data. In the context of healthcare, this adaptability is particularly beneficial when integrated with IoT devices. As patient data continuously flows in, ML models can adapt to evolving patient conditions, treatment responses, and emerging healthcare trends, creating dynamic and learning healthcare systems.

Figure 11.3 illustrates the system architecture for the integration of ML and the IoT in a healthcare setting. It showcases the interconnected components, data flow, and communication pathways, highlighting the seamless integration of ML algorithms with IoT devices for enhanced healthcare outcomes. By exploring the synergies between ML and IoT in healthcare, we uncover a powerful alliance that not only enhances the efficiency of healthcare delivery but also lays the groundwork for innovative and personalized approaches to patient care.

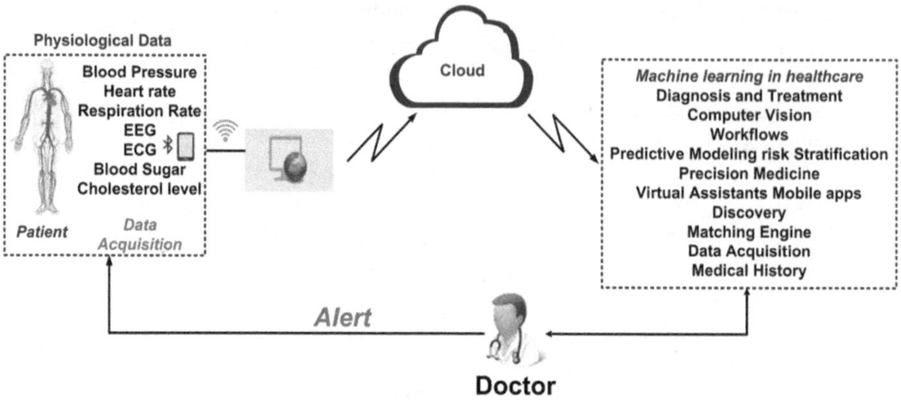

FIGURE 11.3 System architecture for ML and IoT integration in healthcare [15].

11.4.2 Case Studies Highlighting Successful Integration of ML and IoT in Biomedical Projects

11.4.2.1 Remote Monitoring for Chronic Disease Management

- **Objective:** Improve the management of chronic diseases through continuous remote monitoring [16].
- **Solution:** Wearable IoT devices were deployed to monitor vital signs, physical activity, and sleep patterns of patients with chronic conditions, such as diabetes and hypertension. ML algorithms processed the real-time data to identify patterns indicative of health deterioration or non-compliance with treatment plans.
- **Outcome:** Early detection of anomalies led to timely interventions, reducing hospital readmissions and improving overall patient outcomes. ML-driven insights also contributed to personalized treatment plans based on individual patient responses.

11.4.2.2 Smart Prosthetics for Enhanced Mobility

- **Objective:** Enhance the functionality and adaptability of smart prosthetics for individuals with limb loss.
- **Solution:** IoT-enabled prosthetics incorporated sensors to collect data on movement patterns, pressure distribution, and environmental conditions. ML algorithms analyzed this data to adapt the prosthetic's behavior in real-time, providing a more natural and responsive user experience.
- **Outcome:** Users reported improved mobility and comfort, with the smart prosthetics adapting seamlessly to different activities and terrains. The integration of ML and IoT resulted in a personalized and adaptive solution for each user.

11.4.2.3 Predictive Healthcare Analytics for Disease Prevention

- **Objective:** Develop a system for predicting and preventing the onset of chronic diseases [17].

- **Solution:** IoT devices collected health data from a diverse population, including biometric measurements, lifestyle choices, and environmental factors. ML models were trained to analyze this data and predict individuals at high risk of developing specific diseases. Personalized health recommendations were then communicated to users through a mobile app.
- **Outcome:** The system demonstrated success in early disease prediction, empowering individuals to make informed lifestyle choices. The integration of ML and IoT contributed to a proactive approach to healthcare, reducing the overall burden of chronic diseases.

11.4.2.4 Smart Imaging Diagnostics for Radiology

- **Objective:** Improve the accuracy and efficiency of medical imaging diagnostics.
- **Solution:** IoT-connected medical imaging devices, such as MRI scanners and X-ray machines, generate high-resolution images. ML algorithms were employed for image analysis, automating the detection of anomalies and providing quantitative insights. Real-time feedback from the ML models assisted radiologists in making more accurate and efficient diagnoses.
- **Outcome:** Reduced diagnostic time, increased accuracy in detecting subtle abnormalities, and improved overall efficiency in radiology departments. The combination of ML and IoT in imaging diagnostics streamlined workflows and enhanced the diagnostic capabilities of healthcare professionals.

These case studies illustrate the diverse applications and positive outcomes resulting from the synergistic integration of ML and IoT in biomedical projects. From chronic disease management to personalized prosthetics and predictive healthcare analytics, the collaborative power of these technologies is reshaping the landscape of healthcare delivery and patient care.

11.4.3 Advantages of Combining ML and IoT for Real-Time Monitoring, Predictive Analytics, and Personalized Medicine [18]

11.4.3.1 Real-Time Monitoring

- **Continuous Data Streams:** IoT devices generate continuous streams of real-time data, capturing dynamic changes in patient health and environmental conditions.
- **Instantaneous Analysis:** ML algorithms applied to IoT-generated data enable instantaneous analysis, allowing for the detection of anomalies or deviations from normal patterns in real time.
- **Proactive Interventions:** Real-time monitoring, coupled with ML insights, enables healthcare professionals to intervene proactively in response to emergent health issues, minimizing response times and improving patient outcomes.

11.4.3.2 Predictive Analytics

- **Early Disease Detection:** ML models, trained on diverse datasets from IoT devices, excel in predicting the onset of diseases by identifying subtle patterns indicative of health risks.

- **Prognostic Insights:** Predictive analytics empower healthcare providers with prognostic insights, forecasting disease progression, treatment responses, and potential complications.
- **Optimized Resource Allocation:** Anticipating patient admission rates and resource demands through predictive analytics supports optimized resource allocation, ensuring efficient use of healthcare facilities and personnel.

11.4.3.3 Personalized Medicine

- **Holistic Patient Profiles:** Integration of IoT data, including genetic information, lifestyle factors, and real-time physiological data, contributes to the creation of comprehensive and dynamic patient profiles.
- **Tailored Treatment Plans:** ML algorithms analyze diverse datasets to tailor treatment plans based on individual patient characteristics, optimizing therapeutic efficacy and minimizing adverse effects.
- **Adaptive Healthcare Strategies:** Personalized medicine, driven by ML and IoT, enables adaptive healthcare strategies that evolve with changing patient conditions, treatment responses, and emerging healthcare trends.

11.4.3.4 Enhanced Decision-Making

- **Informed Clinical Decision Support:** ML algorithms applied to IoT data provide healthcare professionals with informed clinical decision support, offering insights into diagnosis, treatment planning, and ongoing patient management.
- **Data-Driven Insights:** The combination of ML and IoT transforms raw data into actionable insights, supporting evidence-based decision-making and fostering a more data-driven approach to healthcare.
- **Cross-Disciplinary Collaboration:** Enhanced decision-making is facilitated by cross-disciplinary collaboration, where insights from diverse IoT-generated data sources contribute to a holistic understanding of patient health.

11.4.3.5 Efficiency and Cost Savings

- **Streamlined Workflows:** ML-driven automation of data analysis and decision support streamlines healthcare workflows, reducing manual intervention and improving efficiency.
- **Preventive Healthcare:** Predictive analytics and personalized medicine contribute to preventive healthcare strategies, potentially reducing the long-term burden on healthcare systems and associated costs.
- **Resource Optimization:** Optimized resource allocation, supported by ML and IoT, leads to efficient utilization of healthcare resources, minimizing operational costs and improving overall cost-effectiveness.

The synergies between ML and IoT in real-time monitoring, predictive analytics, and personalized medicine contribute to a paradigm shift in healthcare delivery. These advantages not only improve patient outcomes but also enhance the efficiency, adaptability, and sustainability of healthcare systems.

11.5 CHALLENGES AND SOLUTIONS

11.5.1 Addressing Privacy and Security Concerns in ML and IoT Applications in Healthcare

11.5.1.1 Challenges

11.5.1.1.1 Data Privacy Risks

- **Issue:** Healthcare data, particularly sensitive patient information, is at risk of unauthorized access, leading to privacy breaches and potential misuse of personal health information [19].
- **Solution:** Implement robust encryption methods, access controls, and authentication mechanisms to safeguard patient data. Adherence to data protection regulations, such as HIPAA in the United States or GDPR in Europe, is essential to ensure legal compliance.

11.5.1.1.2 Vulnerabilities in IoT Devices

- **Issue:** IoT devices may have inherent security vulnerabilities, making them susceptible to unauthorized access, data tampering, or exploitation by malicious actors.
- **Solution:** Conduct thorough security assessments of IoT devices, addressing vulnerabilities through regular updates and patches. Employ secure communication protocols, device authentication, and network segmentation to enhance overall IoT device security.

11.5.1.1.3 Inadequate Authentication Mechanisms

- **Issue:** Weak or inadequate authentication mechanisms can compromise the integrity of both ML models and IoT devices, allowing unauthorized users to manipulate data or gain access to sensitive information.
- **Solution:** Implement strong authentication protocols, including multi-factor authentication, biometric verification, and secure credential management. Regularly update authentication mechanisms to adapt to evolving security standards.

11.5.1.1.4 Data Breach Concerns

- **Issue:** The interconnected nature of IoT devices and ML systems increases the risk of data breaches, potentially leading to the exposure of sensitive health information.
- **Solution:** Employ robust intrusion detection systems and real-time monitoring to detect and respond to potential security incidents promptly. Regularly audit and assess the security posture of the entire ML and IoT ecosystem.

11.5.1.1.5 Lack of Standardization

- **Issue:** The absence of standardized security practices across ML and IoT platforms can result in inconsistencies and gaps in security implementations.
- **Solution:** Advocate for and adhere to industry standards for security in ML and IoT applications. Collaborate with regulatory bodies and

industry stakeholders to establish comprehensive security guidelines and best practices.

11.5.1.2 Solutions

11.5.1.2.1 Privacy by Design

- **Approach:** Implement a "privacy by design" approach, integrating privacy measures into the development process from the outset. This involves considering privacy implications at every stage of ML and IoT system design, deployment, and operation.
- **Benefits:** Proactively addressing privacy concerns ensures that privacy measures are an integral part of the system, minimizing the risk of data breaches and fostering user trust.

11.5.1.2.2 Secure Communication Protocols

- **Approach:** Utilize secure communication protocols, such as TLS/SSL, for data transmission between IoT devices, ML models, and healthcare systems. Encryption ensures that data remains confidential during transit.
- **Benefits:** Secure communication protocols protect against eavesdropping and unauthorized access, safeguarding the confidentiality and integrity of healthcare data.

11.5.1.2.3 Regular Security Audits and Updates

- **Approach:** Conduct routine security audits and assessments of both ML models and IoT devices. Implement timely updates and patches to address newly discovered vulnerabilities and maintain a secure environment.
- **Benefits:** Proactive security audits minimize the risk of exploitation, ensuring that the ML and IoT ecosystem remains resilient against emerging threats.

11.5.1.2.4 User Education and Awareness

- **Approach:** Educate users, healthcare professionals, and system administrators about the importance of privacy and security in ML and IoT applications. Promote awareness of best practices for data protection.
- **Benefits:** Informed users are more likely to follow secure practices, reducing the likelihood of security incidents and contributing to a culture of cybersecurity awareness.

11.5.1.2.5 Regulatory Compliance

- **Approach:** Ensure strict adherence to healthcare data protection regulations, like HIPAA, GDPR, or regional equivalents. Establish and enforce policies and procedures that align with regulatory requirements.
- **Benefits:** Regulatory compliance not only mitigates legal risks but also sets a foundation for robust privacy and security practices, instilling confidence in patients and stakeholders.

Addressing privacy and security concerns in ML and IoT applications in healthcare necessitates a multifaceted approach that blends technological measures, regulatory compliance, and user awareness. By prioritizing privacy and security from the inception of system design, healthcare organizations can build a resilient and trustworthy ecosystem for the integration of ML and IoT technologies.

11.5.2 Technical Challenges and Potential Solutions

11.5.2.1 Challenges

- **Data Quality and Variability:** Biomedical data from IoT devices can vary and contain noise, impacting ML model training. Solutions include data preprocessing and quality control measures.
- **Scalability and Resource Constraints:** Resource limitations in IoT devices pose challenges. Solutions involve optimizing models for edge computing, using model compression, and exploring federated learning.
- **Interoperability of Devices and Standards:** Diverse IoT devices and lack of standards hinder interoperability. Solutions include advocating for standards, implementing middleware, and using common data formats.
- **Model Interpretability and Explainability:** Black-box ML models may lack interpretability. Solutions involve using interpretable models, explainability techniques, and prioritizing transparent decision-making.
- **Edge-to-Cloud Integration:** Balancing processing tasks between edge and cloud poses challenges. Solutions include a hierarchical architecture and using edge computing for time-sensitive tasks.
- **Robustness and Security:** ML models and IoT devices are susceptible to security threats. Solutions include robust security measures, regular updates, access controls, and anomaly detection.

11.5.2.2 Solutions

- **Edge AI for Real-Time Processing:** Implement edge AI solutions to enable real-time processing on IoT devices, minimizing latency and enhancing responsiveness.
- **Continuous Model Training:** Implement continuous model training techniques to update models over time with new data, adapting to changing patient conditions.
- **Distributed and Federated Learning:** Explore distributed and federated learning to train models collaboratively across devices while preserving data privacy.
- **Blockchain for Data Integrity:** Utilize blockchain technology to ensure data integrity, providing a decentralized and tamper-resistant ledger.
- **Standardization and Interoperability Protocols:** Advocate for standardized communication protocols and interoperability standards in the healthcare industry, promoting seamless data exchange.

- **Explainable AI Techniques:** Prioritize interpretable ML models and incorporate explainable AI techniques, such as LIME or SHAP, to provide insights into model decisions.

Addressing these technical challenges with the suggested solutions enhances the integration of ML and IoT in biomedical applications, fostering improved patient care and system efficiency.

11.5.3 Regulatory and Ethical Considerations in the Deployment of ML and IoT in Biomedical Settings

11.5.3.1 Regulatory Considerations

- **Compliance with Healthcare Regulations:** Ensure adherence to healthcare regulations such as HIPAA, GDPR, and regional equivalents to safeguard patient data and privacy.
- **Data Security Standards:** Implement robust data security measures, incorporating encryption and access controls, to meet regulatory requirements and protect against unauthorized access [11–20].

11.5.3.2 Ethical Considerations

- **Informed Consent:** Prioritize obtaining informed consent from patients for the collection, processing, and sharing of their health data, respecting individual autonomy.
- **Transparency in AI Decision-Making:** Foster transparency in ML models to help healthcare professionals and patients understand the basis of AI-driven decisions, promoting trust.
- **Bias Mitigation:** Address biases in ML algorithms to ensure fair and unbiased healthcare outcomes, recognizing the ethical implications of biased decision-making.
- **Patient Empowerment:** Promote patient awareness and control over their health data, empowering them to make informed decisions regarding its utilization and sharing.

Balancing regulatory compliance and ethical considerations is crucial for the responsible and trustworthy deployment of ML and IoT in biomedical settings.

11.6 CONCLUSION

In conclusion, the fusion of ML and the IoT marks a transformative phase in biomedical engineering, fundamentally altering healthcare practices and enhancing patient outcomes. This chapter has meticulously examined the synergistic relationship between ML and IoT, unveiling their collective potential and myriad applications within the biomedical sphere.

From laying the groundwork with foundational ML and IoT concepts to showcasing their collaborative prowess in real-time monitoring, predictive analytics, and personalized medicine, this chapter has underscored the substantial progress achieved through their integration. Yet, amid the strides forward, it has also shed light on pressing challenges such as privacy, security, and technical complexities, emphasizing the need for a holistic approach to ensure responsible deployment in healthcare settings.

Navigating regulatory frameworks and ethical considerations remains imperative, advocating for adherence to healthcare regulations, fostering transparency, empowering patients, and mitigating biases. As we traverse the intricate terrain of ML and IoT in biomedical contexts, these considerations serve as linchpins for building trust and upholding ethical standards in data usage.

The provided visual roadmap in Figure 11.4 delineates anticipated future trends, encompassing concepts like edge computing, federated learning, and advancements in remote patient monitoring. This glimpse into the horizon foretells promising developments, with continuous advancements poised to reshape healthcare delivery fundamentally.

Looking forward, the trajectory of ML and IoT biomedical technologies promises a wave of innovation. The evolving landscape, driven by remote patient monitoring, predictive healthcare analytics, and precision medicine, coupled with the emergence of cutting-edge approaches like edge computing and federated learning,

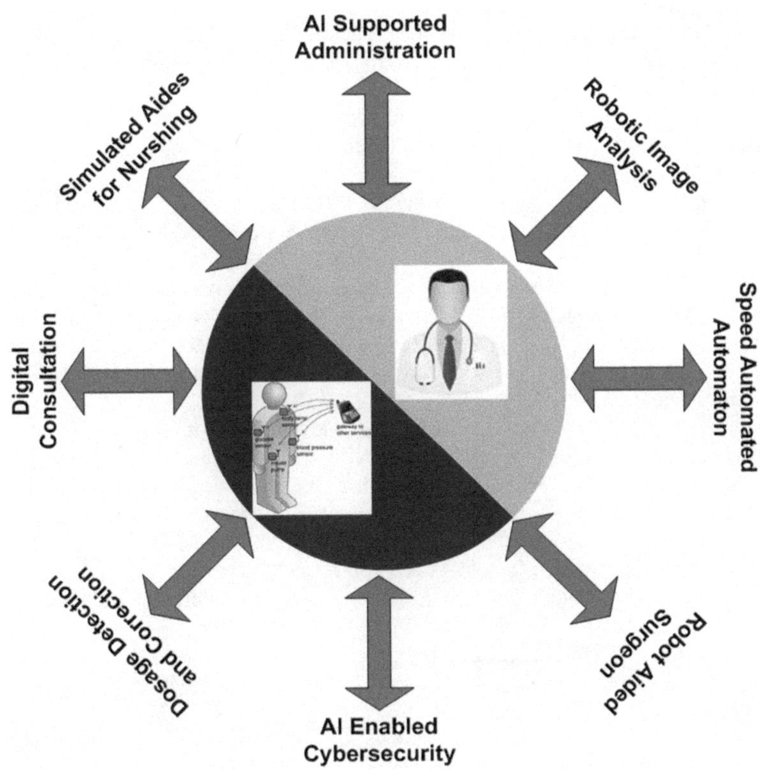

FIGURE 11.4 Future trends in ML and IoT biomedical technologies [21].

holds the potential to usher in more efficient, scalable, and secure healthcare systems.

In summary, this chapter offers an exhaustive overview of current applications, challenges, and future prospects in biomedical engineering. As technological evolution persists, embracing ethical imperatives and staying attuned to emerging trends will be pivotal in harnessing the full transformative potential of ML and IoT to elevate patient care and advance healthcare outcomes.

REFERENCES

1. Wang, W. H., & Hsu, W. S. (2023). Integrating artificial intelligence and wearable IoT system in long-term care environments. *Sensors*, 23(13), 5913.
2. Javaid, M., Haleem, A., Singh, R. P., Suman, R., & Rab, S. (2022). Significance of machine learning in healthcare: Features, pillars and applications. *International Journal of Intelligent Networks*, 3, 58–73.
3. Manickam, P., Mariappan, S. A., Murugesan, S. M., Hansda, S., Kaushik, A., Shinde, R., & Thipperudraswamy, S. P. (2022). Artificial intelligence (AI) and internet of medical things (IoMT) assisted biomedical systems for intelligent healthcare. *Biosensors*, 12(8), 562.
4. Athanasopoulou, K., Daneva, G. N., Adamopoulos, P. G., & Scorilas, A. (2022). Artificial intelligence: The milestone in modern biomedical research. *BioMedInformatics*, 2(4), 727–744.
5. Zhuhadar, L. P., & Lytras, M. D. (2023). The application of AutoML techniques in diabetes diagnosis: Current approaches, performance, and future directions. *Sustainability*, 15(18), 13484.
6. Moubayed, A., Injadat, M., Nassif, A. B., Lutfiyya, H., & Shami, A. (2018). E-learning: Challenges and research opportunities using machine learning & data analytics. *IEEE Access*, 6, 39117–39138.
7. Miraftabzadeh, S. M., Longo, M., Foiadelli, F., Pasetti, M., & Igual, R. (2021). Advances in the application of machine learning techniques for power system analytics: A survey. *Energies*, 14(16), 4776.
8. Galal, A., Talal, M., & Moustafa, A. (2022). Applications of machine learning in metabolomics: Disease modeling and classification. *Frontiers in Genetics*, *13*, 1017340.
9. Javaid, M., Haleem, A., Singh, R. P., Suman, R., & Rab, S. (2022). Significance of machine learning in healthcare: Features, pillars and applications. *International Journal of Intelligent Networks*, 3, 58–73.
10. Taye, M. M. (2023). Understanding of machine learning with deep learning: Architectures, workflow, applications and future directions. *Computers*, 12(5), 91.
11. Verdejo Espinosa, Á., Lopez, J. L., Mata Mata, F., & Estevez, M. E. (2021). Application of IoT in healthcare: Keys to implementation of the sustainable development goals. *Sensors*, 21(7), 2330.
12. Mora, H., Gil, D., Munoz Terol, R., Azorín, J., & Szymanski, J. (2017). An IoT-based computational framework for healthcare monitoring in mobile environments. *Sensors*, 17(10), 2302.
13. Awasthy, N., & Nikhila, V. (2021). Impact of IoT in biomedical applications: Part II. In *Electronic Devices, Circuits, and Systems for Biomedical Applications* (pp. 441–460). Academic Press.
14. Kumar, M., Kumar, A., Verma, S., Bhattacharya, P., Ghimire, D., Kim, S. H., & Hosen, A. S. (2023). Healthcare Internet of Things (H-IoT): Current trends, future prospects, applications, challenges, and security issues. *Electronics*, 12(9), 2050.

15. Aivaliotis, V., Tsantikidou, K., & Sklavos, N. (2022). IoT-based multi-sensor healthcare architectures and a lightweight-based privacy scheme. *Sensors*, 22(11), 4269.
16. Ohashi, C., Akiguchi, S., & Ohira, M. (2022). Development of a remote health monitoring system to prevent frailty in elderly home-care patients with COPD. *Sensors*, 22(7), 2670.
17. Pearson, T. A., Califf, R. M., Roper, R., Engelgau, M. M., Khoury, M. J., Alcantara, & Mensah, G. A. (2020). Precision health analytics with predictive analytics and implementation research: JACC state-of-the-art review. *Journal of the American College of Cardiology*, 76(3), 306–320.
18. Jagatheesaperumal, S. K., Rajkumar, S., Suresh, J. V., Gumaei, A. H., Alhakbani, N., Uddin, M. Z., & Hassan, M. M. (2023). An IoT-based framework for personalized health assessment and recommendations using machine learning. *Mathematics*, *11*(12), 2758.
19. Keshta, I. (2022). AI-driven IoT for smart health care: Security and privacy issues. *Informatics in Medicine Unlocked*, 30, 100903.
20. Rasheed, K., Qayyum, A., Ghaly, M., Al-Fuqaha, A., Razi, A., & Qadir, J. (2022). Explainable, trustworthy, and ethical machine learning for healthcare: A survey. *Computers in Biology and Medicine*, 106043.
21. Mishra, P., & Singh, G. (2023). Internet of medical things healthcare for sustainable smart cities: Current status and future prospects. *Applied Sciences*, 13(15), 8869.

12 Revolutionizing Chronic Kidney Disease Prediction

An Enhanced Semi-Supervised Learning Model

G. Logeswari, J. Deepika Roselind, and G. Sudhakaran

CONTENTS

12.1 INTRODUCTION

Chronic kidney disease (CKD) stands as a formidable public health challenge, affecting millions worldwide and imposing a considerable strain on healthcare systems. The intricate nature of CKD, often latent in its early stages and asymptomatic until advanced, underscores the critical importance of accurate prediction and early intervention [1]. In the pursuit of more effective predictive methodologies, this chapter introduces an innovative paradigm—a sophisticated semi-supervised learning model poised to revolutionize the landscape of CKD prediction [2].

CKD is a progressive condition marked by the gradual deterioration of renal function, presenting a significant threat to global health. Traditional diagnostic approaches, reliant on clinical markers and demographic information, often encounter limitations in discerning subtle patterns indicative of early-stage CKD [3, 4]. The integration of machine learning into healthcare analytics has emerged as a promising

DOI: 10.1201/9781003476207-12

avenue, promising heightened sensitivity and specificity in the prediction of CKD by unraveling complex relationships within vast medical datasets [5, 6].

Amid the burgeoning need for more accurate and early CKD prediction, this research addresses a critical gap by proposing an advanced semi-supervised learning model. The semi-supervised learning paradigm, combining labeled and unlabeled data, presents a unique opportunity to extract nuanced patterns from medical datasets that might elude traditional methodologies. The potential impact of this research lies in its capacity to facilitate early identification of high-risk individuals, enabling timely interventions, personalized treatment strategies, and, ultimately, improving patient outcomes. The primary objective of the chapter is to develop a precise and effective predictive model for CKD. This model aims to facilitate early diagnosis, enhance patient outcomes, and simultaneously decrease the expenses and time associated with data collection and labeling.

The chapter aims to introduce a novel semi-supervised learning model designed specifically for predicting CKD. Using a dataset containing information from 8,819 patients, including essential factors like age, diabetes, and hypertension, the model incorporates both labeled and unlabeled data to improve prediction accuracy. Data preprocessing techniques such as cleaning and normalization are applied, and feature selection methods are utilized to identify key predictors for CKD. The model's performance is then evaluated against traditional supervised methods, employing various classifier models like random forest, K-Nearest Neighbors (KNN), Decision Tree (DT), and AdaBoost ensemble. Results indicate the superiority of the semi-supervised learning approach, particularly with the AdaBoost ensemble model achieving an impressive 93% prediction accuracy. This model holds promise as a valuable tool for healthcare professionals in early CKD detection and prevention, offering proactive management of this critical health condition. Section 2 presents the existing literature focusing on the prediction of CKD. Section 3 elaborates on the proposed semi-supervised learning model designed for CKD prediction. Section 4 explores the presentation of results and subsequent discussion, while Section 5 addresses the conclusion and outlines potential avenues for future work.

12.2 RELATED WORK

CKD poses a significant global health challenge, necessitating innovative approaches for early detection and accurate prognosis. As the prevalence of CKD continues to rise, the exploration of advanced computational techniques, particularly in the realm of machine learning, becomes imperative. In this context, a critical examination of existing literature in CKD prediction lays the foundation for this research. In the study conducted by Priyanka et al. [7] the researchers focused on predicting CKD using the Naive Bayes (NB) classification technique. In their investigation, the researchers not only employed NB but also tested the performance of other machine learning algorithms, including KNN, Support Vector Machines (SVM), DT, and Artificial Neural Networks (ANN). The outcome of their experimentation revealed that the NB model achieved a notably higher accuracy of 94.6% in comparison to the other algorithms tested.

Yashfi [8] introduced a predictive model for assessing the risk of CKD through the utilization of machine learning algorithms. The analysis involved examining data from CKD patients, employing RF and ANN algorithms. From the original set of 25 features, the researcher extracted 20 and applied both RF and ANN. Notably, RF demonstrated the highest accuracy, achieving a noteworthy 97.12%.

Tekale et al. [9] examined 14 distinct attributes associated with CKD patients and assessed the accuracy of various machine learning algorithms, including DT and SVM. The analysis revealed that the DT algorithm achieved an accuracy of 91.75%, while the SVM algorithm demonstrated an accuracy of 96.75%. Rady et al. [10] employed a range of predictive models, including Probabilistic Neural Network (PNN), MLP, SVM, and Radial Basis Function (RBF), for the early-stage prediction of CKD. Their model yielded accuracies of 96.7%, 60.7%, 87%, and 51.5% for PNN, MLP, SVM, and RBF, respectively. It is important to note that certain algorithms, particularly MLP and RBF, may not be well-suited for small dataset sizes, which could impact their performance in the context of CKD prediction.

Alsuhibany et al. [11] introduced an Early Detection and Diagnosis Support System (EDL-CDSS) designed for CKD diagnosis within the Internet of Things (IoT) environment. This innovative technique incorporates the Adaptive Synthetic Sampling (ADASYN) technique for the outlier detection process. The study utilized an ensemble approach, combining three distinct models: Deep Belief Network, Kernelized Extreme Learning Machine, and Convolutional Neural Network with Gated Recurrent Unit (CNN-GRU). This ensemble of models collectively forms the foundation of the proposed EDL-CDSS, showcasing a comprehensive and sophisticated approach to CKD diagnosis within the dynamic context of the IoT environment.

In 2019, Ahmed and Alshebly [12] addressed a medical diagnosis challenge related to CKD using machine learning algorithms, specifically ANN and Logistic Regression (LR). Their analysis focused on 153 cases with 11 attributes of CKD patients. The results indicated that the ANN classifier outperformed the LR model, achieving an accuracy of 84.44%, sensitivity of 84.21%, specificity of 84.61%, and an area under the curve (AUC) of 84.41%. Notably, the study identified creatinine and urea as the most influential factors impacting CKD.

Similarly, Kriplani et al. [13] conducted a comprehensive study using 224 records of CKD from the UC Irvine (UCI) machine learning repository, dating back to 2015. They proposed an algorithm based on deep neural networks for predicting the presence or absence of CKD, achieving an impressive accuracy of 97%. Employing cross-validation techniques ensured that the model was resilient against overfitting, and the results demonstrated superior performance compared to other existing algorithms.

12.3 PROPOSED SYSTEM

The proposed Semi-Supervised Learning Model presented in Figure 12.1 is designed to predict the occurrence of CKD. The primary objective is to pre-process the data by addressing null values and completing the dataset through the imputation of missing values. This ensures a comprehensive dataset for the development of an enhanced prediction model. Upon receiving user-provided data, the proposed system promptly

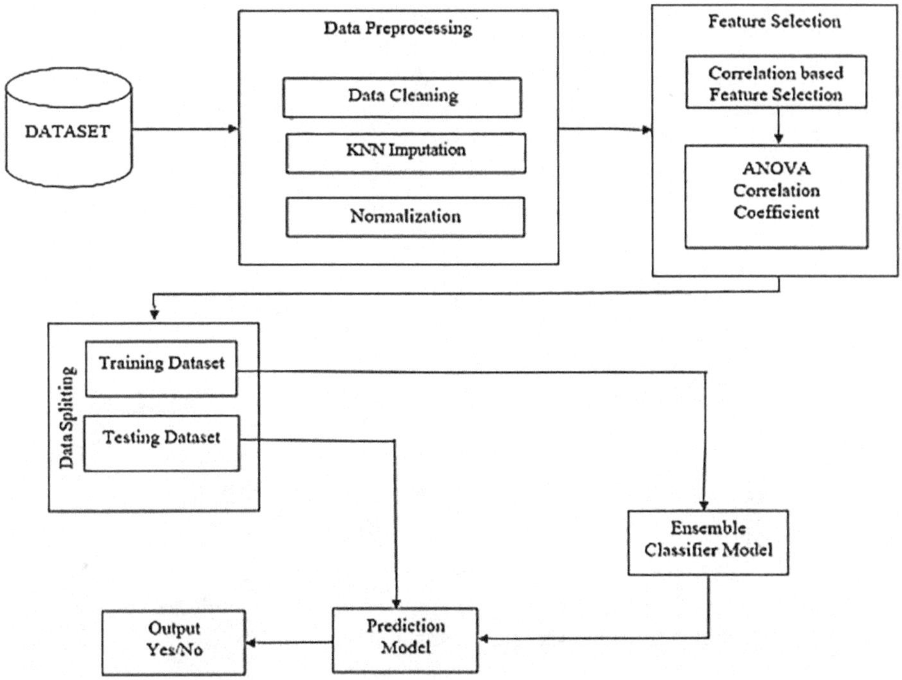

FIGURE 12.1 Architectural diagram of the proposed system.

indicates whether the individual is affected by CKD. The system relies on medical records as the dataset source. The initial step involves data preprocessing, encompassing tasks such as data cleaning, KNN imputation, and normalization methods. The subsequent step entails feature selection using the correlation feature selection (CFS) technique, specifically the analysis of variance (ANOVA) correlation coefficient method. The dataset is then divided into training and testing sets. A classifier model is constructed utilizing algorithms such as RF, KNN, and DT. To enhance classifier performance, an ensemble technique, AdaBoost, is implemented. The boosting technique is applied, resulting in the acquisition of a refined prediction model. The model's efficacy is evaluated using the test data, which is input into the trained model for predicting CKD status. Ultimately, the final output is generated by inputting user-provided data into the model, which in turn predicts whether the individual is affected by CKD. This multifaceted approach ensures a robust and accurate prediction process for CKD detection.

12.3.1 Data Preprocessing and Feature Selection

The Data Preprocessing technique undergoes various procedures, encompassing data cleaning, data imputation, and normalization. The Data Cleaning method is implemented to address missing values within the dataset. In this system, the Data Imputation method employs KNN imputation, filling missing values with the mean value derived from the K-neighbors identified in the dataset. KNN Imputer, being a distance-based imputation method, necessitates data normalization to ensure unbiased replacements for missing values. To achieve this, MinMaxScaler and StandardScaler methods are employed for normalizing the dataset. In the subsequent stage of the algorithm, features are chosen by assessing their correlation with one another. This is accomplished by utilizing a CFS technique referred to as the ANOVA correlation coefficient method. The principal objective of employing this method is to recognize and preserve optimal features characterized by a substantial F-score. The dataset is subsequently partitioned into training data and test data, wherein the training data is employed for model training, and the test data is employed for predicting the outcomes of the trained model. Additionally, the test data serves as a means to assess the performance and effectiveness of the model.

ALGORITHM 1: DATA PREPROCESSING AND FEATURE SELECTION

Input: A dataset comprising medical records of patients.

Output: Obtaining a preprocessed dataset devoid of any null values and optimal features after the feature selection method.

Data Preprocessing:

1. Load the dataset from a (.csv) file.
2. Check for null values in the dataset.
3. If the dataset contains categorical attributes, convert them into numerical attributes.
4. Label Encoding method for numerical attribute conversion, replacing categorical values ranging from 0 to −1.
5. Scale the dataset using the MinMaxScaler method.
6. Employ the KNN Imputation method to fill in missing values in the dataset.
7. After filling in missing values, verify null values and scale the dataset using the StandardScaler method.
8. Obtain the preprocessed data as the output.

FEATURE SELECTION ALGORITHM:

1. Utilize the preprocessed data obtained from the Data Preprocessing step.
2. Separate independent (x) and dependent (y) variables from the data.
3. Construct the feature selection model with parameters such as the score function and k (number of features to be selected)
4. Fit the feature selection model using x and y variables.
5. Calculate the feature scores based on the selected model.
6. Choose features with the largest scores.
7. Obtain the optimal features as the final output.

12.3.2 Ensemble Classification Model

The next stage in the process involves constructing a classifier model, and several algorithms such as RF, KNN, and DT are considered for this purpose. The utilization of diverse algorithms in this context aims to harness the strengths of each individual algorithm while mitigating their respective weaknesses. This diversity is beneficial for capturing complex patterns and relationships within the data.

To further enhance the predictive power of the model, an ensemble technique known as the AdaBoost method is employed. The rationale behind using ensemble methods is to combine the predictions from multiple base models (the individual classifiers) in a way that collectively improves the overall accuracy and robustness of the model. AdaBoost, short for Adaptive Boosting, assigns weights to the instances in the dataset, emphasizing the misclassified instances in each iteration. This iterative process focuses on improving the model's performance by giving more attention to challenging instances, leading to a more resilient and accurate ensemble classifier.

ALGORITHM 2: ENSEMBLE CLASSIFIER MODEL

Input: Training data
Output: Obtain the prediction model
Algorithm:

1. Implement cross-validation on the training data to ensure robust model assessment.
2. Employ multiple learning algorithms such as RF, KNN, and DT to enhance prediction performance.
3. Train models with distinct algorithms to capture varied patterns in the data.
4. Construct an AdaBoost Ensemble Model, amalgamating the strengths of diverse learning algorithms to improve overall predictive accuracy.
5. Evaluate each model's performance metrics.
6. Identify and choose the best-performing prediction model based on predefined criteria (e.g., accuracy, precision, recall).

In the prediction model, user data, encompassing attributes like age, hypertension, Spontaneous bacterial peritonitis (SBP), cardiovascular diseases (CVD), and congestive heart failure (CHF), undergoes processing to determine whether the individual is affected by CKD or not.

12.4 RESULTS AND DISCUSSION

The dataset used in this research comprises 8,819 instances and has been sourced from Darden Business Publishing. These instances represent individual data points or records within the dataset, and each instance likely contains a set of features or variables related to CKD. The dataset, with its substantial number of instances, serves as the foundational source of information for the analysis, modeling, or research conducted in the given context. In Table 9.1, a comprehensive evaluation of performance metrics is presented, encompassing key indicators such as accuracy, precision, recall, and F1 score for the proposed model. These metrics provide a detailed insight into the effectiveness and reliability of the models under consideration. Accuracy gauges the overall correctness of the model's predictions, precision assesses the accuracy of positive predictions, recall measures the model's ability to capture all relevant instances, and the F1 score is a harmonized metric that balances precision and recall. Figure 12.2 offers a visual summary of the models' performance across these crucial metrics, aiding in a nuanced understanding of their overall efficacy. Table 12.1 shows performance metrics analysis.

Figure 12.3 illustrates the range of the AUC and the Receiver Operating Characteristic (ROC) curve for various models.

12.5 CONCLUSION AND FUTURE ENHANCEMENTS

A highly effective semi-supervised learning model is proposed for predicting CKD). This model optimally utilizes both labeled and unlabeled data, contributing to heightened accuracy in CKD prediction, thereby assisting clinicians in prompt and precise diagnoses. The incorporation of a meticulous feature selection process and the utilization of diverse classification models further augment the predictive capabilities of the model. Evaluation of the model, using a publicly available CKD dataset, reveals that the AdaBoost ensemble model surpasses the other three classification models, achieving a remarkable accuracy of 93%. Additionally, this ensemble model exhibits superior sensitivity, specificity, and F1-score. The potential impact of the proposed model extends to improving patient outcomes, curbing healthcare costs, and aiding in the early detection and prevention of CKD. Moreover, a prospective avenue for future work involves the development of a Recommendation System for CKD diagnosis, leveraging the insights from the predictive model. This system, based on the

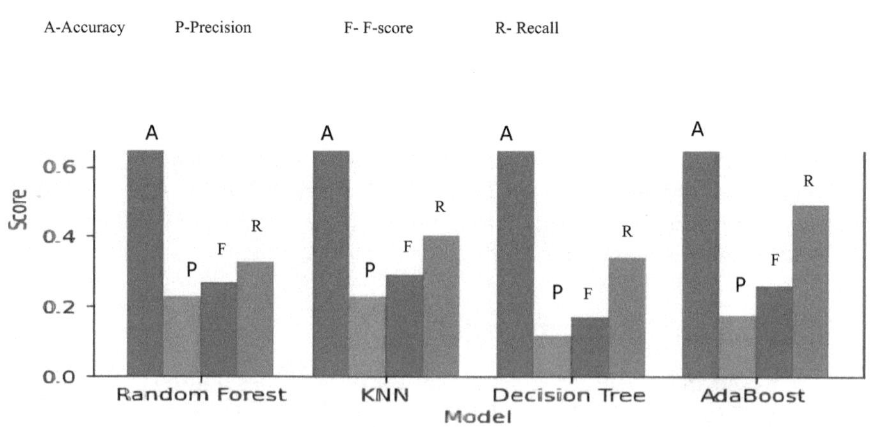

FIGURE 12.2 Performance analysis of various models.

TABLE 12.1
Performance Metrics Analysis

	ACC	FPR	Precision	Recall	F1_Score
Random Forest	0.908889	0.0037170	0.227273	0.326087	0.267857
KNN	0.918333	0.026978	0.227273	0.400000	0.289655
Decision Tree	0.918889	0.017386	0.113636	0.340909	0.170455
AdaBoost	0.926111	0.014388	0.174242	0.489362	0.256963

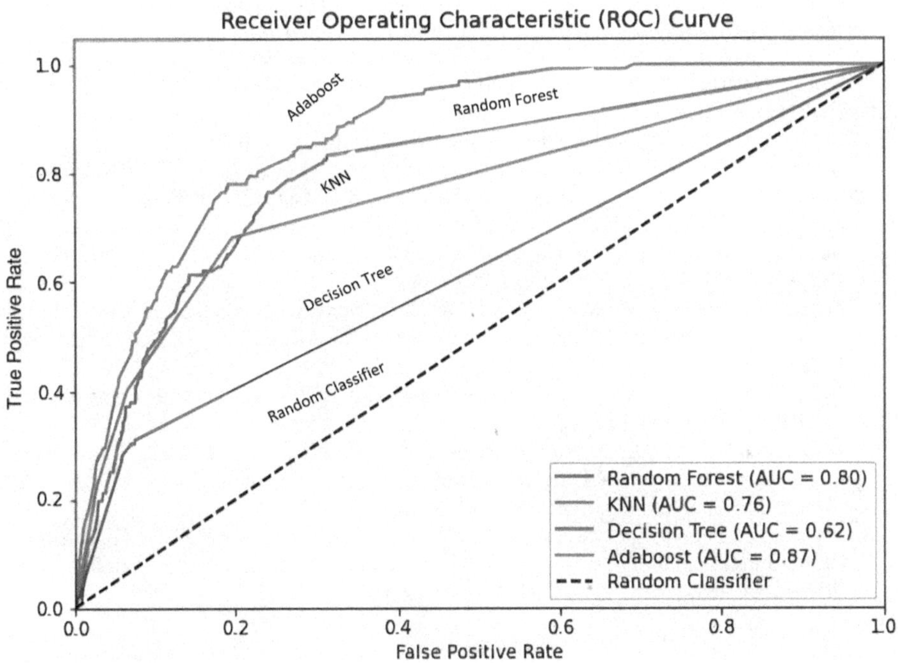

FIGURE 12.3 AUC–ROC curve.

calculated glomerular filtration rate and zone attributes, categorizes the stages of CKD. Tailored food recommendations are then provided, aligning with the severity of the condition, and offering valuable support to individuals affected by CKD.

REFERENCES

1. Qin, J., Chen, L., Liu, Y., Liu, C., Feng, C., & Chen, B, "A machine learning methodology for diagnosing chronic kidney disease," *IEEE Access*, Vol. 8, pp. 20991–21002, 2019.
2. Deepika, B., Rao, V. K. R., Rampure, D. N., Prajwal, P., & Gowda, D. G, "Early prediction of chronic kidney disease by using machine learning techniques," *American Journal of Computer Science and Engineering: The Survey*, Vol. 8, No. 2, p. 7, 2020.

3. Alsuhibany, S. A., Abdel-Khalek, S., Algarni, A., Fayomi, A., Gupta, D., Kumar, V., & Mansour, R. F, "Ensemble of deep learning based clinical decision support system for chronic kidney disease diagnosis in medical internet of things environment," *Computational Intelligence and Neuroscience*, Vol. 11, p. 22, 2021.
4. Chimwayi, K. B., Haris, N., Caytiles, R. D., & Iyengar, N. C. S, "Risk level prediction of chronic kidney disease using neuro-fuzzy and hierarchical clustering algorithm (s)," *Journal of Translational Medicine*, Vol. 16, No. 1, pp. 10–23, 2017.
5. Xiao, J., Ding, R., Xu, X., Guan, H., Feng, X., Sun, T.,. . . Ye, Z, "Comparison and development of machine learning tools in the prediction of chronic kidney disease progression," *Journal of Translational Medicine*, Vol. 17, No. 1, pp. 1–13, 2017.
6. Kriplani, H., Patel, B., & Roy, S, "Prediction of chronic kidney diseases using deep artificial neural network technique," in *Computer aided intervention and diagnostics in clinical and medical images*, pp. 179–187, Springer International Publishing, 2019.
7. Molla, M. D., Degef, M., Bekele, A., Geto, Z., Challa, F., Lejisa, T., . . . Seifu, D, "Assessment of serum electrolytes and kidney function test for screening of chronic kidney disease among Ethiopian Public Health Institute staff members," *Addis Ababa*, Ethiopia. *BMC Nephrology*, Vol. 21, pp. 1–11, 2020.
8. Priyanka K, "Chronic kidney disease prediction using machine learning," *International Journal of Computer Science and Information Security (IJCSIS)*, Vol. 16, No. 4, 2018.
9. Yashfi, S. Y., Islam, M. A., Sakib, N., Islam, T., Shahbaaz, M., & Pantho, S. S, "Risk prediction of chronic kidney disease using machine learning algorithms," In *2020 11th International Conference on Computing, Communication and Networking Technologies (ICCCNT)*, pp. 1–5, Springer, Rom, 2020.
10. Tekale, S., Shingavi, P., Wandhekar, S., & Chatorikar, A, "Prediction of chronic kidney disease using machine learning algorithm," *International Journal of Advanced Research in Computer and Communication Engineering*, Vol. 7, No. 10, pp. 92–96, 2018.
11. Rady, E. H. A., & Anwar, A. S, "Prediction of kidney disease stages using data mining algorithms," *Informatics in Medicine Unlocked*, Vol. 15, pp. 100178, 2019.
12. Ma, F., Sun, T., Liu, L., & Jing, H, "Detection and diagnosis of chronic kidney disease using deep learning-based heterogeneous modified artificial neural network," *Future Generation Computer Systems*, Vol. 111, pp. 17–26, 2020.
13. Poonia, R. C., Gupta, M. K., Abunadi, I., Albraikan, A. A., Al-Wesabi, F. N., & Hamza, M. A, "Intelligent diagnostic prediction and classification models for detection of kidney disease. In Healthcare," *MDPI*, Vol. 10, No. 2, pp. 371, 2022.

13 Analyzing the Seamless Integration of Machine Learning and Internet of Things in the Daily Dynamics of Contemporary Living

Kanchan Naithani, Y. P. Raiwani, and Shrikant Tiwari

CONTENTS

13.1 INTRODUCTION TO SEAMLESS INTEGRATION OF ML AND IoT IN THE DAILY DYNAMICS OF CONTEMPORARY LIVING

The seamless integration of machine learning (ML) and the Internet of Things (IoT) has become a transformative force in the daily dynamics of contemporary living. This convergence is revolutionizing how we interact with our surroundings, making our environments smarter, more efficient, and more responsive to our needs. From smart homes and wearable devices to intelligent transportation systems and healthcare applications, the convergence of ML and IoT is meant to make everyday activities more efficient, convenient, and tailored to individual preferences. This convergence not only revolutionizes daily dynamics but also marks a significant advancement in

DOI: 10.1201/9781003476207-13

technology's ability to adapt to human behavior, preferences, and needs [1]. ML algorithms, integrated with IoT devices, enable a high degree of personalization in various aspects of daily life. For instance, smart homes can learn and adapt to residents' habits, adjusting lighting, temperature, and other settings automatically. Wearable devices equipped with ML capabilities can provide personalized health insights and recommendations based on individual data patterns [2]. ML algorithms integrated into IoT-enabled devices also enable proactive maintenance, predictive analytics, and efficient resource management. This chapter scrutinizes various aspects where ML and IoT are integrated into different aspects of daily life dynamics. The basic idea for the integration of ML and IoT in the everyday flux of modern life can be visualized in Figure 13.1.

The subsequent sections of the chapter are outlined after the basic introduction as Section 13.2 presents a literature review on the integration of ML and the IoT in everyday life. Section 13.3 discusses the challenges and solutions related to integrating ML with IoT. Section 13.4 elaborates on algorithmic advancements for daily operations, while Section 13.5 delves into a quantitative analysis of the impact of ML and IoT. Sections 13.6 and 13.7 explore future trends, developments, and ethical considerations. The chapter concludes with a summary in Section 13.8.

13.2 LITERATURE REVIEW OF ML AND IoT INTEGRATION IN DAILY LIVING

Globally, IoT is expanding rapidly. Nowadays, wearables and smartphones are just two examples of the many IoT gadgets that people are surrounded by in their daily lives. Furthermore, sensors and actuators connected via the IoT are advantageous for smart environments, including smart cities, smart industries, and smart healthcare systems [3]. However, with the rise of IoT devices, the difficulty of identifying

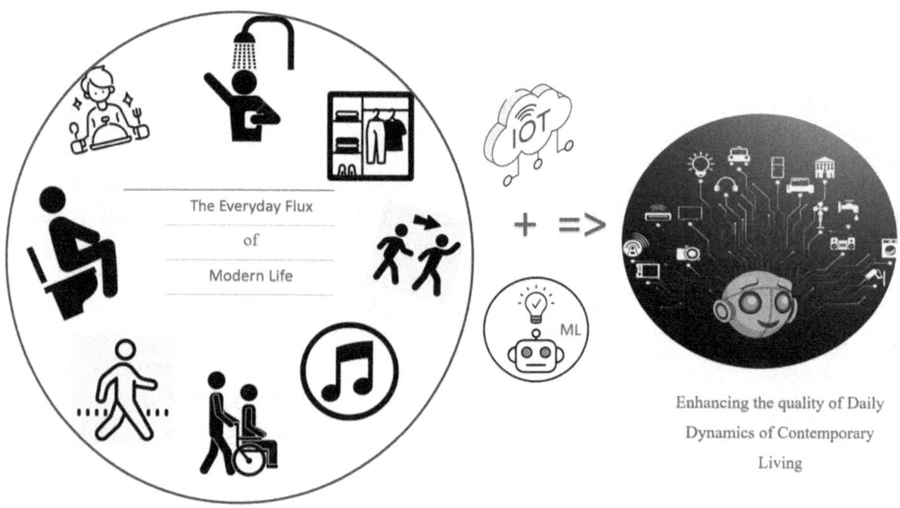

FIGURE 13.1 Integration of ML and IoT in the daily dynamics of contemporary living.

and countering cybersecurity risks and assaults that target them, such as malware, privacy violations, and denial-of-service attacks, has also increased. The research conducted by various scholars highlights the transformative impact of integrating ML and IoT on daily living dynamics [4].

As research continues to evolve, addressing challenges and exploring emerging trends has become crucial for harnessing the full potential of ML and IoT integration in enhancing the quality of daily life. Research work conducted by various researchers is shown in Table 13.1 along with their respective outcomes for corresponding design considerations.

Conducting a wide-ranging review of existing literature is imperative in gaining a distinct understanding of the current state of ML and IoT integration in the context of daily living. This endeavor has tried to delve into a diverse array of scholarly articles, research papers, and industry reports to distill key insights, trends, and challenges at the intersection of ML and IoT [11].

The first facet of this literature review involves scrutinizing studies that explore the theoretical frameworks underpinning ML–IoT integration. Understanding the foundational concepts and principles guiding this amalgamation is crucial for discerning the intricacies of how these technologies collaborate to enhance daily living dynamics [11].

Next, attention can be directed toward empirical studies and real-world implementations. Whether it be in smart homes, healthcare systems, urban environments, or industrial settings, a thorough review of the literature has unveiled the successes, challenges, and lessons learned from these practical deployments [12]. Understanding the existing frameworks and protocols is crucial for assessing interoperability, security, and ethical considerations [13]. Additionally, the societal implications of ML–IoT integration have explored how these technologies influence human behavior, impact job markets, and contribute to digital inclusion or exclusion. Moreover, understanding the economic ramifications, market trends, and potential disruptions in various sectors due to the integration of ML and IoT is vital for a holistic perspective.

Examining the impact of ML and IoT on real-world applications within the realms of smart homes and transportation unveils a transformative landscape that is reshaping the way we live and move. This can be visualized with the help of Figure 13.2.

This analysis encompasses various facets, including traffic management, personalized healthcare monitoring, and predictive maintenance in vehicles and advancements in autonomous vehicles, discussed as follows:

- **Smart Homes:** In the domain of smart homes, ML and IoT integration has redefined the concept of modern living. Home automation systems leverage ML algorithms to learn user preferences, optimize energy consumption, and enhance security. From intelligent thermostats that adapt to occupants' routines to smart lighting systems that respond to changing daylight conditions, ML–IoT synergy brings unprecedented convenience and efficiency to daily life.
- **Transportation and Traffic Management:** ML and IoT play pivotal roles in revolutionizing transportation, particularly in traffic management.

TABLE 13.1
Year-wise Research Overview for ML and IoT Integration in Daily Living

Reference	The Approach in Daily Dynamics of Contemporary Living	Design Considerations	Outcome
[5]	Radio-frequency identification technology, sensors, actuators, GPS devices and mobile devices, near-field communications, ICT	Energy, Latency, Throughput, Topology, Scalability, Security & Safety	The review analysis of major IoT techniques used in Industries helped in identifying various research trends and challenges.
[6]	Widget with wizard functionality and a wide range of data visualization elements, including gauges, charts, maps, etc.	Virtual Factory environment over a user interface such as "dashboard."	Visualization provides crucial key performance indicator (KPIs) for managing virtual factories. Partners can monitor processes, make collaborative decisions, and create their own dashboards using a user-friendly wizard and diverse visualization components.
[7]	Growing holistic learning systems and practices, actively fostering a common global knowledge and dimensions of action required to encourage changes in patterns	Extensive participation of society in knowledge creation; restructuring of incentives and financing; and comprehensive methods and systems of education	Major findings lead to conclusions that already known knowledge systems possess ideas about what needs to be achieved and how it could be encouraged.
[8]	Social life cycle assessment (S-LCA) methodology	A prosthesis and an orthosis	Value chain actors experienced a negative social impact.
[9]	Daily experiences of routines being broken and re-made in reaction to the epidemic	Time, practice, and consumption	Institutional arrangement of the temporal relationships between behaviors in terms of how they coexist, coordinate, or vie for the attention of the family.
[10]	Enhanced high-resolution space-based satellite monitoring, manual monitoring of local ground-based sensors, deep learning analysis methods, and high-resolution sensing systems	Satellite-based atmospheric imagery and datasets and the use of different kinds of computational intelligence/soft-computing techniques for analysis, forecasting and modeling, giant leaps	Remote sensing coupled with the techniques of ML/DL has the most impact in shaping the modern trends in air quality (AQ) research.

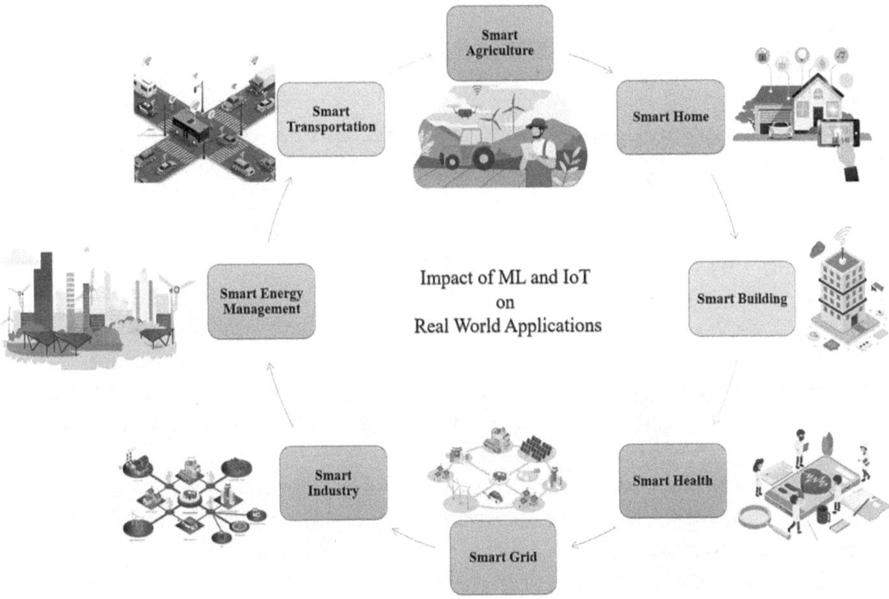

FIGURE 13.2 Impact of ML and IoT on real-world applications.

Through the deployment of IoT sensors and ML algorithms, traffic patterns are analyzed in real time, leading to dynamic adjustments and optimized traffic flow. This not only reduces congestion but also contributes to fuel efficiency and environmental sustainability. Additionally, ML algorithms are employed in predictive modeling to anticipate traffic patterns and optimize routes for vehicles, improving overall efficiency in urban mobility.

- **Personalized Healthcare Monitoring:** In the healthcare sector, ML and IoT are instrumental in personalized healthcare monitoring. Wearable devices equipped with sensors collect real-time health data, while ML algorithms analyze this information to provide personalized insights and early detection of potential health issues. This not only facilitates proactive healthcare management but also empowers individuals to take control of their well-being.
- **Advancements in Autonomous Vehicles:** The synergy between ML and IoT is a driving force behind advancements in autonomous vehicles. IoT sensors gather real-time data from the vehicle's surroundings, while ML algorithms process and interpret this data to make informed decisions. From recognizing pedestrians and other vehicles to navigating complex traffic scenarios, ML–IoT integration is propelling the development of safe and efficient autonomous driving technology.

The ongoing advancements in these domains underscore the transformative potential of combining ML and IoT technologies, paving the way for a smarter, safer, and more connected future.

13.3 CHALLENGES AND SOLUTIONS IN INTEGRATING ML WITH IoT

The integration of ML with IoT presents a plethora of opportunities for innovation and efficiency. However, this convergence is not without its challenges, and identifying issues such as data interoperability and device management is crucial for successful implementation [14].

A major obstacle to ML integration with IoT is the variety of data formats and protocols produced by various devices. IoT devices may produce data in various structures and standards, making it challenging for ML algorithms to seamlessly analyze and derive meaningful insights. Achieving data interoperability involves establishing standardized formats and protocols, ensuring that diverse datasets can be harmoniously integrated and processed by ML algorithms. Lack of interoperability can hinder the scalability and effectiveness of ML–IoT solutions, limiting their potential impact across diverse environments.

The intricate and diverse landscape of IoT devices introduces intricate challenges as shown in Figure 13.3, in the administration and coordination of interactions within an ML-driven ecosystem.

Device management encompasses critical tasks, including software updates, security patching, and ensuring seamless compatibility across a spectrum of hardware variations. ML models frequently rely on real-time data from IoT devices, demanding streamlined mechanisms for tasks such as device discovery, authentication, and communication. Discrepancies or inefficiencies in device management can result in systemic inefficiencies and security vulnerabilities and compromise the overall reliability of ML–IoT applications. The integration of ML with IoT introduces security and privacy

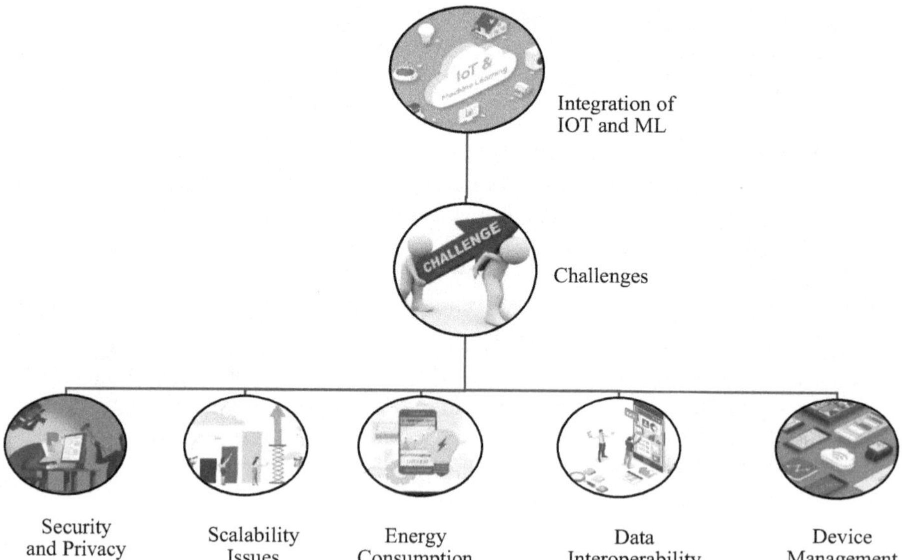

FIGURE 13.3 Challenges faced while integrating machine learning with IoT.

challenges, including the potential compromise of sensitive data. ML models trained on IoT-generated data may inadvertently expose vulnerabilities and the communication between devices and ML systems must be secured to prevent unauthorized access. Additionally, ensuring data privacy becomes paramount, especially when dealing with personal or sensitive information collected by IoT devices. Establishing robust security measures and privacy safeguards is crucial to building trust in ML–IoT ecosystems.

Ensuring that ML algorithms can adapt and scale efficiently without compromising performance is essential for the long-term success of integrated ML–IoT solutions. IoT devices often operate on constrained resources, including limited processing power and energy. ML algorithms, especially complex models, may demand significant computational resources, leading to increased energy consumption.

Balancing the computational requirements of ML with the energy constraints of IoT devices is a critical consideration for sustainable and practical implementations. To tackle these obstacles, a multidisciplinary strategy combining cooperation across ML, IoT, and cybersecurity professionals is needed. Standardization efforts, robust security protocols, and advancements in device management technologies are essential for creating a foundation that facilitates the seamless and secure integration of ML with IoT, unlocking the full potential of this powerful convergence.

To deal with the difficulties posed by the integration of ML and the IoT, it is crucial to propose effective remedies. Implementing advanced data integration techniques and enhancing device management can significantly contribute to a more seamless and efficient ML–IoT integration [15]. Here are key proposals for remedying the identified issues:

a) Advanced Data Integration Techniques
   - **Standardized Protocols:** Develop and promote standardized data formats and communication protocols within IoT ecosystems. Establishing industry-wide standards ensures compatibility, enabling diverse devices to communicate and share data effectively.
   - **Data Preprocessing and Normalization:** Implement advanced data preprocessing techniques to grip the heterogeneity of information generated by different IoT devices. Normalizing data formats and cleaning noisy datasets enhance the compatibility and consistency required for ML algorithms.
   - **Edge Computing:** Leverage edge computing to process data closer to the source, reducing latency and optimizing bandwidth. This approach not only enhances real-time processing capabilities but also minimizes the burden on centralized ML models, improving scalability.
   - **Federated Learning:** Implement federated learning techniques to train ML models collaboratively across distributed IoT devices. This approach allows models to learn from decentralized data without centralizing sensitive information, addressing privacy concerns.

b) Improved Device Management
   - **Dynamic Device Discovery**: Develop dynamic device discovery mechanisms that adapt to changes in the IoT ecosystem. Automated discovery

protocols can facilitate seamless integration with ML models, ensuring that new devices are identified and incorporated efficiently.

- **Over-the-Air (OTA) Updates:** Implement robust OTA update mechanisms for IoT devices, enabling seamless software updates and security patching. This ensures that devices remain up-to-date with the latest features and security measures, enhancing the overall reliability of the ML–IoT system.
- **Unified Device Management Platforms:** Integrate unified device management platforms that provide a centralized interface for monitoring, configuring, and maintaining IoT devices. This approach streamlines device management tasks and enhances the overall control and coordination of the interconnected ecosystem.
- **Security by Design:** Implement a security-first approach in device management, incorporating encryption, authentication, and access control measures. Proactive security measures reduce the potential for unauthorized access and protect sensitive data, fostering trust in the ML–IoT integration.
- **Energy-Efficient Device Management:** Develop energy-efficient device management strategies to mitigate the impact of increased computational requirements on IoT device batteries. This includes optimizing communication protocols and implementing energy-saving modes when feasible.

As the synergy between ML and IoT continues to evolve, these proactive solutions contribute to creating resilient and adaptive ecosystems that harness the full potential of these transformative technologies. The gist of the solutions for integrating ML with IoT can be seen in Figure 13.4.

13.4 ALGORITHMIC INNOVATIONS FOR DAILY DYNAMICS

Investigating cutting-edge ML algorithms is essential for understanding their pivotal role in shaping the daily dynamics of contemporary living. Principal component

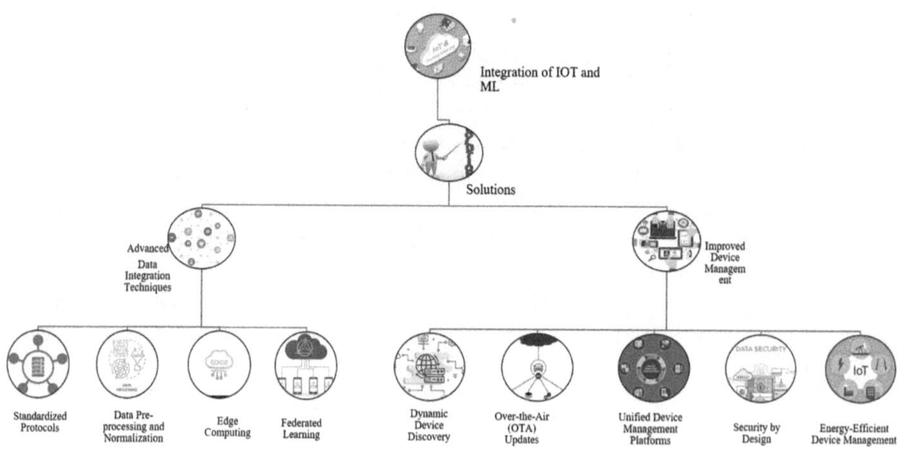

FIGURE 13.4 Solutions for integrating machine learning with IoT.

analysis (PCA) stands out as one such algorithm that has garnered significant attention due to its versatility and applications across various domains. This exploration delves into the significance of PCA in the context of modern living, elucidating its impact on diverse aspects of our daily lives.

- **Dimensionality Reduction and Data Compression**: PCA is a powerful algorithm used for dimensionality reduction, a crucial process in handling high-dimensional datasets. In contemporary living, where the volume of data generated is immense, PCA plays a key role in compressing and summarizing information. This not only aids in efficient data storage but also accelerates processing times, contributing to the seamless functioning of applications that permeate daily life.
- **Image and Signal Processing**: In the realm of contemporary living, image, and signal processing are ubiquitous, from facial recognition in smartphones to audio processing in smart home devices. PCA is instrumental in feature extraction, enhancing the efficiency of these processes. By identifying and retaining essential information, PCA contributes to improved image and signal analysis, ultimately enhancing user experiences in applications ranging from photography to voice recognition.
- **Enhanced Predictive Modeling**: Contemporary living is increasingly influenced by predictive modeling, shaping areas such as personalized recommendations, financial forecasting, and healthcare diagnostics. PCA aids in identifying the most influential features in datasets, improving the accuracy and interpretability of predictive models. This, in turn, enhances the efficacy of applications that predict user preferences, financial trends, or potential health issues.
- **Anomaly Detection and Cybersecurity**: In the digital age, cybersecurity is paramount. PCA is employed for anomaly detection, identifying deviations from normal patterns in large datasets. This is crucial for safeguarding daily digital interactions, from online transactions to protecting personal information. By detecting unusual patterns, PCA contributes to fortifying the cybersecurity infrastructure that underpins contemporary living.

The real-world applications of innovative ML algorithms, such as PCA, have had a profound impact on various domains, significantly contributing to enhanced efficiency, personalization and improved user experiences [16].

In healthcare, PCA is utilized for dimensionality reduction in medical data. By extracting relevant features from complex datasets, PCA aids in medical image analysis, enabling more accurate diagnostics. Additionally, it contributes to personalized medicine by identifying crucial factors for treatment responses, optimizing drug regimens, and tailoring medical interventions to individual patient profiles. Principle components, a new set of uncorrelated features that represent the largest variation in the data, are created from the original features by algorithms such as PCA. The mathematical formulation includes finding the eigenvectors and eigenvalues of the covariance matrix of the original data.

Let M be the matrix representing the original data, where each row corresponds to an observation and each column corresponds to a feature. The covariance matrix C of X is given by Equation 13.1 [17].

$$C = \frac{1}{n-1}\left(M - \bar{M}\right)^{T}\left(M - \bar{M}\right) \tag{1}$$

- where n is the number of observations and $\bar{M}$ is the mean vector of the columns of M.

We can also use eigenvectors and eigenvalues of the covariance matrix C as shown in Equation 13.2. Let D_m be the diagonal matrix of matching eigenvalues, and let V_m be the matrix whose columns are the eigenvectors of C.

$$CV_m = VD_m \tag{13.2}$$

The columns of V are the principal components and the eigenvalues in D represent the amount of variance captured by each principal component.

To perform the dimensionality reduction, you can select the top k eigenvectors corresponding to the k largest eigenvalues. The new data matrix Y is obtained by projecting the original data onto these k principal components as given by Equation 13.3.

$$Y = XV_k \tag{13.3}$$

- where V_k contains the top k eigenvectors.

In the realm of computer vision and natural language processing, singular value decomposition (SVD) is employed for dimensionality reduction and feature extraction. SVD is a generalization of PCA and is used to factorize a matrix into three other matrices. In the context of dimensionality reduction, it is used to find the principal components. The SVD decomposition of a matrix X is given by Equation 13.4.

$$X = U \Sigma V^{T} \tag{13.4}$$

- where U and V are orthogonal matrices and Σ is a diagonal matrix with singular values.

In image recognition applications, it helps identify key patterns and features, contributing to improved object recognition and classification. Similarly, in speech recognition systems, PCA aids in processing and extracting relevant features from audio data, enhancing the accuracy of voice-based interactions and user experiences.

Similarly, Social media platforms leverage ML algorithms, like linear discriminant analysis (LDA), to enhance content personalization. By analyzing user engagement patterns and preferences, PCA helps tailor content recommendations, advertisements and news feeds. This contributes to a more personalized and engaging user experience, fostering user satisfaction and retention as it focuses on preserving local relationships between data points, making it useful for clustering and visualization. Apart from LDA, t-SNE (t-Distributed Stochastic Neighbor Embedding) can be used to visualize the distribution of users based on their interactions with content, identifying clusters of users who exhibit similar behavior. The algorithm is particularly effective for visualizing clusters and capturing local structures. The high-level objective of t-SNE can be expressed as Algorithm 13.1.

ALGORITHM 13.1

1. In the high-dimensional space, compute the pairwise similarities Pij between the data points.
2. In the lower-dimensional space, compute the pairwise similarities, or Qij, between the data points.
3. Reduce the two distributions' Kullback-Leibler divergence.
4. A Gaussian kernel is frequently utilized to define the pairwise similarities in the original space:

$$P_{ij} = \frac{\exp(-\| x_i - x_j \|^2)/(2\sigma_i^2)}{\sum_{k \neq 1} \exp\left(-\| x_k - x_1 \|^2 /(2\sigma_i^2)\right)}$$

- where y_i and y_j are the mapped points in the lower-dimensional space.

13.5 QUANTITATIVE ANALYSIS OF ML AND IoT IMPACT

Conducting a quantitative analysis to measure the impact of ML and IoT integration is essential for gaining actionable insights into the performance of such systems. This analytical approach allows organizations to evaluate the effectiveness of ML–IoT deployments across various metrics, including efficiency, cost-effectiveness, and user satisfaction [18]. Here is an overview of the key components involved in this quantitative analysis:

Begin by clearly defining the key metrics that align with the objectives of ML–IoT integration. Metrics may include:

- **Efficiency Metrics**: Evaluate the system's performance in terms of speed, accuracy, and resource utilization. This can involve measuring response times, processing speeds, and the overall efficiency of data processing.
- **Cost-Effectiveness Metrics**: Assess the financial impact of ML–IoT integration by considering factors such as reduced operational costs, optimized resource utilization, and potential return on investment.
- **User Satisfaction Metrics**: Gauge user experiences through metrics like user engagement, satisfaction surveys, and feedback mechanisms. Consider aspects such as system responsiveness, reliability, and ease of use.

- **Data Collection**: Gather relevant data to feed into the quantitative analysis. This involves collecting data from integrated ML and IoT systems, which may include performance logs, user interactions, cost-related information, and any other relevant metrics identified during the planning phase.

Apart from these, benchmarks can be established to measure the performance of ML–IoT systems against predefined standards or industry benchmarks. This involves comparing the current system performance with baseline metrics to quantify improvements or identify areas for optimization. Statistical analysis techniques can be applied to the collected data. This may involve using regression analysis, correlation studies or hypothesis testing to identify patterns, relationships, and statistical significance in the metrics being measured. Then ML models can be evaluated to assess their performance using standard evaluation metrics such as precision, recall, accuracy, and F1 score. Evaluation can be achieved against predefined criteria to ensure they meet the desired objectives.

By systematically conducting a quantitative analysis, organizations can gain valuable insights into the tangible impact of ML and IoT integration on key metrics. This approach enables informed decision-making, iterative improvements, and the optimization of integrated systems for greater efficiency and user satisfaction.

13.6 FUTURE TRENDS AND DEVELOPMENTS

Several emerging technologies are significantly influencing the landscape of ML and IoT, contributing to innovative applications and transformative advancements. Following are major new technologies that could influence ML and the IoT in the future [12]:

- **Edge Computing**: Edge computing involves processing data closer to the source of generation, reducing latency, and improving real-time decision-making. In the context of ML and IoT, edge computing is pivotal. By deploying ML models directly on edge devices, organizations can enhance efficiency, reduce bandwidth usage, and address privacy concerns by processing sensitive data locally.
- **5G Technology**: The rollout of 5G networks is revolutionizing connectivity and communication. In the realm of ML and IoT, 5G enables faster data transfer, lower latency, and increased device density. This facilitates the seamless integration of ML algorithms with IoT devices, enabling more responsive and data-intensive applications such as autonomous vehicles, augmented reality, and smart cities.
- **Federated Learning**: Federated learning is a technique that maintains localized data while training ML models across dispersed devices or servers. This aligns with privacy concerns and regulatory requirements. In the IoT context, federated learning allows devices to collaboratively train ML models without sharing raw data, making it suitable for applications in healthcare, finance, and other sensitive domains.

- **Explainable AI (XAI)**: Explainable AI is gaining prominence, especially in critical applications where understanding the decision-making process of ML models is essential. In IoT scenarios, particularly in healthcare and finance, XAI ensures transparency and accountability, enabling users to comprehend the reasoning behind ML-driven recommendations or decisions.
- **Quantum Computing**: By addressing difficult issues that are currently computationally impossible, quantum computing has the potential to completely transform ML. In the IoT domain, quantum computing can enhance security protocols, enabling the development of quantum-resistant cryptographic algorithms for safeguarding sensitive data transmitted between devices.
- **Blockchain Technology**: Blockchain technology is impacting both ML and IoT by providing a decentralized and secure way to manage data. In IoT, blockchain ensures data integrity, traceability, and secure transactions. In ML, blockchain can be employed for the secure sharing of models and for fostering trust in collaborative learning environments.
- **Neuromorphic Computing**: Neuromorphic computing mimics the architecture and functionality of the human brain, enabling more efficient and parallel processing. In the context of ML and IoT, neuromorphic computing can lead to energy-efficient algorithms and hardware, allowing for more powerful and intelligent edge devices.
- **Swarm Intelligence**: In IoT applications, swarm intelligence can optimize resource allocation, enhance network efficiency, and improve scalability in decentralized systems.
- **Synthetic Data Generation**: Synthetic data generation involves creating artificial datasets that mimic real-world scenarios. In ML and IoT, synthetic data can be used to augment limited datasets, improve model training, and address privacy concerns by generating representative data without revealing sensitive information.

These emerging technologies are not only influencing the development and deployment of ML and IoT solutions but are also paving the way for novel applications and use cases. As these technologies continue to evolve, their integration with ML and IoT is expected to shape a future where intelligent, efficient and secure connected systems play a central role in various industries and aspects of daily life. A gist of emerging technologies influencing ML and IoT is shown in Figure 13.5.

Predicting the future evolution of ML and IoT integration involves anticipating trends and developments based on current trajectories. Some predictions for the continued evolution of ML and IoT integration [19]. These predictions reflect the ongoing trajectory of ML and IoT integration, driven by technological advancements, industry demands and evolving user expectations. As these technologies continue to mature, their convergence is expected to shape a future where intelligent, secure and efficient systems play a central role in reshaping industries and daily life.

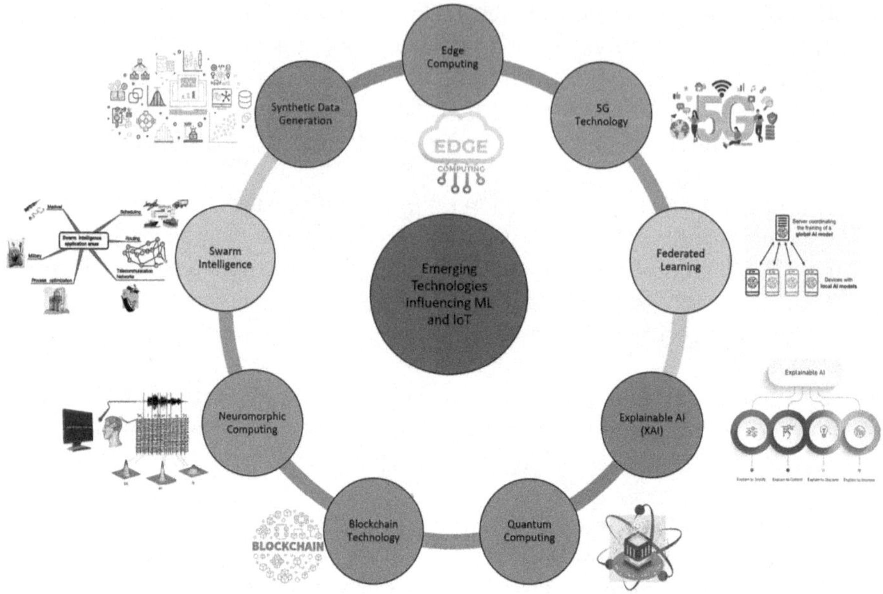

FIGURE 13.5 Emerging technologies influencing ML and IoT.

13.7 ETHICAL CONSIDERATIONS

The integration of ML and the IoT brings forth numerous benefits, but it also raises significant ethical challenges. To ensure responsible development and implementation of ML and IoT technologies, addressing key moral questions is imperative [20]:

- **Privacy Concerns**: IoT devices generate vast amounts of data, often including personal and sensitive information. As ML algorithms process this data to derive insights, there is a risk of unauthorized access, data breaches, and the potential for surveillance, leading to serious privacy infringements.
- **Data Security**: ML models heavily depend on diverse datasets for training and inference. Insecure data storage, transmission, or processing could lead to data manipulation, unauthorized access, and compromising the integrity of the ML algorithms, with implications for user trust and safety.
- **Bias and Fairness**: ML algorithms are susceptible to biases present in the training data. In the context of IoT, biased data may lead to discriminatory outcomes, disproportionately affecting certain demographic groups. Addressing bias in ML models is an ethical imperative to ensure fair and equitable treatment, particularly in applications like predictive policing, hiring processes, and healthcare.
- **Lack of Transparency**: The complexity of ML algorithms, especially deep learning models, can result in a lack of transparency. Understanding how these models make decisions is crucial, especially in applications where human lives or significant resources are at stake. Lack of transparency can

hinder accountability and raise ethical concerns regarding the opacity of decision-making processes.
- **Security Vulnerabilities in IoT Devices**: The security of IoT devices themselves is a major ethical concern. Insecure devices can be exploited for malicious purposes, leading to unauthorized access, data breaches, and potentially endangering user safety. Ensuring robust security measures in IoT devices is essential for preventing ethical lapses.

Addressing these ethical challenges requires collaboration among technologists, policymakers, ethicists, and the broader society. Developing ethical guidelines, regulatory frameworks and promoting responsible practices are essential steps toward ensuring that ML and IoT technologies are developed and deployed in ways that align with societal values, principles, and norms. We can observe some key considerations for fostering responsible AI and IoT practices in Table 13.2.

13.8 CONCLUSION AND FUTURE SCOPE

The seamless integration of ML and IoT holds immense promise in reshaping the daily dynamics of contemporary living. Through our analysis, we have witnessed the transformative impact of this integration across various domains, from smart homes to transportation, healthcare, and beyond. ML's ability to process vast datasets and

TABLE 13.2
Key Considerations for Fostering Responsible AI and IoT Practices

Ethical Design and Development	Informed Consent	Privacy by Design
Embed ethical considerations into the start of AI and IoT projects, adopting transparent, fair, and accountable design principles that address biases, privacy, and inclusivity.	Transparently communicate data practices, obtain informed consent for IoT and AI systems involving user data.	Integrate privacy into AI and IoT design with encryption, anonymization, and minimal necessary data collection.
Transparent Decision-Making	**Bias Mitigation**	**Security Measures**
Promote AI transparency by using Explainable AI (XAI) techniques to clarify decision-making processes for users and stakeholders.	Proactively identify and address biases in AI models through regular dataset audits and fairness-enhancing techniques for equitable treatment.	Prioritize IoT security with robust protocols, regular updates, and patches to prevent unauthorized access and data breaches.
User Empowerment and Control	**Lifecycle Management**	**Collaboration and Accountability**
Empower users with control over data and interactions in AI/IoT. Offer customizable privacy settings, opt-out choices, and transparent data usage insights through user-friendly interfaces.	Adopt ethical practices across the entire AI/IoT lifecycle, from design to retirement. This ensures sustained ethical behavior and addresses issues proactively.	Encourage collaboration among stakeholders for ethical AI/IoT. Establish clear accountability lines, fostering ongoing dialogue to address emerging challenges.

derive meaningful insights, coupled with the interconnected nature of IoT devices, has ushered in a new era of efficiency, personalization, and connectivity. This book chapter offers significant insights into recent techniques integrating IoT with ML, focusing on the daily dynamics of contemporary living. Initially seamless integration of ML and IoT was defined. This chapter provides background and research on ML and IoT integration in daily living, emphasizing fundamental technologies. It introduces key industrial IoT applications and analyzes associated challenges and future trends. A unique contribution is its focus on industrial applications, outlining research opportunities. In conclusion, the seamless integration of ML and IoT not only enhances the efficiency and convenience of daily activities but also brings about a fundamental shift in how technology adapts to human behavior and needs. This convergence is propelling us into an era where our surroundings are not just connected but also intelligent, responding dynamically to our preferences and contributing to a more sustainable, secure, and personalized way of living.

The future scope for the seamless integration of ML and the IoT is vast and holds promising advancements across various industries. As the volume of data generated by IoT devices continues to grow, there will be an increased emphasis on edge computing. ML algorithms will be deployed directly on edge devices, enabling real-time processing of data, and reducing the need for transmitting large amounts of data to centralized servers. This approach enhances efficiency and responsiveness in applications such as smart homes, industrial automation, and autonomous vehicles.

REFERENCES

1. Rai, P., & Maharjan, S., "Empowering south Asian agricultural communities: A comprehensive approach to IoT-driven agriculture through awareness, training and collaboration", *Quarterly Journal of Emerging Technologies and Innovations*, Vol. 8(3), pp. 18–32, 2023.
2. Kasula, B. Y., "Harnessing machine learning for personalized patient care", *Transactions on Latest Trends in Artificial Intelligence*, Vol. 4(4), 2023.
3. Chataut, R., Phoummalayvane, A., & Akl, R., "Unleashing the power of IoT: A comprehensive review of IoT applications and future prospects in healthcare, agriculture, smart homes, smart cities and industry 4.0.", *Sensors*, Vol. 23(16), pp. 7194, 2023.
4. Tyagi, A. K., Fernandez, T. F., Mishra, S., & Kumari, S., "Intelligent automation systems at the core of Industry 4.0.", in *International conference on intelligent systems design and applications* (pp. 1–18), 2020. Cham: Springer International Publishing.
5. Da Xu, L., He, W., & Li, S., "Internet of things in industries: A survey", *IEEE Transactions on Industrial Informatics*, Vol. 10(4), pp. 2233–2243, 2014.
6. Shamsuzzoha, A., Ferreira, F., Azevedo, A., & Helo, P. "Collaborative smart process monitoring within virtual factory environment: An implementation issue", *International Journal of Computer Integrated Manufacturing*, Vol. 30(1), pp. 167–181, 2017, DOI: 10.1080/0951192X.2016.1185156
7. Fazey, I., Schäpke, N., Caniglia, G., Hodgson, A., Kendrick, I., Lyon, C.,. . Saha, P., "Transforming knowledge systems for life on Earth: Visions of future systems and how to get there", *Energy Research & Social Science*, Vol. 70, 101724, 2020.
8. Soares, B., Ribeiro, I., Cardeal, G., Leite, M., Carvalho, H., & Peças, P., "Social life cycle performance of additive manufacturing in the healthcare industry: The orthosis and prosthesis cases", *International Journal of Computer Integrated Manufacturing*, Vol. 34(3), pp. 327–340, 2021, DOI: 10.1080/0951192X.2021.1872100

9. Greene, M., Hansen, A., Hoolohan, C., Süßbauer, E., & Domaneschi, L., "Consumption and shifting temporalities of daily life in times of disruption: Undoing and reassembling household practices during the COVID-19 pandemic", *Sustainability: Science, Practice and Policy*, Vol. 18(1), pp. 215–230, 2022.
10. Tahir Bahadur, F., Rasool Shah, S., & Rao Nidamanuri, R., "Air pollution monitoring and modelling: An overview", *Environmental Forensics,* pp. 1–28, 2023.
11. Allioui, H., & Mourdi, Y., "Exploring the full potentials of IoT for better financial growth and stability: A comprehensive survey", *Sensors*, Vol. 23(19), pp. 8015, 2023.
12. Khalil, R. A., Saeed, N., Masood, M., Fard, Y. M., Alouini, M. S., & Al-Naffouri, T. Y., "Deep learning in the industrial internet of things: Potentials, challenges and emerging applications", *IEEE Internet of Things Journal*, Vol. 8(14), pp. 11016–11040, 2021.
13. Manheim, K., & Kaplan, L., "Artificial intelligence: Risks to privacy and democracy", *Yale Journal of Law & Technology*, Vol. 21, pp. 106, 2019.
14. Raptis, T. P., Passarella, A., & Conti, M., "Data management in industry 4.0: State of the art and open challenges", *IEEE Access*, Vol. 7, pp. 97052–97093, 2019.
15. Rani, S., Mishra, R. K., Usman, M., Kataria, A., Kumar, P., Bhambri, P., & Mishra, A. K., "Amalgamation of advanced technologies for sustainable development of smart city environment: A review", *IEEE Access*, Vol. 9, pp. 150060–150087, 2021.
16. Zhang, S., Zhang, S., Wang, B., & Habetler, T. G., "Deep learning algorithms for bearing fault diagnostics-A comprehensive review", *IEEE Access*, Vol. 8, pp. 29857–29881, 2020.
17. Akewar, M., "Classification of EEG signals utilizing DWT for feature extraction and evolutionary algorithms for feature selection", *TechRxiv*, Vol. 55, p. 560, 2023. DOI: 10.36227/techrxiv.24633585.v1
18. Tyagi, A. K. (Ed.), *Privacy Preservation of Genomic and Medical Data*, John Wiley & Sons, 2023.
19. Din, I. U., Guizani, M., Rodrigues, J. J., Hassan, S., & Korotaev, V. V., "Machine learning in the Internet of Things: Designed techniques for smart cities", *Future Generation Computer Systems*, Vol. 100, pp. 826–843, 2019.
20. Khan, J. I., Khan, J., Ali, F., Ullah, F., Bacha, J., & Lee, S., "Artificial intelligence and internet of things (AI-IoT) technologies in response to COVID-19 pandemic: A systematic review", *IEEE Access*, Vol. 10, 62613–62660, 2022.

14 Convergence of AR, VR, IoT with Artificial Intelligence to Train Surgeons for Medical Surgeries

Rishabh Jha, Amrita Singh, and Arun Kumar Rana

CONTENTS

In the recent decade, the cases of brain-related fatalities have increased, although the medical sciences are constantly upgrading themselves, especially in low-income countries. One thing that has not been remarkably upgraded is related to the training of the surgeons who are still using the older prosthesis methods which have a low efficiency and high cost. Medical sciences have benefited from the advancement of cutting-edge technologies like augmented reality (AR), virtual reality (VR), the Internet of Things (IoT), and artificial intelligence (AI). AI and VR can help with the simulation of real-world case studies whereas sensor-based IoT can help execute the training to work in real time for these problems. The learnings can be even improved when the feedback is generated by an AI-based model. In this research, we are proposing a novel method in which an AR/VR-based learning tool for surgeons will be added up with sensors and IoT and later retrained with an AI-based platform. The main objective of this research is to increase the efficiency of surgeons. This will help to uplift the way brain surgeries, how they are performed, and how efficient they become!

 DOI: 10.1201/9781003476207-14

14.1 INTRODUCTION

The capacity of computers to carry out activities that ordinarily need human intelligence is known as AI, and its importance in the world is continually growing [1–7]. The medical field was slow to adopt AI. But AI in medicine is growing quickly, and, in the years to come, it promises to completely transform patient care. Moreover, technology has the power to democratize and make accessible top-notch medical care to everyone on the planet. Certain medical fields, like radiology, adopted AI rather quickly, whereas others, like pathology (and surgical pathology in particular), are only now starting to do so. AI holds great promise for improving cancer diagnosis, prognosis, and treatment. This chapter first defines the broad concepts of AI and then goes into great detail about how AI is now used in medicine. The current and future use of AI in surgical pathology is covered in depth in the second half of this thorough analysis, along with an explanation of the practical challenges and pathologists' concerns about being supplanted by computer algorithms. The benefits of AI in surgical pathology are emphasized [8–11].

14.1.1 Use of AR for Medical Applications

AR is that domain of digital technologies that combines digital information with a real-time environment made artificially for a surreal experience. This technology is used by medical professionals for various applications effectively for finding any hidden patterns in the visceral parts of the body which is otherwise hard to view using existing technologies. There are three potential applications in the case of surgeries: preoperative planning, intraoperative navigation, and surgical training. Preoperative planning is used to create 3D models of a patient's internal anatomy using medical imaging data. By using this surgeons [7] can understand the medical case better and plan the surgery better. Intraoperative navigation can be used during the time of surgery to understand the activities in real time in an even more advanced way. Similarly, actual surgery simulation can be given to trainees to provide an actual surgery environment and a better feedback system can be developed for the trainees [12–18].

14.1.2 Use of VR for Medical Applications

A rapidly evolving technology, VR has a wide range of potential uses in the medical field. VR is mostly used in three ways in surgery. Using data from medical imaging, VR can be used to build 3D reconstructions of a patient's anatomy [8]. Before making a single incision, this enables physicians to see the patient's unique anatomy and plan the procedure in great detail. This might lessen the possibility of complications and enhance the surgical procedure's overall result. VR can be utilized to produce accurate simulations of surgical operations for use in surgical training [19–24]. As a result, surgeons can practice difficult procedures without endangering patients. Surgical abilities can be evaluated and enhanced through VR training.

14.1.3 Use of IoT for Medical Applications

Healthcare is one of several industries being transformed by the IoT. IoT devices and technologies [8] are being used in surgery to increase patient safety, effectiveness,

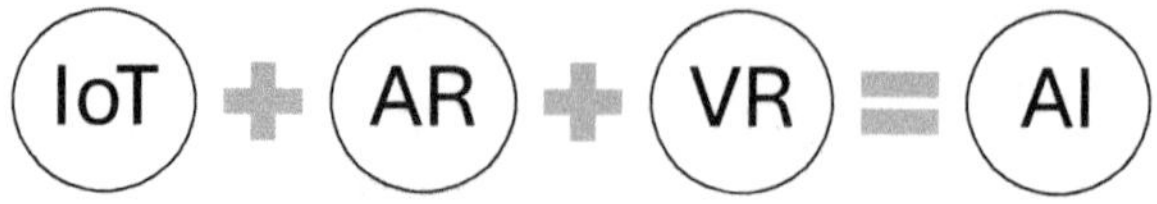

FIGURE 14.1 Convergence of AR, VR, and IoT with artificial intelligence.

and results. IoT-enabled robotic surgery equipment lets surgeons carry out intricate operations with more accuracy and precision. These systems give surgeons a magnified view of the surgical site and real-time feedback on their motions using cameras, sensors, and other gadgets. Surgery can be performed remotely on patients who are in remote or underserved locations thanks to IoT-enabled telemedicine technologies. These devices have sensors that record information on the force exerted, the properties of the tissue, and the temperature. This information can be utilized to give surgeons immediate feedback and aid in their decision-making during surgery. IoT-enabled platforms for surgical data analytics can be used to gather and examine information from many sources, including patient monitors, surgical robots, and smart surgical equipment. This information can be utilized to spot patterns, enhance surgical methods, and create novel surgical approaches [25–30]. Figure 14.1 shows the convergence of AR, VR, and IoT with AI.

14.2 EXISTING PROBLEMS IN NEUROSURGERY

Neurosurgery now faces a number of issues. Among the most typical are:

Complex Structure:

The brain and spine are complicated organs, and to operate on them safely, neurosurgeons must have a thorough understanding of their anatomy and function.

Complication Risk:

Neurosurgery is a high-risk field, and even minor issues can have severe effects on patients.

Access to care is restricted because neurosurgery is a specialized discipline, and there is a global lack of neurosurgeons. Patients may find it challenging to obtain neurosurgical care as a result, particularly in remote or underdeveloped locations.

High Cost of Care:

Due to the high expense of training neurosurgeons and the specific tools and supplies that they need, neurosurgery is an extremely expensive specialty.

The following are some actions being taken to solve the current issues in neurosurgery:

Research: To create novel and more effective techniques to treat neurological diseases, neurosurgeons, and other researchers are always working. New surgical procedures, new medications, and new medical equipment are all being developed as a result of this research.

Education: Medical schools and residency programs are working to increase the number of neurosurgeons. This will assist in solving the neurosurgeon shortage and improve patient access to neurosurgical care.

Technology: New tools are being created to assist neurosurgeons in operating more skillfully and securely. For instance, robotic surgery devices enable neurosurgeons to carry out intricate surgeries with increased accuracy and precision.

14.3 LITERATURE REVIEW

For the past two centuries imaging technologies have been used to understand the general anatomy of the human body. Especially in the case of trauma CT [2] is used to understand the nature of the wound and understand the condition better as described by Villarraga-Gómez, H et al in their research. This research has now evolved from medical imaging to the dimensional metrology. At present CT scans are not only used for dimensional inspection but also for geometric analysis so that any malformation inside the anatomy can be detected and further proceeded for the treatment.

A recent study by F. Cutolo has proposed the use of cutting-edge AR tools for image-guided surgeries. Human eyes and traditional tomography and imaging technologies have certain limitations which can be improved using the three-dimensional real-time image rendering capabilities of AR [3]. This imaging can not only be used for training purposes but also can act as surgical guidance in real time. This brings the concept of integrating in situ the surgeon's perceptive efficiency by using the AR tools and can heavily contribute toward medical surgeries which are mostly vulnerable at times.

Similarly, a relatively newer framework is also proposed at times: Medical Imaging in Extended Reality (MIXR) [4]. Extended reality is the combination of AR and mixed reality. Research by B. Allison et al. proposed an architecture of MIXR where they tried to utilize the power of AI, IoT, AR, mixed reality, and IoT.

AR has a clear efficiency when it comes to plastic surgeries [5] as explained by Y. Kim et. al. in their research. Various devices like head-mounted displays, haptic devices, and AR glasses were used to conduct the studies to study the patterns inside the skin tissues to conduct plastic surgeries. Moreover, research by G. Quero [6] conducted the use case of AR/VR tools and technologies on oncological liver cases which demonstrated the capability of these tools to understand the condition of hepatic tissues of the liver well.

14.4 RESEARCH METHODOLOGY

In this proposed research, first of all, the affected brain parts are to be digitally imagined by the existing tomography and medical imaging tools. A fine replication of the exact anatomy is to be obtained, which will require a fine reprinting into a completely new environment of AR/VR. Based on the imprint available, an architecture of MIXR is to be developed with clear interpretations. These interpretations are then divided into various regions based on the complexities and complications of surgeries. Figure 14.2 shows the proposed model.

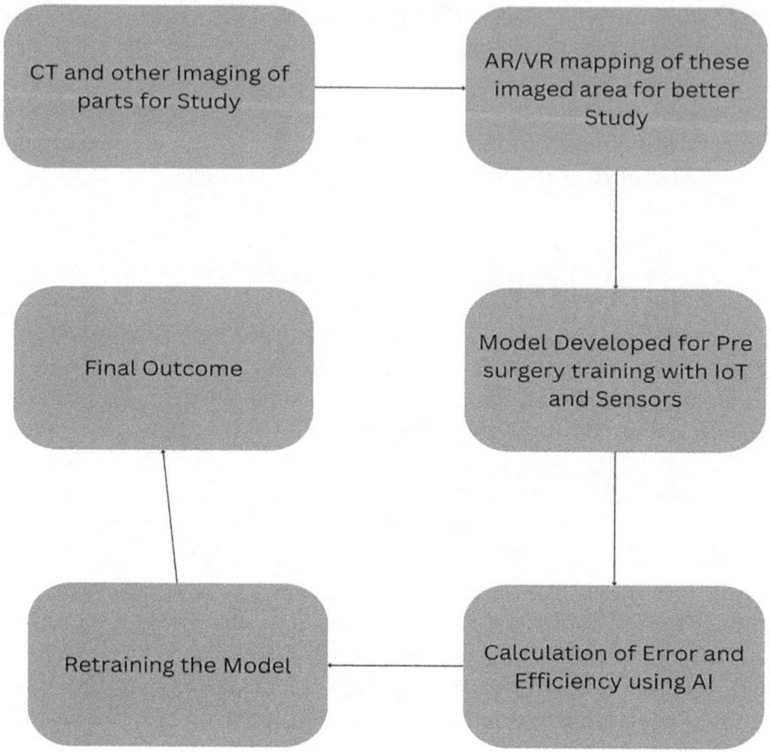

FIGURE 14.2 Proposed model.

This architecture is then supported by various AR/VR devices as well as IoT devices and sensors. This architecture should provide feedback and analysis in real time, which is the reason why IoT and the sensor-based system are used. This system then employs the use of AI and machine learning at two different levels. The first level will make use of a convolutional neural network to analyze the imaging and action by the surgeon during the period of training whereas a simple regression model will be used to find the actual efficiency at various jobs during surgery of the designated surgeon at another level. This model will then be used to retrain till a satisfying efficiency of the surgeon is not met.

14.5 CONCLUSION

The primary purpose of this research is to develop a system that could help surgeons to practice complex surgeries using the simulations beforehand. The complex jobs of surgeries can be benefited by using cutting-edge tools as mentioned in the research. It can also be a great learning method to train the resident surgery students as well as existing surgeons. In the near future, this system can help to increase the efficiency of surgeons as well as save many patients whose cases are complicated, and no conclusive evidence is available beforehand the surgery.

REFERENCES

1. Feigin, V. L., Vos, T., Nichols, E., *et al.*, 2020, March. The global burden of neurological disorders: Translating evidence into policy. *Lancet Neurology*, *19*(3), pp. 255–265. https://doi.org/10.1016/S1474-4422(19)30411-9. Epub 2019 Dec 5. PMID: 31813850; PMCID: PMC9945815.
2. Villarraga-Gómez, H., Herazo, E. L. and Smith, S. T., 2019. X-ray computed tomography: From medical imaging to dimensional metrology. *Precision Engineering*, *60*, pp. 544–569.
3. Cutolo, F., 2019. *Augmented Reality in Image-Guided Surgery.* IEEE.
4. Allison, B., Ye, X. and Janan, F., 2020, December. MIXR: A standard architecture for medical image analysis in augmented and mixed reality. In *2020 IEEE International Conference on Artificial Intelligence and Virtual Reality (AIVR)* (pp. 252–257). IEEE.
5. Kim, Y., Kim, H. and Kim, Y. O., 2017. Virtual reality and augmented reality in plastic surgery: A review. *Archives of Plastic Surgery*, *44*(03), pp. 179–187.
6. Quero, G., Lapergola, A., Soler, L., *et al.*, 2019. Virtual and augmented reality in oncologic liver surgery. *Surgical Oncology Clinics*, 28(1), pp. 31–44.
7. Dennler, C., Bauer, D. E., Scheibler, A. G., *et al.*, 2021. Augmented reality in the operating room: A clinical feasibility study. *BMC Musculoskeletal Disorder*, *22*, p. 451. https://doi.org/10.1186/s12891-021-04339-w
8. Khan, F. and Taekeun, W., 2022. Application of internet of things and sensors in healthcare. *Sensors (*Basel, Switzerland*)*, 22(15). https://doi.org/10.3390/s22155738
9. Rana, A., Sharma, S., Nisar, K., *et al.*, 2022. The Rise of Blockchain Internet of Things (BIoT): Secured, device-to-device architecture and simulation scenarios. *Applied Sciences*, 12(15), p. 7694.
10. Kumar, A., Sharma, S., Goyal, N., Singh, A., Cheng, X. and Singh, P., 2021. Secure and energy-efficient smart building architecture with emerging technology IoT. *Computer Communications*, *176*, pp. 207–217.
11. Kumar, A., Sharma, S., Singh, A., *et al.*, 2021. Revolutionary strategies analysis and proposed system for future infrastructure in internet of things. *Sustainability*, 14(1), p. 71.
12. Rana, A., Chakraborty, C., Sharma, S., Dhawan, S., Pani, S. K. and Ashraf, I., 2022. Internet of medical things-based secure and energy-efficient framework for health care. *Big Data*, 10(1), pp. 18–33.
13. Kumar, A. and Sharma, S., 2021. Internet of robotic things: Design and develop the quality of service framework for the healthcare sector using CoAP. *IAES International Journal of Robotics and Automation*, 10(4), p. 289.
14. Dhawan, S., Chakraborty, C., Frnda, J., Gupta, R., Rana, A. K. and Pani, S. K., 2021. SSII: Secured and high-quality steganography using intelligent hybrid optimization algorithms for IoT. *IEEE Access*, *9*, pp. 87563–87578.
15. Rana, S. K., Kim, H. C., Pani, S. K., Rana, S. K., Joo, M. I., Rana, A. K. and Aich, S., 2021. Blockchain-based model to improve the performance of the next-generation digital supply chain. *Sustainability*, 13(18), p. 10008.
16. Rana, A. K. and Sharma, S., 2021. Internet of things based stable increased-throughput multi-hop protocol for link efficiency (IoT-SIMPLE) for health monitoring using wireless body area networks. *International Journal of Sensors Wireless Communications and Control*, 11(7), pp. 789–798.
17. Kumar, A., Sharma, S., Goyal, N., Gupta, S. K., Kumari, S. and Kumar, S., 2022. Energy-efficient fog computing in Internet of Things based on Routing Protocol for Low-Power and Lossy Network with Contiki. *International Journal of Communication Systems*, 35(4), p. e5049.

18. Pandit, M., Gupta, D., Anand, D., *et al.*, 2022. Towards design and feasibility analysis of DePaaS: AI based global unified software defect prediction framework. *Applied Sciences*, 12(1), p. 493.
19. Lilhore, U. K., Imoize, A. L., Lee, C. C., *et al.*, 2022. Enhanced convolutional neural network model for cassava leaf disease identification and classification. *Mathematics*, 10(4), p. 580.
20. Rana, S. K., Rana, S. K., Nisar, K., Ag Ibrahim, A. A., Rana, A. K., Goyal, N. and Chawla, P., 2022. Blockchain technology and artificial intelligence based decentralized access control model to enable secure interoperability for healthcare. *Sustainability*, 14(15), p. 9471.
21. Rana, A. K. and Sharma, S., 2019. Enhanced energy-efficient heterogeneous routing protocols in WSNs for IoT application. *IJEAT*, 9(1), pp. 4418–4415.
22. Rana, A. K. and Sharma, S., 2021. Industry 4.0 manufacturing based on IoT, cloud computing, and big data: Manufacturing purpose scenario. In *Advances in Communication and Computational Technology* (pp. 1109–1119). Springer, Singapore.
23. Rana, A. K., Krishna, R., Dhwan, S., Sharma, S. and Gupta, R., 2019, October. Review on artificial intelligence with internet of things-problems, challenges and opportunities. In *2019 2nd International Conference on Power Energy, Environment and Intelligent Control (PEEIC)* (pp. 383–387). IEEE.
24. Negi, A. S., Gupta, P., Srivastava, R. and Rana, A. K., 2024, COVID-19 detection and pandemic prevention system using data science. In *Convergence of Blockchain and Internet of Things in Healthcare* (pp. 210–222). CRC Press.
25. Singh, I., Singh, B. and Rana, A. K., 2024, Role and impact of blockchain–IoT-enabled supply chain management model for medical supply. In *Convergence of Blockchain and Internet of Things in Healthcare* (pp. 54–67). CRC Press.
26. Dhawan, S., Bhuyan, H. K., Pani, S. K., Ravi, V., Gupta, R., Rana, A. and Al Mazroa, A., 2024. Secure and resilient improved image steganography using hybrid fuzzy neural network with fuzzy logic. *Journal of Safety Science and Resilience*, *5*(1), 91–101.
27. Bonkra, A., Bhatt, P. K., Rosak-Szyrocka, J., *et al.*, 2023. Apple leave disease detection using collaborative ML/DL and artificial intelligence methods: Scientometric analysis. *International Journal of Environmental Research and Public Health*, *20*(4), p. 3222.
28. Dhawan, S., Gupta, R., Bhuyan, H. K., Vinayakumar, R., Pani, S. K. and Rana, A. K., 2023. An efficient steganography technique based on S2OA & DESAE model. *Multimedia Tools and Applications*, 82(10), pp. 14527–14555.
29. Chahal, N., Bisht, R., Rana, A. K. and Srivastava, A., 2023. Robotic arm: Impact on industrial and domestic applications. In *Handbook of Computational Sciences: A Multi and Interdisciplinary Approach* (pp. 323–339). Wiley.
30. Jain, R., Dhingra, S., Joshi, K., Rana, A. K. and Goyal, N., 2023. Enhance traffic flow prediction with real-time vehicle data integration. *Journal of Autonomous Intelligence*, 6(2), p. 574.

15 An Overview of IoT and Machine Learning Approach in Healthcare

Niva Tripathy, Subhranshu Sekhar Tripathy, and Subhendu Kumar Pani

CONTENTS

15.1 INTRODUCTION

Nowadays, the Internet of Things (IoT) is transforming society in various aspects of society. This technology connects businesses and enables the optimization of systems across multiple industries [1]. There has been an increase in deployed IoT services in the past few years, bringing much value to operations and society [2]. Several areas have benefited from the use of IoT. For example, in transportation systems, there is the Internet of Vehicles (IoV) concept [3, 4]. In addition, several solutions have been proposed in the context of smart logistics [5]. Finally, there are other successful IoT applications in areas such as education [6] and agriculture [7]. In the last several years, the healthcare IT community has been very enthusiastic about the IoT. IoT offers an extensive range of options to improve the healthcare industry, which is a subject of tremendous practical importance. Many modern medical sensors and devices may connect to one another over a variety of networks, giving access to important information regarding patients' status. The aforementioned data can be employed for many functions, including remote patient monitoring, predicting disease and recovery by gaining a better understanding of symptoms and enhancing the diagnosis and treatment procedure through enhanced automation and mobility. An important component of the IoT is machine learning (ML), which gives IoT devices

DOI: 10.1201/9781003476207-15

intelligence, data processing, and information inference. ML is a potential technology that may be applied to several IoT application areas, ranging from embedded intelligence to cloud-based big data processing. Several surveys on ML and IoT were presented recently each of which covers a different aspect of ML in IoT as summarized in Table 15.1.

Thus, reviewing the literature on ML solutions for IoT security in healthcare is the primary objective of this study. In addition, this analysis is carried out with a dataset perspective, emphasizing resources, applications, and open challenges that are now available. Figure 15.1 describes the concept of a smart healthcare system. We want to draw attention to the state of the art in terms of IoT security datasets in

TABLE 15.1
Existing Work on IoT and ML for Smart Healthcare System

Ref	Concept Used	Description
[7]	Big data analytics	Using the concept of context-aware computing the changes in environmental conditions is identified
[8]	Deep learning	Basic concept of smart healthcare system using deep learning methodology
[9]	ML	Developing a reliable, secure, and energy-efficient ML model
[10]	IoT with big data	Developing deep learning model and streaming data for IoT-enabled healthcare system
[11]	Deep learning	Designing hardware model and algorithm for embedded deep learning method
[13]	ML	For image classification designing hardware-friendly and mixed-signal circuits using ML techniques

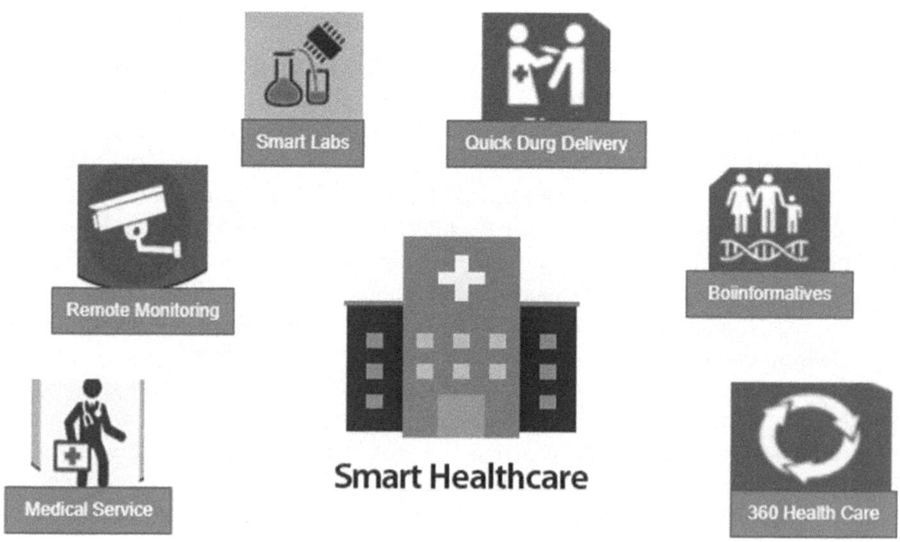

FIGURE 15.1 Concept of smart healthcare system.

healthcare [12] and the urgent need for new datasets to facilitate the creation of innovative solutions.

The main contributions of this research are:

- A comprehensive review of efforts on ML-based solutions for IoT security in healthcare.
- The unique methods, resources, future directions, data requirements, and supportive resources available (e.g., existing datasets, potential features, attacks, tools).
- An extensive investigation of open challenges regarding the proposal of new IoT security datasets in healthcare based on the data requirements of new endeavors.
- The opportunities are categorized into diversity, threats, reproducibility, and behavior and emphasize the current demand for extensive test beds, realistic scenarios (e.g., collection and data transmission), execution of attacks, and profiling experiments.

The rest of the sections are arranged as Section 15.2 illustrates the related work done on the IoT ML approach used in the healthcare domain; Section 15.3 describes the application, operation, and benefits of IoT in healthcare; Section 15.4 briefly describes the ML approach in healthcare and different ML algorithms used in prediction and classification; Section 15.5 describes the conclusion and future scope.

15.2 RELATED WORK

In this section we will give a detail of related work related to smart healthcare using IoT and ML. Different security considerations in smart healthcare systems were addressed by Habibzadeh et al. [14], along with their implications and preventative strategies. Latif et al. [15] analyze security and privacy concerns in IoT applications in smart cities using graph theory, and they also suggest remedies. Additionally, the author outlined problems since traditional methods do not yield the best outcomes for systems that are crucial to security and safety. The practical experiences and difficulties encountered by implementers globally have been explained by Arasteh et al. [16]. To improve the overall intelligence of smart cities based on data collection, privacy, security, public safety, disaster management, energy consumption, and quality of life in smart cities, Alsamhi et al. [17] presented an in-depth analysis of potential techniques and applications of collaborative drones with the IoT. These tools have recently been used. Based on fog computing, Kharel et al. [18] presented a model for a smart health monitoring system. According to the proposed architecture, a smart patient-centric healthcare system will replace the clinic-centric one by addressing its fundamental issues. An evaluation of the functions of deep reinforcement learning, ML, and artificial intelligence in the development of smart cities was conducted by Ullah et al. [19]. An efficient system for potential loss monitoring, traffic management, smart city innovations, digitalized and interconnected systems, and software was developed by Jha et al. [20]. For the future generation web and the IoT, Singh et al. [21] presented a distributed large data analysis framework for

ML and showed that it is more effective than other existing frameworks. Hathaliya et al. [22] review security and privacy issues in Healthcare 4.0. The authors focus on blockchain-based solutions and different taxonomies used in this context. Bharadwaj et al. [23] proposed a review of the role of ML in IoT applications in healthcare is presented. The authors focus on multiple aspects, including prognosis, diagnosis, and assistive systems. Security aspects are also considered alongside the constraints and drawbacks of each application. The authors Yempally et al. [24] present an overview of ML solutions in IoT medical data and suggest that model selection is vital to solve problems related to critical healthcare data. The authors Aldahiri et al. [25] present an overview of health monitoring systems using IoT and deep learning. Multiple sensors are listed alongside DL models, including the analysis of frameworks (e.g., tensorflow and keras). Bhuiyan et al. [26] present a review of applications, standards, protocols, and market opportunities from an IoT security standpoint in the context of healthcare. The authors classify existing IoT-based healthcare networks, analyze widely used IoT healthcare protocols, investigate aspects of IoT healthcare security, and propose a model for IoT healthcare security.

15.3 IoT IN HEALTHCARE

The IoT concept has been widely adopted recently. Furthermore, healthcare IoT solutions can potentially enhance medical treatments. IoT supports healthcare solutions in several ways. This technology can improve the accuracy of procedures [27], improve the decision-making process [28], and create new models of healthcare solutions. In addition, the benefits include the relationship between smart homes and the medical center.

Figure 15.2 shows the structure of IoT healthcare systems like bed management, BP checking, sugar control steps, smartwatch monitoring health, and Wi-Fi devices used for keeping track of the data. For example, using healthcare devices, real-time capturing, motion tracking, and emergency monitoring enable novel remote monitoring capabilities. They can also support the use of analytics and improve overall communication.

Figure 15.3 describes the operational steps used in healthcare systems. There are basically three common steps: data collection, which collects data from different sources, and data storage, which stores the large amount of data used for transmission. The last step is data preprocessing, which is used for analyzing data through different computing algorithms.

15.3.1 Technologies Used for IoT Healthcare System

- **Identification Technique**: Basically unique identifier is used to identify the node in the network. The information then can be accessed and communicated securely.
- **Communication Techniques**: The healthcare system needs both short- and long-distance communication. Short-term communication requires wireless communication like Bluetooth, zigbee, and RFID. Long-distance communication uses conventional ways like Internet.

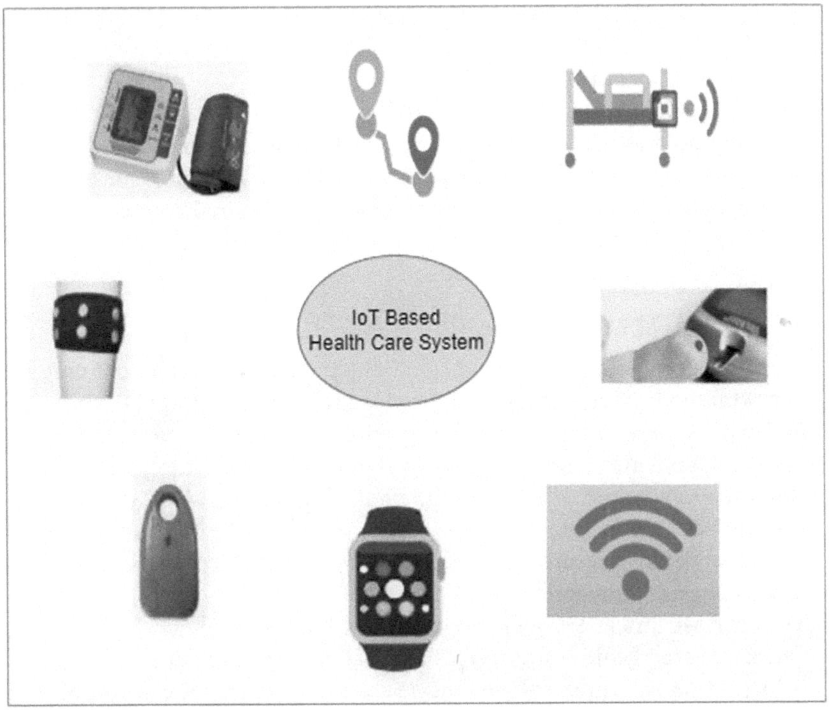

FIGURE 15.2 IoT healthcare system.

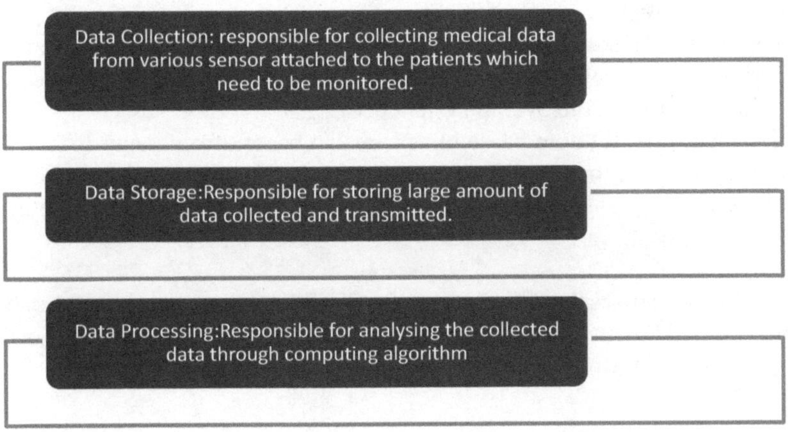

FIGURE 15.3 Operation steps of IoT healthcare system.

- **Location Technique**: To accurately track GPS is used to identify the location in a healthcare monitoring system.
- **Sensing Technique**: Real-time processing of a large volume of data, including alterations in the body in patients' bodies, is required. A wide range of

sensors can be used to collect this kind of data; these include gyroscopes, which measure angular velocity, accelerometers, which detect linear acceleration, and electrocardiogram (ECG) sensors, which record electrical activity in the heart.

- **Application-Level Technique**: The healthcare system allows various devices in the system to independently represent the state transfer. Each device's operations are mentioned clearly and can be altered as and when required without compromising the interoperability of the system.

15.3.2 Application of IoT Healthcare System

- **Remote Monitoring**: IoT healthcare system enables constant communication with medical centers. This system is more informed, quick, and effective in decision-making in different treatments and procedures.
- **Special Care**: IoT healthcare system for children and elderly people to be continuous and more effective with remote monitoring.
- **Health Record**: IoT healthcare system can support healthcare systems by providing detailed information about patients through continuous and more comprehensive data collection approaches.
- **Mobile Assistance**: Through the presence of multiple devices, IoT can enable customized healthcare services and availability to patients.
- **Information Systems**: IoT healthcare system can support the optimization of storage, access, and use of primary healthcare data in different ways.
- **Integrated Solutions**: Multimodal scenarios can also be considered, in which healthcare IoT healthcare applications can be part of an ecosystem composed of other applications (e.g., transportation and logistics).
- **Knowledge Resources**: In an IoT healthcare system, professionals can rely on wider awareness, short response times, and continuous data collection. This can improve the overall system performance.
- **Telemedicine**: Remote procedures can also benefit from using IoT healthcare systems. Although different mechanisms can be adopted depending on the procedure considered, IoT can potentially transform telemedicine in the next few years.

Figure 15.4 visualizes the different benefits of IoT healthcare systems. It can be used for rapid disease identification, smart treatment, proactive medical care, drug and medical equipment management, and error reduction in treatment at low cost.

15.4 ML IN SMART HEALTHCARE

ML is a phenomenon related to artificial intelligence. It gives a system the capacity to autonomously understand and evaluate a variety of inputs as an experience without further assistance [29]. Training and testing are two essential stages in the development of a successful predictive model. Providing labeled or unlabeled inputs to the system is part of the training phase, which is a highly research-intensive phase. For use in upcoming predictions, the system then keeps records of these training inputs

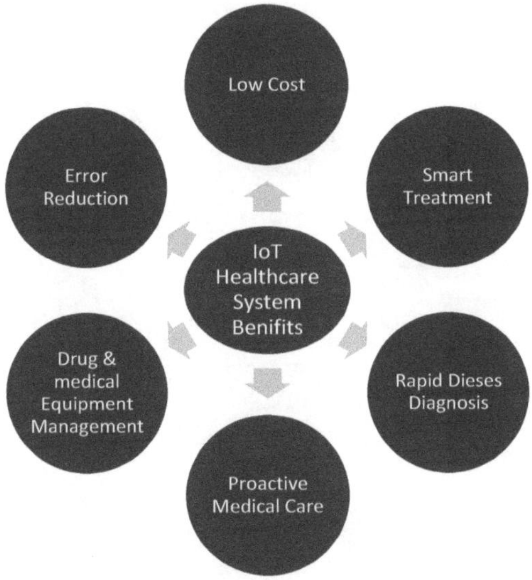

FIGURE 15.4 Benefits of IoT healthcare system.

in the feature space. The system must finally predict the proper output when it is fed an unlabeled input during the testing phase. Applications for ML in healthcare services have become increasingly common in recent years. Additionally, a lot of clinical decision support systems use these ML techniques to create refined learning models that improve applications for healthcare services. Applications of ML in healthcare services include Support Vector Machines (SVM) and artificial neural networks. To accurately diagnose the kind of cancer, these models are employed in a variety of cancer classification applications. The algorithms function by assessing the information gathered from various data sources and sensor devices. These algorithms determine a patient's behavioral patterns and medical issues.

Figure 15.5 shows the classification of different ML algorithms. It can be broadly divided into supervised, unsupervised, and reinforcement learning approaches.

a) Supervised Learning:
 In the supervised ML approach developer provides a prepared set of data to the training source. The model only recognizes the pattern. The objective of training data is to predict the value of one or many outcomes through the input features. The supervised learning approach uses to generate the data which latter work on its own way to generalizing the learning pattern. It needs larger-scale labeled data to be generated. The supervised learning approach is basically used for classification and regression purposes. In classification if the value does not fall in any group the missing value negatively affects the classification and prediction process. The teaching methods that need to be used can be decided based on the task. Figure 15.6 shows the detailed process of the supervised ML approach.

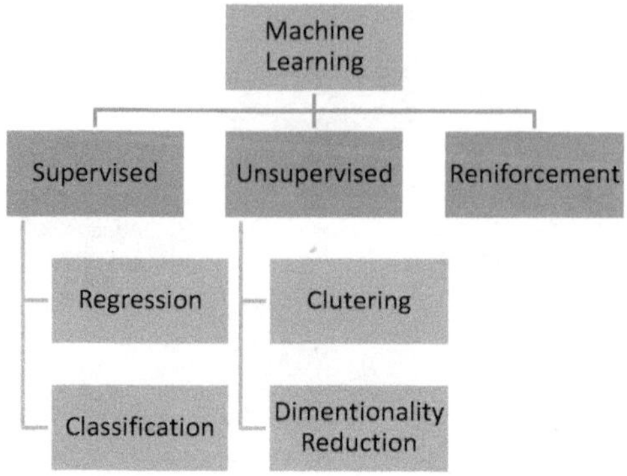

FIGURE 15.5 Classification of ML.

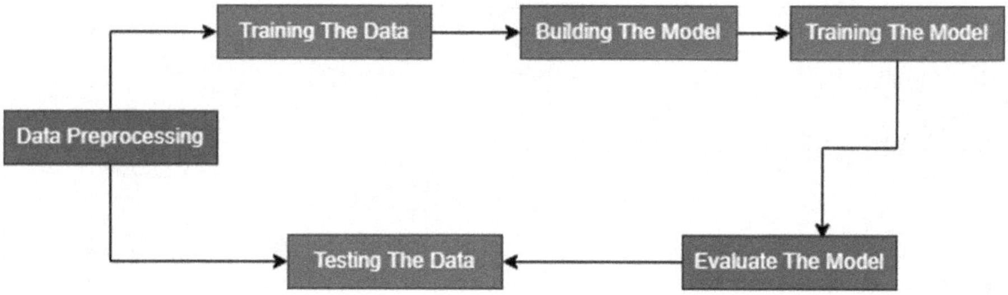

FIGURE 15.6 Supervised learning process.

b) Unsupervised learning
The unsupervised learning approach is used to identify the hidden structure of the unmarked data in the list. This approach is beneficial, but sometimes it is difficult to evaluate due to the lack of training dataset unavailability. So the model produces errors in such cases. It includes data transformation and clustering. In transformation process, the given data can be altered and presented in different ways so that it can be understood easily. In clustering the data can be grouped into relatable objects. The problem of the unsupervised approach is to evaluate the success of the algorithm, that is, whether it is useful or not. Figure 15.7 shows the unsupervised ML approach followed by a dataset to interpret the result.

c) Reinforcement learning
The reinforcement learning approach does not require any data before head. It follows trial and error method for output generation. Learning through interaction is the main basis of this approach. The main aim is to maximize the number of rewards generated. This approach executes the action, and in every step it received the feedback from environment. Due to this the system learns the consequences and can follow a long-term strategy to maximize the reward. Figure 15.8 shows the detailed process used in the reinforcement ML approach.

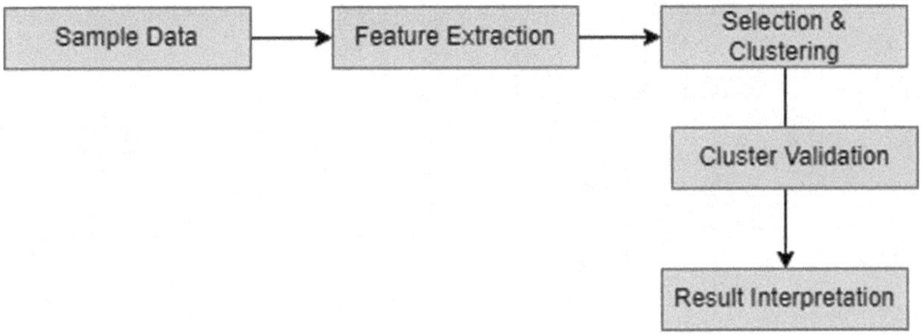

FIGURE 15.7 Unsupervised learning process.

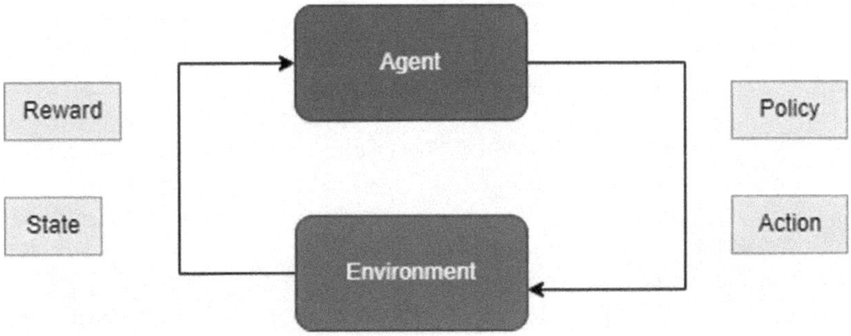

FIGURE 15.8 Reinforcement learning process.

Table 15.2 describes the comparative analysis of different learning approaches. It compares different data types used, the accuracy level of different approaches, and the cost of implementation.

Table 15.3 describes the commonly used ML algorithms. The uses of the algorithm and the methodology they are using for classification and working principle are clearly mentioned.

15.4.1 Application of ML in Healthcare

- **Medical Imaging**: It refers to the process of creating images of body parts for diagnostic purposes. Basically, it uses MRI and X-ray radiology [30]. Using ML and other emerging tools computer-aided disease prediction and video analysis are possible.
- **Disease Diagnostic**: using ML [31] it is easy to examine and find the physiological factors for disease diagnosis. It creates models that identify the risk factors associated with the signs and symptoms of disease.
- **Research in Clinical Trial**: ML allows the healthcare professionals to examine a large amount of data and the effectiveness involve in the extraction [32] of features from the data.
- **Electronic Health Record**: This can evaluate the vast amount of data to quantify and facilitate highlighting the improvement required [33]. Input data can be in the format of text, images, tables, and time series.

TABLE 15.2
Comparison of ML Approach

Learning Approach	Data Type Used	Accuracy	Cost
Supervised	Labeled	Low	Expensive
Unsupervised	Unlabeled	High	Inexpensive
Semi Supervised	Both labeled and unlabeled	Moderate	Moderate

TABLE 15.3
Commonly Used ML Algorithm

Algorithm	Used For	Method Used	Working
KNN	Classification, regression	Euclidian and Hamming distance	Non-parametric approach
NB	Classification	Continuous variables	Scanning of record by seeing individual feature
Decision Tree	Prediction	Continuous target variable	Handle categorial and continuous attributes
Random Forest	Classification, regression	Bagging	Correlation
Gradient-boosted Decision Tree	Classification, regression	Prepruning	Prediction performance iteratively increase
SVM	Binary and Nonlinear Classification	Decision boundary	Kernel trick used for effective high dimensional space

- **Pandemic Outbreak Prediction**: Using long short-term memory (LSTM) and DNN [34] model, it is easy to regulate and administrate healthcare data for pandemic outbreak prediction. This input data can feed to the ML model, and the ML model can learn from that to predict future trends.
- **Prediction of Heart Disease Rate**: ML has the capability to provide a protective strategy and evaluate patient data to forecast heart disease. Several ML algorithms like NB, SVM, and KNN [35] are used for managing heart disease prediction.
- **Personalized Care**: It provides patient-centric care. ML plays an important role in enabling personalized healthcare provision and discovering person-specific [36] diagnostics.
- **Chronic Illness Treatment**: ML has developed potential diagnostic care that uses a model that uses various AL [37] networks to recognize changes in certain patterns in patients.

15.4.2 Challenges and Opportunities

In this section we discussed challenges related to IoT ML-based healthcare systems. Further it is easy to identify the new domain in designing the systems:

a) **Resource Scarcity**: In IoT the devices used are sensors, smartphones, gateway, and so on having limited energy and computational capacity. Resource starvation is an issue. It can be resolved by integrating IoT with the cloud or fog computing paradigm. Several optimizations can be used to design the model that is lightweight and energy efficient.
b) **Security and Privacy**: As the healthcare domain is providing personalized facilities, there must be a provision in context to security privacy. Several underlying data aggregation techniques can be used. Designing a lightweight energy-efficient data management approach is useful for increasing the privacy of the domain.
c) **Interoperability**: In healthcare several hardware and software are used, which need global standardization. The domain must adopt the interoperability nature. It increases the throughput, minimizes unplanned outage, and reduces maintenance costs.
d) **Energy Management**: As healthcare devices are equipped with a limited energy supply, the cost of maintenance is high. For that a low-power, liable supply is preferable.
e) **Big Data Analytics**: As it contains a large amount of data, for any innovative IoT application, the data required are redundant and adversely affect the network performance. Using an optimal data storage location must emerge for a wide range of IoT applications.

15.5 CONCLUSION AND FUTURE SCOPE

This chapter briefly describes the IoT and ML approach in healthcare domain. The various advantages are described. The availability of smart devices adds value to healthcare domain. The patient can easily monitor their disease and diagnosis pattern to develop a quick and responsive cure. Several challenges associated with healthcare platforms are identified and solutions to overcome these challenges are studied. Moreover, computing paradigms like cloud computing and fog commuting can be a part of the efficient IoT healthcare domain. Further we can study several optimization approaches used in IoT-based healthcare.

REFERENCES

1. K. Rose, S. Eldridge, L. Chapin, The internet of things: An overview, *Internet Soc. (ISOC)* 80 (2015) 1–50.
2. L. Tan, N. Wang, Future internet: The internet of things, in: *2010 3rd International Conference on Advanced Computer Theory and Engineering (ICACTE)*, Vol. 5, IEEE, 2010, pp. V5–376.
3. F. Yang, S. Wang, J. Li, Z. Liu, Q. Sun, An overview of internet of vehicles, *China Commun.* 11 (10) (2014) 1–15.
4. B. Kaur, S. Dadkhah, F. Shoeleh, E.C.P. Neto, P. Xiong, S. Iqbal, P. Lamontagne, S. Ray, A.A. Ghorbani, Internet of Things (IoT) security dataset evolution: Challenges and future directions, *Internet Things* (2023) 100780.
5. Y. Ding, M. Jin, S. Li, D. Feng, Smart logistics based on the internet of things technology: An overview, *Int. J. Logist. Res. Appl.* 24 (4) (2021) 323–345.

6. D.D. Ramlowat, B.K. Pattanayak, Exploring the internet of things (IoT) in education: A review, in: *Information Systems Design and Intelligent Applications: Proceedings of Fifth International Conference* INDIA *2018*, Vol. 2, Springer, 2019, pp. 245–255.
7. C. Verdouw, S. Wolfert, B. Tekinerdogan, Internet of Things in agriculture, *CABI Rev.* (2016) (2016) 1–12.
8. R. De Michele, M. Furini, IoT healthcare: Benefits, issues and challenges, in: *Proceedings of the 5th EAI International Conference on Smart Objects and Technologies for Social Good*, IEEE, 2019, pp. 160–164.
9. Sundas, S. Badotra, S. Bharany, A. Almogren, E.M. Tag-ElDin, A.U. Rehman, Health-Guard: An intelligent healthcare system security framework based on ML, *Sustainability* 14 (19) (2022) 11934.
10. E.C.P. Neto, S. Dadkhah, R. Ferreira, A. Zohourian, R. Lu, A.A. Ghorbani, CICIoT2023: A real-time dataset and benchmark for large-scale attacks in IoT environment, *IEEE Access* 7 (2021) 106576–106584.
11. S. Dadkhah, H. Mahdikhani, P.K. Danso, A. Zohourian, K.A. Truong, A.A. Ghorbani, Towards the development of a realistic multidimensional IoT profiling dataset, in: *2022 19th Annual International Conference on Privacy, Security & Trust (PST)*, IEEE, 2022, pp. 1–11.
12. A.A. Hady, A. Ghubaish, T. Salman, D. Unal, R. Jain, Intrusion detection system for healthcare systems using medical and network data: A comparison study, *IEEE Access* 8 (2020) 106576–106584.
13. F. Hussain, S.G. Abbas, G.A. Shah, I.M. Pires, U.U. Fayyaz, F. Shahzad, N.M. Garcia, E. Zdravevski, A framework for malicious traffic detection in IoT healthcare environment, *Sensors* 21 (9) (2021) 3025.
14. H. Habibzadeh, T. Soyata, Toward uniform smart healthcare ecosystems: A survey on prospects, security, and privacy considerations, in: *Connected Health in Smart Cities*, Springer, 2019; ISBN: 9783665545.
15. S. Latif, N.A. Zafar, A survey of security and privacy issues in IoT for smart cities, in: *Proceedings of the 5th International Conference on Aerospace Science and Engineering ICASE*, Islamabad, Pakistan, 14–16 November 2017; pp. 1–5.
16. H. Arasteh, V. Hosseinnezhad, V. Loia, A. Tommasetti, O. Troisi, M. Shafie-Khah, P. Siano, IoT-based smart cities: A survey, in: *Proceedings of the EEEIC 2016 International Conference on Environment and Electrical Engineering*, Florence, Italy, 7–10 June 2016; pp. 2–7.
17. S.H. Alsamhi, O. Ma, M.S. Ansari, F.A. Almalki, Survey on collaborative smart drones and internet of things for improving smartness of smart cities, *IEEE Access* 7 (2019) 128125–128152.
18. J. Kharel, H.T. Reda, S.Y. Shin, An architecture for smart health monitoring system based on fog computing, *J. Commun.* 12 (2017) 228–233.
19. Z. Ullah, F. Al-Turjman, L. Mostarda, R. Gagliardi, Applications of artificial intelligence and ML in smart cities, *Comput. Commun.* 154 (2020) 313–323.
20. S. Jha, L. Nkenyereye, G.P. Joshi, E. Yang, Mitigating and monitoring smart city using internet of things, *Comput. Mater. Contin.* 65 (2020) 1059–1079.
21. S.K. Singh, J. Cha, T.W. Kim, J.H. Park, ML based distributed big data analysis framework for next generation web in IoT, *Comput. Sci. Inf. Syst.* 18 (2021).
22. J.J. Hathaliya, S. Tanwar, An exhaustive survey on security and privacy issues in Healthcare 4.0, *Comput. Commun.* 153 (2020) 311–335.
23. H.K. Bharadwaj, A. Agarwal, V. Chamola, N.R. Lakkaniga, V. Hassija, M. Guizani, B. Sikdar, A review on the role of ML in enabling IoT based healthcare applications, *IEEE Access* 9 (2021) 38859–38890.
24. S. Yempally, S.K. Singh, S. Velliangiri, Analytical review on deep learning and IoT for smart healthcare monitoring system, *Int. J. Intell. Unmanned Syst.* (ahead-of-print) (2022)

25. A. Aldahiri, B. Alrashed, W. Hussain, Trends in using IoT with ML in health prediction system, *Forecasting* 3 (1) (2021) 181–206.
26. M.N. Bhuiyan, M.M. Rahman, M.M. Billah, D. Saha, Internet of things (IoT): A review of its enabling technologies in healthcare applications, standards protocols, security, and market opportunities, *IEEE Internet Things J.* 8 (13) (2021) 10474–10498.
27. M. Javaid, I.H. Khan, Internet of Things (IoT) enabled healthcare helps to take the challenges of COVID-19 pandemic, *J. Oral Biol. Craniofac. Res.* 11 (2) (2021) 209–214.
28. P. Keikhosrokiani, IoT for enhanced decision-making in medical information systems: A systematic review, in: *Enhanced Telemedicine and e-Health: Advanced IoT Enabled Soft Computing Framework*, Springer, 2021, pp. 119–140.
29. H.U. Dike, Y. Zhou, K.K. Deveerasetty, Q. Wu, Unsupervised learning based on artificial neural network: A review, in: *Proceedings of the 2018 IEEE International Conference on Cyborg and Bionic Systems (CBS)*, Shenzhen, China, 25–27 October 2018; pp. 322–327.
30. M. Kim, J. Yun, Y. Cho, K. Shin, R. Jang, H.-J. Bae, N. Kim, Deep learning in medical imaging, *Neurospine* 16 (2019) 657–668.
31. J. Xu, K. Xue, K. Zhang, Current status and future trends of clinical diagnoses via image-based deep learning, *Theranostics* 9 (2019) 7556–7565.
32. S. Michie, J. Thomas, S.-T. John, P. Mac Aonghusa, J. Shawe-Taylor, M.P. Kelly, L.A. Deleris, A.N. Finnerty, M.M. Marques, E. Norris, et al. The human behaviour-change project: Harnessing the power of artificial intelligence and ML for evidence synthesis and interpretation, *Implement. Sci.* 12 (2017) 1–12.
33. P. Shah, F. Kendall, S. Khozin, R. Goosen, J. Hu, J. Laramie, M. Ringel, N. Schork, Artificial intelligence and ML in clinical development: A translational perspective, *NPJ Digit. Med.* 2 (2019) 1–5.
34. S. Chae, S. Kwon, D. Lee, Predicting infectious disease using deep learning and big data, *Int. J. Environ. Res. Public Health* 15 (2018) 1596.
35. Y. Yan, J.-W. Zhang, G.-Y. Zang, J. Pu, The primary use of artificial intelligence in cardiovascular diseases: What kind of potential role does artificial intelligence play in future medicine? *J. Geriatr. Cardiol. JGC* 16 (2019) 585–591.
36. J. Wilkinson, K.F. Arnold, E.J. Murray, M. van Smeden, K. Carr, R. Sippy, M. de Kamps, A. Beam, S. Konigorski, C. Lippert, et al., Time to reality check the promises of ML-powered precision medicine, *Lancet Digit. Health* 2 (2020) e677–e680.
37. S. Bloch-Budzier, NHS using Google technology to treat patients, *BBC News*, 22 November 2016; p. 22.

16 Healthcare Unbound

Navigating Emerging Trends and Future Applications in IoT-Based Innovations for Daily Well-Being

Mrunalini H. Kulkarni and Poonam R. Inamdar

CONTENTS

16.1 INTRODUCTION

The Internet of Things (IoT) represents a network of interconnected and Internet-enabled objects designed to autonomously collect and exchange data across global wireless networks, eliminating the need for human intervention. This transformative technology has undergone remarkable growth, propelled by continuous technological advancements that cater to the escalating demand for real-time insights in the realm

DOI: 10.1201/9781003476207-16

of digital transformation solutions. The pervasive digitalization of various aspects of our lives has seen a significant surge, facilitated by the widespread availability of affordable resources, ensuring accessibility to a broad spectrum of individuals. Projections indicate a staggering 64 billion IoT devices by 2025, underscoring the profound impact and widespread adoption of this technology. In the realm of the latest IT industry technologies, artificial intelligence (AI) and the IoT frequently take the forefront, seamlessly complementing each other. This powerful duo has spearheaded a revolution in traditional industrial and corporate solutions, ushering in a new era of innovation and efficiency. The chapter focuses mainly on applications of Health-IoT (H-IoT) in daily healthcare (1).

16.2 H-IoT AND HEALTHCARE SYSTEM

The key steps in harnessing the potential of healthcare-specific IoT products. The steps involved in the development of robust architecture include interconnected devices, such as sensors, monitors, actuators, detectors, and camera systems, which are deployed in healthcare settings. These devices gather a diverse range of data, including patient vitals, environmental conditions, and other relevant parameters. Data Aggregation and Conversion, the data collected by devices is often in analog form, and this step involves aggregating and converting it into a digital format. It is crucial for standardization and compatibility across different devices and systems. Preprocessing and Standardization to ensure that the data is consistent and ready for further analysis, reducing variability and enhancing reliability. The standardized data is then transferred to a data center or cloud environment. Cloud storage and computing resources offer scalability, accessibility, and centralization, enabling efficient management of large volumes of healthcare data. The integration of IoT technologies in healthcare brings forth comprehensive support for patients, physicians, hospitals, caregivers, and insurance providers. This transformative approach enhances various facets of the healthcare ecosystem, fostering improved patient care, streamlined medical processes, and enhanced communication among stakeholders. From remote patient monitoring and smart medical devices to hospital asset management and predictive maintenance, IoT applications contribute to a more efficient and personalized healthcare experience (2). Additionally, the incorporation of IoT facilitates advancements in telehealth services, medication adherence, data analytics, and decision support, ultimately leading to better patient outcomes. Furthermore, the utilization of IoT in insurance and risk management ensures a more tailored approach to healthcare coverage. As the healthcare industry embraces these technologies, considerations for security and privacy remain paramount to safeguard sensitive patient information. In essence, the adoption of IoT in healthcare is a multifaceted strategy that positively impacts the entire healthcare ecosystem.

16.3 H-IoT IN BIG DATA ANALYTICS

The H-IoT framework plays a pivotal role in H-IoT analytics in the diagnosis and prediction of diseases in prescriptive and descriptive analytics (3). With an unprecedented proliferation of IoT objects, the ensuing deluge of data poses both a challenge and an opportunity. The need for effective decision-making and knowledge discovery in this data-rich environment has paved the way for the development of cognitive IoT frameworks. As large-scale industrial automation burgeons, the quantity of IoT objects is set to reach astronomical figures, potentially generating trillions of data points amounting to thousands of exabytes. Managing this colossal volume of data becomes a pivotal aspect of deriving actionable insights and making informed decisions. Traditional data storage and processing mechanisms often fall short of addressing the real-time requirements of applications, necessitating the advent of advanced frameworks. Cognitive IoT frameworks are designed to meet the dynamic demands of large-scale industrial automation by incorporating intelligent decision-making processes. These frameworks go beyond mere data storage and retrieval, actively engaging in real-time data collection and information extraction. By leveraging machine learning algorithms and AI, cognitive IoT frameworks enable systems to adapt, learn, and evolve, thereby enhancing the decision-making capabilities required for complex industrial scenarios. By embracing information management frameworks and incorporating ontology-based modeling mechanisms, organizations can navigate the complexities of IoT data and unlock a new realm of possibilities in the pursuit of efficiency, innovation, and sustainable growth. Different machine learning algorithms are used for the prediction of acute and chronic diseases. Table 16.1 highlights various tools used in big data analytics applied to H-IoT architecture (4, 5).

16.4 H-IoT IN SOFTWARE-DEFINED NETWORKING

In the realm of network management, a software-defined approach has revolutionized the conventional administration model by allowing the regulation of network nodes through language programming. This departure from traditional methods addresses various limitations of the IoT by leveraging Software-Defined Networks (SDNs). SDNs contribute to network virtualization, efficient network management, energy optimization, resource utilization, as well as addressing privacy and security concerns through the separation of hardware device control.

The primary function of an SDN lies in the separation of the configuration plane from the user plane, streamlining network performance. In a notable work by the authors of, a secured framework was proposed for IoT Device Verification using endpoint platforms equipped with a lightweight authentication system. Following verification, these devices retrieve data from respective patients and transmit it to end user for accumulation, computation, and evaluation. The interconnected endpoint platforms are coordinated by a Network Virtualization Controller, responsible for bandwidth optimization, traffic distribution and utilization efficiency improvement. Evaluation through computer simulations demonstrated superior outcomes.

In the context of medical data security, particularly for confidential reports stored in the cloud, the system is designed to combat network security attacks. Immediate alerts are sent to medical workers, enabling control over various diseases. The proposed SDN-based framework ensures that each patient has an exclusive Virtual Server, capable of being released to disseminated to Permitted Users furthermore, the server is safeguarded by a Secure Software-Defined Network Channel acting as a firewall, guaranteeing privacy and permitted to consumer via virtual machines

TABLE 16.1
Tools Used in Big Data Analytics Applied to H-IoT Architecture (4, 5)

S. No	Tools	Application
1	Apache Hadoop	It serves as a robust solution for managing extensive datasets.
2	Apache Pig	Its functionality contributes to the seamless handling and manipulation of data flows.
3	Apache HBase	An open-source, and NoSQL database written in Java, serves as a scalable solution tailored for large datasets. It provides a robust and flexible framework for managing and storing data efficiently.
4	Apache Spark	A sophisticated programming interface designed for managing clusters. It incorporates implicit data parallelism and fault tolerance, making it a valuable tool for distributed computing tasks.
5	Splunk	It features a user-friendly interface, making it an asset for effectively interpreting and utilizing data.
6	Map reduce	MapReduce provides a versatile interface for distributing sub-tasks and collecting outputs. It plays a pivotal role in tracking the computation of machine-interconnected units during execution, contributing to efficient parallel processing.
7	PIG	PIG is a programming language designed to consolidate diverse Information. It comprises the Pig Latin language and a runtime version for seamless execution of code.
8	Hive	Hive leverages Structured Query Language within the Hadoop platform. It streamlines data processing tasks efficiently.
9	Jaql	Jaql is a functional query language designed for processing huge data repositories, facilitating concurrent computing for enhanced efficiency.
10	Zookeeper	It enables Complex Data Interpretation Platforms to use this assistance to coordinate simultaneous processing over extensive clusters.
11	HBase	It is particularly well-suited for scenarios involving real-time data processing or the need for random read/write access to substantial volumes of data. The design allows for rapid access to particular data points, optimizing the performance of retrieving individual rows and columns.
12	Cassandra	NoSQL databases demonstrate exceptional capabilities in real-time data processing, a pivotal necessity in the healthcare sector. Healthcare providers can harness the power of these databases to handle streaming data emanating from wearable devices. This allows them to closely monitor the vital signs of patients in real-time and promptly initiate alerts in the case of critical conditions.
13	Oozie	It integrates with the Hadoop stack and allows for streamlined workflow management, enhancing the overall efficiency of data processing tasks within the Hadoop ecosystem. Oozie acts as an orchestration tool, enabling the coordination and execution of diverse jobs in a structured sequence, contributing to a more organized and manageable data processing workflow.
14	Avro	It can be integrated with other AI tools like Hadoop for generating E-Health records, and radiology for diagnosis and treatment.

(*Continued*)

TABLE 16.1 (*Continued*)
Tools Used in Big Data Analytics Applied to H-IoT Architecture (4, 5)

S. No	Tools	Application
15	Mahout	This powerful toolset encompasses a wide range of libraries and algorithms, making it an invaluable resource for leveraging machine learning techniques to tackle intricate business challenges. With Mahout, users gain access to tools that facilitate the analysis of large volumes of data, enabling the extraction of meaningful insights and the development of solutions for complex problems. It finds application in data processing, analysis, or optimization to predict the outcomes and early detection of diseases.

with unique Network Identifiers. This innovative approach aims to enhance overall network security and privacy, especially in the critical domain of healthcare.

The application of SDN in healthcare has brought about transformative advancements, impacting various facets of the industry. One prominent area is the facilitation of remote patient monitoring, telemedicine, and telehealth services, wherein SDN plays a pivotal role in ensuring efficient and secure connectivity. The integration of Healthcare IoT further benefits from SDN, encompassing device connectivity and management, as well as network automation to streamline resource management. In the realm of hospital network management, SDN proves instrumental in traffic prioritization, network resource optimization, and the establishment of a scalable infrastructure tailored for telemedicine applications. The centralized management of medical devices and equipment is streamlined, ensuring efficient data transfer and storage for electronic health records (EHR). Notably, SDN's contribution extends to Quality of Service management, offering granular control over parameters. This allows prioritization of critical healthcare applications, including EHR systems and diagnostic imaging services. Furthermore, SDN optimizes unified communications systems, facilitating seamless communication among medical staff while prioritizing essential voice and video traffic. In disaster recovery planning, SDN's dynamic rerouting capabilities prove invaluable, ensuring continuous access to critical healthcare applications in emergencies or network failures. This comprehensive integration of SDN in healthcare underscores its role in enhancing efficiency, security, and resilience within the healthcare ecosystem.

16.5 H-IoT IN NETWORK FUNCTION VIRTUALIZATION (6)

Network Functions (VNFs). This strategic decoupling brings forth a host of advantages, foremost among them being a momentous decline in both financial funding and running costs. Moreover, Network Function Virtualization (NFV) introduces a heightened level of service flexibility, enabling more elastic and adaptable service provisioning.

The advent of NFV has sparked a remarkable development and, in some cases, a technological revolution in the realm of network-based services. Notably, it contributes to a substantial decrease in deployment costs for network operators. This cost reduction is attributed to the lowering of hardware tool costs, decreased energy consumption, and an overall enhancement of operational performance, where network configuration becomes a focal point of optimization.

Despite these substantial benefits, the implementation of NFV does not come without its challenges, particularly in the realm of security. The focus in NFV research and development is dedicated to addressing potential security issues that may arise from the virtualization of network functions. As NFV continues to advance, addressing and mitigating these security concerns will be imperative to fully harness its revolutionary potential in optimizing network infrastructure and services.

16.6 H-IoT IN INTERNET OF NANO THINGS (IONT) (7–15)

One pivotal driver behind the adoption of IoNT in healthcare is the escalating urgency for rapid and miniaturized Portable Diagnostics. The breakthroughs facilitated by IoNT could transform healthcare practices, allowing doctors to monitor patients in real-time and eliminating the need for manual measurements as in traditional approaches.

A noteworthy example of IoNT application is the Body Sensor Network (BSN), wherein various embedded Physiological Monitors provide invaluable insights and diagnostically relevant data. These data points often transcend the capabilities of traditional diagnostic methods. The utilization of nanoscale biosensors in BSN not only grants surgeons access to previously inaccessible aspects of the human body's internal workings but also opens avenues for monitoring and tracking vital signs, diagnosing, and treating diseases, and delivering targeted therapies to specific areas. Moreover, nanodevices have the potential to detect the early stages of diseases, prompting appropriate responses such as releasing therapeutic agents and enhancing smart medication management. The IoNT's transformative impact on healthcare holds the promise of ushering in a new era of precision diagnostics and personalized patient care.

16.7 H-IoT IN EDGE COMPUTING AND BLOCKCHAIN TECHNOLOGY (16, 17)

The integration of edge-computing processors directly into medical devices represents a pivotal advancement in healthcare technology, enabling simultaneous data collection and processing at the source. This approach significantly reduces latency, thereby enhancing the performance and accuracy of applications utilizing health data. In the healthcare industry, the implementation of edge intelligence has paved the way for a variety of applications and services, notably including real-time monitoring and analysis of patient data from wearable devices such as smartwatches and fitness trackers. This facilitates the early detection of signs of illness or disease, as well as applications like telesurgery.

Recent trends in edge computing have played a crucial role in developing effective healthcare applications, particularly in the domain of distant patient surveillance through master cloud servers. This paradigm necessitates patient treatment excellence, with elevated recognition sensitivity, and precise imagery, with a particular emphasis on prioritizing the latter. Algorithms Window-based Rate Control Algorithm (W-RCA) is a promising solution and optimizes patient treatment excellence in edge computing. Comparative evaluations, including benchmarking against prevailing algorithms like the Battery Smoothing Algorithm, demonstrated the superior performance of the suggested W-RCA in optimizing applications such as telesurgery.

The integration of cutting-edge edge-computing architectures, exemplified by the Highly Intelligent Cloud Healthcare (HiCH) framework, and the utilization of comprehensive datasets like mHealth rapidly evolving landscape in E-healthcare. This transformative synergy is marked by the application of machine learning techniques, ushering in a new era of precision and efficiency in healthcare monitoring. The HiCH architecture, with its intelligence-driven approach, stands as a paradigm for intelligent healthcare, offering innovative solutions for continuous health monitoring.

The mHealth dataset, renowned for its richness and diversity, emerges as a crucial asset, providing a robust foundation for training machine learning models. The application of machine learning techniques within the HiCH architecture, fuelled by the mHealth dataset, enhances the capabilities of health monitoring systems, enabling tasks such as anomaly detection, predictive analysis, and personalized health insights. (18–20)

16.8 APPLICATIONS OF IoT IN HEALTHCARE

16.8.1 Remote Patient Monitoring in Chronic Diseases (21)

The intersection of innovative wireless communication technologies with internal body sensing and the proliferation of the IoT has given rise to a paradigm shift in healthcare. These technological advancements are instrumental in introducing modern healthcare schemes aimed at providing personalized health management and preventing acute and chronic diseases. The seamless integration of IoT, cloud computing and intelligent machines has ushered in a new era of healthcare innovation, particularly in the realm of remote patient monitoring. Various illnesses, ranging from metabolic disorders like diabetes, obesity, coronary heart disease, neurological disorders melanoma and other cancers, and blood disorders to vital parameters, can now be monitored and managed remotely with unprecedented precision. The utilization of smart sensors and intelligent decision-making technologies facilitates the remote monitoring of patients, not only during the post-operative phase but also for elderly patients. These transformative technologies not only enhance the efficiency of healthcare delivery but also contribute significantly to preventive care and the overall well-being of individuals, marking a substantial leap forward in the evolution of healthcare practice.

16.8.2 Wearable Fitness Healthcare Trackers and Connected Medical Devices (22, 23)

The integration of the IoT into the healthcare sector has manifested significantly in the domain of fitness tracking through wearable devices, readily available in the consumer electronics market. This application primarily revolves around smart wristbands, which serve as comprehensive health monitors capable of tracking motion, physical exercise, calories burned, vision recovery, visualization of the digestive tract, as well as monitoring pulse and cardiac activity. In the architecture of these wearables, the device layer acts as the input interface, facilitating communication between the individual and the proximal compute engine in a tripartite framework. The on-site processed information is then seamlessly transmitted data repository for retention. Users can distantly access this database to monitor and manage their vital signs. The devices employed in this framework encompass a range of health-related metrics, including pulse, temperature, SpO_2 monitoring, slumber stage analysis, stress level assessment, emotional well-being tracking, implanted devices for drug delivery, and even menstrual cycle tracking. Recognizable brands in this realm, such as Apple, Samsung Galaxy, Fitbit Charge, and Garmin Venu, have contributed to the popularity and widespread adoption of IoT-enabled fitness tracking devices, fostering a paradigm shift in personalized healthcare management.

16.8.3 Smart Pill Dispensers (24)

Dose non-compliance or mismanagement, including missing doses, incorrect dosage, or improper timing of medication intake, poses a significant concern, particularly among elderly patients or those grappling with serious illnesses, and can potentially result in severe outcomes. To address this issue, medicine dispensers play a crucial role in ensuring adherence to prescribed medication schedules. Smart Pill dispensers, equipped with special alarms, serve as advanced solutions to remind patients when it is time to take their medication or alert them to renew their prescriptions. A notable example is the Smart Medication Dispenser, which seamlessly connects to Bluetooth and features an Automatic Lock Box with 28 sealed pill compartments. This innovative technology not only provides timely reminders but also ensures secure and accurate medication delivery, enhancing patient adherence and ultimately contributing to improved health outcomes. Examples include Comfytemp, MedCenter 4 Alarm Medication Reminder, Fullicon Electronic Pill Reminder, T.O.G. Electronic Pill Dispenser Smart Alarm Vibration for Vitamins Elderly Blue, e-pill Medication Reminders, e-Pill MedSmart Voice Bluetooth Locked Automatic Pill Dispenser, Premsons 7 Days Pill Medicine Organizer with 28 Compartments with Reminder Alarm, and Generic Lcd Digital Pill Medicine Case Box Alarm Reminder Container Timer.

16.8.4 Telemedicine with Virtual Consultations with Healthcare Providers (25–29)

The application of telemedicine spans a diverse range of uses, significantly transforming the healthcare landscape. This innovative approach includes online patient consultations, remote control functionalities, telehealth nursing services, and remote physical and psychiatry rehabilitation. The prominence of virtual consultations through telemedicine gained widespread recognition during the COVID-19 pandemic. Among the myriad advantages, time savings became evident due to reduced travel and waiting times, coupled with improved accessibility and convenience. Telemedicine proved to be cost-efficient, enabling easier monitoring of discharged patients and effective management of their recovery processes. This approach facilitates services to disabled patients and proves particularly effective for disorders that do not necessitate laboratory examinations. Moreover, it aids in digital health monitoring, enabling the tracking of patients' medication adherence and providing a secure means of care for immune-compromised individuals. The multifaceted benefits of telemedicine underscore its potential to revolutionize healthcare delivery and accessibility.

16.8.5 Smart Home Healthcare Devices for Elderly Care (30–32)

The healthcare landscape for elderly patients is evolving, emphasizing the importance of immediate medical intervention and continuous monitoring of their physiological parameters and activities to avert potential emergencies. In emergency cases, the traditional approach involves seeking in-patient care, which, while effective, can impose a substantial financial burden, particularly with extended hospital stays. The emergence of remote health monitoring within smart home platforms presents a transformative solution, allowing individuals to age comfortably in their familiar home environments rather than being confined to expensive and often limited nursing homes or hospitals. Smart homes, equipped with unobtrusive environmental and physiological sensors and actuators, facilitate remote monitoring of both the home environment and essential physiological signs. This includes features such as fall detection systems, motion awareness, and specialized considerations for disabled patients. Various platforms, such as Dexter Net, EnViBo, and Closer, showcase the diversity of applications within smart homes. Numerous wireless technologies, ranging from RFID and Bluetooth to BLE, ZigBee, WiFi, and more, provide insights in connection with the overall fitness status and sustained vigilance over the aging Population. The integration of these technologies not only enhances the quality of care for elderly occupants but also promotes independence and cost-effective alternatives to traditional in-patient care.

16.8.6 IoT-Enabled Medical Imaging and Diagnostics (33–37)

Machine learning algorithms play a pivotal role in the diagnosis and prediction of various chronic diseases, contributing significantly to advancements in healthcare. An intelligent Internet of Medical Things framework has been widely implemented, particularly in the analysis of medical images for conditions such as blood cancer and lung diseases, notably during the COVID-19 pandemic. Multi-sensor platforms further enhance diagnostic capabilities by extracting vital physiological parameters, such as blood pressure, and capturing patterns in electrocardiogram (ECG) recordings to predict heart diseases. Emotion recognition patterns have also been extracted using various AI tools like MapReduce and Spark, particularly in the context of analyzing brain images (EEG) for epilepsy detection and sleep disorders and utilizing CT, MRI, and PET scans for the detection of bone-related issues and tumors. The integration of multi-sensor fusion and a cross-domain incremental classifier approach further refines medical human–robot interactions, highlighting the diverse applications of AI in the healthcare domain.

16.8.7 Intelligent Hospitals and Remote Surgery and Robot-Assisted Procedures (38–44)

The landscape of minimally invasive surgery has witnessed a transformative shift with the emergence of surgical robots, which have become a benchmark for excellence in medical centers. Despite the current challenges associated with practical applications, surgical robots are increasingly viewed as essential tools for achieving excellence in minimally invasive procedures. Notable FDA-approved robotic systems such as Prodoc, ROBODOC, da Vinci, Zeus, Mako, OMNIBot, Mazor X Stealth, NEOCIS, CARLO, Avatera, Symani system, EPIONE, TiRobot, Canady Flex RoboWrist, R-One, Niobe, MUSA Galen Robotics Platform, LBR Med are at the forefront of this technological evolution, facilitating video-assisted surgeries and telesurgeries. The advantages of surgical robots include their capacity for good geometric accuracy, stability, untiring precision, diverse control centers, sterilization capabilities, and resistance to infection. These robotic systems have found applications in a variety of surgical procedures, ranging from antireflux procedures, cholecystectomies, hysterectomy, and cardiac surgeries to hernia repair, orthopedic surgeries, neurosurgery, dental surgery, prostate, kidney, and liver tumors, diabetic foot surgery, ENT surgery, and appendectomy. The integration of surgical robots not only enhances the precision and efficiency of minimally invasive surgeries but also establishes medical centers as pioneers in embracing cutting-edge technology for advanced patient care.

16.9 CONCLUSION

In conclusion, the IoT has emerged as a transformative force in the healthcare sector, offering innovative solutions and unlocking a realm of possibilities. The evolving applications of IoT and H-IoT signal a paradigm shift in patient monitoring and diagnosis, laying the foundation for Medicine 4.0. This new era, powered by automated platforms and advanced connectivity, presents immense opportunities for healthcare. Despite the promising potential, the widespread adoption of H-IoT faces challenges, yet the chapter highlights novel solutions to overcome these obstacles. The imminent introduction of 5G technology is anticipated to accelerate the large-scale adoption of H-IoT, propelling the evolution of healthcare delivery. Tactile Internet, a leading paradigm shift in H-IoT communication, is paving the way for revolutionary advancements in healthcare. The projected market size, reaching USD 289.2 billion by 2028, underscores the substantial momentum behind IoT's role in reshaping healthcare globally. As we delve into the future, the continuous exploration of research directions promises to further enhance H-IoT's impact, contributing to improved patient outcomes and addressing current challenges in the healthcare landscape.

BIBLIOGRAPHY

1. Zou, N., Liang, S., He, D. Issues and challenges of user and data interaction in healthcare-related IoT: A systematic review. *Library Hi Tech* 2020, 38(4), 769–782. https://doi.org/10.1108/LHT-09-2019-0177
2. Kaur, J., Jaskaran, Sindhwani, N., Anand, R., Pandey, D. Implementation of IoT in various domains. In: Sindhwani, N., Anand, R., Niranjanamurthy, M., Chander Verma, D.,

Valentina, E. B. (eds) *IoT Based Smart Applications. EAI/Springer Innovations in Communication and Computing*. Springer, Cham, 2023. https://doi.org/10.1007/978-3-031-04524-0_10

3. Kumar, M., Kumar, A., Verma, S., Bhattacharya, P., Ghimire, D., Kim, S.-H., Sanwar Hosen, A. S. M. Healthcare Internet of Things (H-IoT): Current trends, future prospects, applications, challenges, and security issues. *Electronics* 2023, 12(9), 2050. https://doi.org/10.3390/electronics12092050.
4. Asri, H., Jarir, Z. Toward a smart health: Big data analytics and IoT for real-time miscarriage prediction. *Journal of Big Data* 2023, 10, 34. https://doi.org/10.1186/s40537-023-00704-9
5. Raghupathi, W. Big data analytics in healthcare: Promise and potential. *Health Information Science and Systems* 2014, 2(3) http://www.hissjournal.com/content/2/1/3
6. Jawdhari, H. A., Abdullah, A. A. The application of network functions virtualization on different networks, and its new applications in blockchain: A survey. *Webology*, Special Issue on Computing Technology and Information Management 2021, 18, September. https://doi.org/10.14704/WEB/V18SI04/WEB18179
7. Miraz, M. H., Ali, M., Excell, P. S., Picking, R. A review on Internet of Things (IoT), Internet of Everything (IoE) and Internet of Nano Things (IoNT). In *Proceedings of the* 2015 *Internet Technologies and Applications (I.T.A.)*, Wrexham, UK, 8–11 September 2015; pp. 219–224. [Google Scholar] [CrossRef]
8. ER Internet of Nano Things Market Share | IoNT Industry Forecast 2020–2028. Available online: https://www.emergenresearch.com/amp/industry-report/internet-of-nanothings-market (accessed on 6 January 2023).
9. Senturk, S., Kok, I., Senturk, F. Internet of nano, bio-nano, biodegradable and ingestible things: A survey. *arXiv* 2022, arXiv:2202.12409. [Google Scholar]
10. El-Fatyany, A., Wang, H., Abd El-atty, S. M., Khan, M. Biocyber interface-based privacy for internet of bio-nano things. *Wireless Personal Communications* 2020, 114, 1465–1483. [Google Scholar] [CrossRef]
11. Lee, S. J., Jung, C., Choi, K., Kim, S. Design of wireless nanosensor networks for intrabody application. *International Journal of Distributed Sensor Networks* 2015, 11, 176761. [Google Scholar] [CrossRef]
12. Akyildiz, I. F., Jornet, J. M. Electromagnetic wireless nanosensor networks. *Nano Communications Network* 2010, 1, 3–19. [Google Scholar] [CrossRef]
13. Stelzner, M., Dressler, F., Fischer, S. Function centric networking: An approach for addressing in in-body nano networks. In *Proceedings of the 3rd A.C.M. International Conference on Nanoscale Computing and Communication*, New York, NY, USA, 28–30 September 2016; pp. 1–2. [Google Scholar] [CrossRef]
14. Al-Turjman, F. Intelligence and security in big 5G-oriented IoNT: An overview. *Future Generation Computer Systems 2019*, 102, 357–368. [Google Scholar] [CrossRef]
15. Ali, N. A., Abu-Elkheir, M. Internet of nano-things healthcare applications: Requirements, opportunities, and challenges. In *Proceedings of the* 2015 *IEEE 11th International Conference on Wireless and Mobile Computing, Networking and Communications (WiMob)*, Abu Dhabi, United Arab Emirates, 19–21 October 2015; pp. 9–14. [Google Scholar] [CrossRef]
16. Aazam, M., Zeadally, S., Harras, K. A. Fog computing architecture, evaluation, and future research directions. *IEEE Communications Magazine* 2018, 56, 46–52. [CrossRef]
17. Hamdan, S., Ayyash, M., Almajali, S. Edge-computing architectures for internet of things applications: A survey. *Sensors* 2020, 20, 6441. https://doi.org/10.3390/s20226441
18. Yang, M., Zhu, T., Liu, B., Xiang, Y., Zhou, W. Machine learning differential privacy with multifunctional aggregation in a fog computing architecture. *IEEE Access* 2018, 6, 17119–17129. [CrossRef]

19. Azimi, I., Anzanpour, A., Rahmani, A. M., Pahikkala, T., Levorato, M., Liljeberg, P., Dutt, N. Hich: Hierarchical fog-assisted computing architecture for healthcare IoT. *ACM Transactions on Embedded Computing System (TECS)* 2017, 16, 174. [CrossRef]
20. Sharma, P. K. Chen, M. Y., Park, J. H. A software defined fog node based distributed blockchain cloud architecture for IoT. *IEEE Access* 2017, 6, 115–124. [CrossRef]
21. Negra, R., Jemili, I., Belghith, A. Wireless body area networks: Applications and technologies. *Procedia Computer Science* 2016, 83, 1274–1281.
22. Tricás-Vidal, H. J., Lucha-López, M. O., Hidalgo-García, C., Vidal-Peracho, M. C., Monti-Ballano, S., Tricás-Moreno, J. M. Health habits and wearable activity tracker devices: Analytical cross-sectional study. *Sensors* 2022, 22(8), 2960. https://doi.org/10.3390/s22082960.
23. L. Bell. The best health tech and fitness innovations at CES 2019. *Forbes*, 17 January 2019. Available online: https://www.forbes.com/sites/leebelltech/2019/01/11/the-best-health-tech-and-fitness-innovations-of-ces2019/#6faea5574c87 (accessed on 7 February 2019).
24. Nasir, A., Asif, A., Nawaz, M., Ali, M. Design of a smart medical box for automatic pill dispensing and health monitoring. *Engineering Proceedings* 2023, 32(1), 7. https://doi.org/10.3390/engproc2023032007.
25. Stipa, G., Gabbrielli, F., Rabbito, C., Di Lazzaro, V., Amantini, A., Grippo, A., Carrai, R., Pasqui, R., Barloscio, D., Olivi, D., Lori, S. The Italian technical/administrative recommendations for telemedicine in clinical neurophysiology. *Neurological Sciences* 2021, 42(5), May, 1923–1931. [PMC free article] [PubMed] [Google Scholar]
26. Jnr, B. A. Use of telemedicine and virtual care for remote treatment in response to COVID-19 pandemic. *Journal of Medical Systems* 2020, 44(7), July, 1–9. [PMC free article] [PubMed] [Google Scholar]
27. Fernández, C. E., Maturana, C. A., Coloma, S. I., Carrasco-Labra, A., Giacaman, R. A. Teledentistry and mHealth for promotion and prevention of oral health: A systematic review and meta-analysis. *Journal of Dental Research* 2021, 7, March 26, 890. [PubMed] [Google Scholar]
28. Schwalb, P., Klecun, E. The role of contradictions and norms in the design and use of telemedicine: Healthcare professionals' perspective. *AIS Transactions on Human-Computer Interaction* 2019, 11(3), 117–135. [Google Scholar]
29. Abdellatif, M. M., Mohamed, W. Telemedicine: An IoT based remote healthcare system. *International Journal of Online & Biomedical Engineering* 2020, 16(6), 1 June [Google Scholar]
30. Deen, M. J. Information and communications technologies for elderly ubiquitous healthcare in a smart home. *Personal and Ubiquitous Computing* 2015, 19, 573–599. [CrossRef]
31. Majumder, S., Mondal, T., Deen, M. J. Wearable sensors for remote health monitoring. *Sensors* 2017, 17, 45.[CrossRef] [PubMed]
32. Van Hoof, J., Demiris, G., Wouters, E. J. M. *Handbook of Smart Homes, Health Care and Well-Being;* Springer: Basel, Switzerland, 2017.
33. Karar, M. E., Alotaibi, B., Alotaibi, M. Intelligent medical IoT-enabled automated microscopic image diagnosis of acute blood cancers. *Sensors* 2022, 22(6), 2348. https://doi.org/10.3390/s22062348
34. Yang, F., Zhao, X., Jiang, W., Gao, P., Liu, G. Multi-method fusion of cross-subject emotion recognition based on high dimensional EEG features. *Frontiers in Computational Neuroscience* 13, 53. Available online: https://www.ncbi.nlm.nih.gov/pmc/articles/PMC6714862 (accessed on 1 July 2020).
35. Muzammal, M., Talat, R., Sodhro, A. H., Pirbhulal, A. A multi-sensor data fusion enabled ensemble approach for medical data from body sensor networks. *Information Fusion* 2020, 53, January, 155–164.

36. Van Steenkiste, T., Deschrijver, D., Dhaene, T. Sensor fusion using backward shortcut connections for sleep apnea detection in multi-modal data. *arXiv preprint* arXiv:1912.06879, 2019. Available online: http://arxiv.org/abs/1912.06879
37. Lin, K., Li, Y., Sun, J., Zhou, D., Zhang, Q. Multi-sensor fusion for body sensor network in medical human–robot interaction scenario. *Information Fusion* 2020, 57, May, 15–26.
38. Hu, T., Castellanos, A., Tholey, G., et al. Real-time haptic feedback laparoscopic tool for use in gastro-intestinal surgery. *Fifth International Conference on Medical Image Computing and Computer Assisted Intervention (MICCAI)*, Tokyo, Japan, September 2002.
39. Kennedy, C., Hu, T., Desai, J. P., et al. A novel approach to robotic cardiac surgery using haptics and vision. *Cardiovascular Engineering: An International Journal* 2002, 56, 4562.
40. Biswas, P., Sikander, S., Kulkarni, P. Recent advances in robot-assisted surgical systems. *Biomedical Engineering Advances* 2023, 6, November, 100109. https://doi.org/10.1016/j.bea.2023.100109
41. Tholey, G. Understanding the surgeon's behaviour during robot-assisted surgery: Protocol for the qualitative Behav' Robot study. *BMJ Open* 2022, 12(4), April, Article e056002. https://doi.org/10.1136/BMJOPEN-2021-056002
42. A robot with improved absolute positioning accuracy for CT guided stereotactic brain surgery. *IEEE Transactions on Biomedical Engineering* 1988, 35(2), 153–160. https://doi.org/10.1109/10.1354
43. NEOCIS. Yomi robotic system for dental implant surgery. *Neocis Inc*, 2022. Available online: https://www.neocis.com/ (accessed on 14 September 2022).

17 Image-Guided Surgery Through ML and IoT

Pallavi Pandey and Priyanka Gauniya

CONTENTS

DOI: 10.1201/9781003476207-17

17.1 INTRODUCTION

Image-guided surgery (IGS) is a computer-assisted navigation approach that allows surgeons to use real-time imaging technologies during surgical procedures. This method has seen to be experiencing steady growth, with a compound annual growth rate of 5.4%, projected to reach USD 5.5 billion by 2028. By facilitating precise navigation and targeting of specific areas, IGS enhances surgical accuracy and safety. Widely employed across various medical domains such as neurosurgery, orthopedics, and oncology, it aids in tasks like tumor resection and implant placement, supporting complex surgical procedures.[1, 2] Placing images directly within the surgeon's view, IGS facilitates the identification of malignant cells or tissues and ensures the attainment of tumor-free margins during the procedure. This aspect is vital for the patient's prognosis, as complete surgical removal of the tumor is imperative.[3] IGS employs cutting-edge imaging technologies to generate virtual representations of the body's internal structures. These models can be superimposed onto the surgical site, offering live visual guidance Figure 17.1 shows application associated with the ML algorithms. This enhances accuracy and reduces complications across different surgical specialties.[4]

17.1.1 Significance of ML and IoT in Augmenting IGS

Machine learning (ML) and the IoT in IGS systems signify a notable progression in surgical technology, elevating precision, safety, and surgical outcomes. These advancements foster the creation of intelligent surgical instruments, refined imaging modalities, and enhanced patient monitoring, thereby enabling more efficient and tailored surgical interventions.

(i) ML in IGS

- **Improved Image Analysis:** ML algorithms have the ability to greatly enhance the analysis of medical images such as MRI and CT scans, providing more precise and comprehensive insights into patient anatomy and the precise localization of lesions or tumors.[5]
- **Predictive Analytics for Surgical Outcomes:** ML models can predict potential complications and outcomes of surgeries, enabling personalized patient care plans and optimizing surgical strategies.[6]

(ii) IoT in IGS

- **Real-Time Data Collection and Monitoring:** IoT devices can help monitor patient vital signs and intraoperative conditions, providing real-time data to surgeons. This information can guide intraoperative decisions and adjustments, enhancing surgical safety and outcomes.[7]

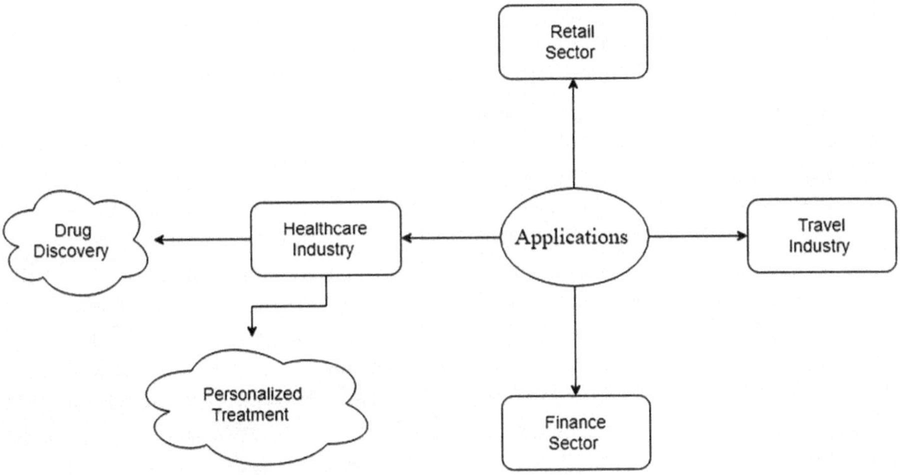

FIGURE 17.1 Application associated with the ML algorithms.

- **Smart Surgical Instruments:** IoT-enabled surgical instruments can offer feedback on their position, force, and motion, allowing for more precise manipulations and minimizing the risk of inadvertent damage to surrounding organs.[8]

(iii) Combining ML and IoT in IGS

- The combination of ML and IoT technologies in IGS systems can lead to the development of adaptive and intelligent surgical environments. These systems can analyze data from IoT devices using ML algorithms to make predictions or recommendations, adjust surgical plans in real-time, and improve the overall safety and efficacy of surgical procedures.[5]

17.1.2 Objectives of the Chapter

- To explore the advantages of ML and IoT for enhancing the capabilities and effectiveness of IGS systems.
- To highlight the diverse applications and substantial benefits of IGS in modern healthcare settings, demonstrating its critical role in improving surgical outcomes.
- To introduce key ML algorithms and discuss their application in the processing and recognition of surgical images.
- To understand how IoT devices and sensors can revolutionize surgical instrumentation and the management of medical imaging systems.
- To propose a conceptual framework for ML-enabled IGS and outline the advantages of this integration.

17.2 ESSENTIALS OF IGS

The fundamentals of IGS include various elements such as image acquisition, planning, registration, and visualization. Image acquisition is the preoperative planning in which surgeons can plan the surgery in detail by studying the high-resolution, 3D images of the patient's anatomy by loading the image in the image guidance software such as MRI, CT, ultrasound, and sometimes fluoroscopy to create a comprehensive, real-time visualization of the anatomy. These images are then merged for comprehensive surgical planning. Utilizing the acquired images, planning software enables the merging of different sequences for a detailed surgical plan. Registration is the process that connects the actual coordinates of the patient's anatomy with the digital image space. It can be achieved via point merge systems, where selected points on the patient are matched with their counterparts in the preoperative images using optical tracking technology. Subsequently, surgical instruments are monitored in real-time through technologies such as infrared light or electromagnetic fields, a crucial step in ensuring the precision of the surgical procedure according to the preoperative plan. This can include traditional axial, coronal, and sagittal views, as well as more advanced options like 3D reconstruction and fiber tracking, depending on the system used.[9]

17.2.1 History

17.2.1.1 Early Developments and Conceptual Foundations

Late 19th to Early 20th Century: The discovery of X-rays by Wilhelm Conrad Roentgen in 1895 marked the inception of medical imaging. Further developments in imaging techniques, such as CT and MRI in the 1970s and 1980s, respectively, laid the groundwork for image-guided procedures.[10, 11]

17.2.1.2 Introduction of Computer-Assisted and Stereotactic Surgery

1980s: The advent of computer-assisted tomography facilitated the creation of three-dimensional anatomical models, heralding the era of computer-assisted surgery. Early applications were primarily in neurosurgery, leveraging the brain's relatively stable anatomy for precise interventions.[12]

17.2.1.3 Advancements in Real-Time Imaging

1990s: Innovations in real-time imaging technologies, including optical and electromagnetic tracking systems, significantly advanced IGS. The introduction of intraoperative MRI and ultrasound also emerged during this period, allowing for updates to navigational maps during procedures.[13,14]

17.2.1.4 Integration of Robotics and Minimally Invasive Techniques

2000s to Present: The integration of robotic systems with IGS, exemplified by da Vinci Surgical System, has enhanced the precision and capabilities of surgical procedures. Developments in augmented reality and virtual reality for surgical planning and guidance represent the latest frontier in IGS technology.[15,16]

17.2.2 Applications and Benefits of IGS in Modern Healthcare

IGS has revolutionized modern healthcare by enhancing the precision, safety, and outcomes of surgical methodology across a wide spectrum of specialties. The applications of IGS cover neurosurgery, orthopedics, ENT (ear, nose, and throat), and oncologic surgery, among others. The integration of advanced imaging techniques with surgical practice offers numerous benefits, including minimally invasive approaches, improved accuracy, and better patient outcomes. Some of the applications of IGS are mentioned in the following subsection.

17.2.2.1 Applications of IGS

(i) **Neurosurgery:** IGS is extensively used in neurosurgery for tumor resection, epilepsy surgery, and vascular malformations, allowing for precise navigation and minimization of damage to critical brain structures.[13,17]

(ii) **Orthopedic Surgery:** In orthopedics, IGS facilitates the accurate placement of implants in joint replacement surgeries and the precise alignment and fixation in spinal surgery, contributing to improved long-term outcomes.[18]

(iii) **ENT Surgery:** IGS is beneficial in sinus surgery and procedures involving the skull base, helping to avoid vital structures such as the optic nerve and brain.[19]

(iv) **Oncologic Surgery:** In oncology, IGS aids in the resection of tumors, especially those located in challenging or critical areas, by distinguishing between healthy tissue and tumors.[20]

17.2.2.2 Benefits of IGS

- **Minimally Invasive Approaches**: IGS technologies facilitate minimally invasive procedures, which are associated with smaller incision pressure, reduced pain, shortening the hospital stays, and faster recovery times compared to traditional open surgery.[20]
- **Enhanced Accuracy and Safety**: By providing real-time visual guidance, IGS improves the accuracy of surgical interventions, reducing the risk of complications and damage to adjacent healthy tissues.[21]
- **Improved Surgical Outcomes**: The precision and efficiency of IGS contribute to better surgical outcomes, including higher success rates in tumor removal and improved functionality in orthopedic and neurosurgical procedures.
- **Customized Surgical Planning**: IGS also allows the preoperative planning and simulation of surgical procedures based on individual patient anatomy, leading to more personalized and effective treatment strategies.[20]

17.3 ML IN IMAGE ANALYSIS

ML has had a profound influence on image analysis, providing robust tools that improve accuracy, efficiency, and capabilities in interpreting images across diverse applications. Within medical imaging, ML algorithms enable automated analysis, disease detection, and the extraction of quantitative data, thereby assisting in diagnosis, treatment planning, and patient monitoring.

- **Automated Disease Detection and Diagnosis**
- ML models, particularly deep learning (DL) algorithms like convolutional neural networks (CNNs), have shown exceptional success in autonomously

recognizing and diagnosing diseases from medical imagery. These models excel at identifying patterns and abnormalities in images such as X-rays, MRIs, and CT scans, potentially signaling conditions like cancer, pneumonia, or neurological disorders.[22]

- **Image Segmentation**
  Image segmentation includes dividing an image into various segments or pixels to streamline its representation. ML algorithms, especially CNNs, have proven highly successful in segmenting medical images to isolate areas of interest, such as tumors or organs. This process aids in achieving more precise diagnoses and treatment planning.[23]
- **Image Registration**
  Image registration is the method of aligning two or more images of the same scene, typically captured at various times, angles, or by distinct sensors. ML has enhanced the precision and effectiveness of image registration methods, which is vital for tasks such as monitoring disease advancement over time or integrating data from diverse imaging techniques.[24]
- **Image Reconstruction**
  ML algorithms have been applied to reconstruct high-quality images from lower-quality inputs, such as to enhance the resolution of medical images or reconstruct images from sparse data in tomography. This can significantly reduce imaging time and patient exposure to radiation.[25]
- **Predictive Modeling**
  ML models can analyze medical images alongside other patient data to predict the likelihood of disease development, progression, and treatment outcomes. This holistic approach supports personalized medicine by tailoring treatment plans to individual patient profiles.[26]

17.3.1 Introduction to ML Algorithms

ML algorithm is the core of AI applications, enabling systems to learn from data and improve over time. These algorithms can be broadly classified into several categories: supervised learning, unsupervised learning, semi-supervised learning, and reinforcement learning. Each category serves different purposes and is suited for different types of data and learning tasks. Figure 17.2 shows schematic classification of machine learning.

17.3.1.1 Supervised Learning

Supervised learning algorithms build models that make predictions based on a set of input-output pairs. These algorithms learn a mapping from inputs to outputs, aiming to predict the output for new, unseen data. This model relies on having all necessary input values available; without them, it becomes impossible to deduce any information about the outcomes. This method is widely used for training both neural networks and Decision Trees.

- **Linear Regression**: It is the most common ML technique, among all techniques. It is a basic algorithm for regression tasks, predicting a continuous

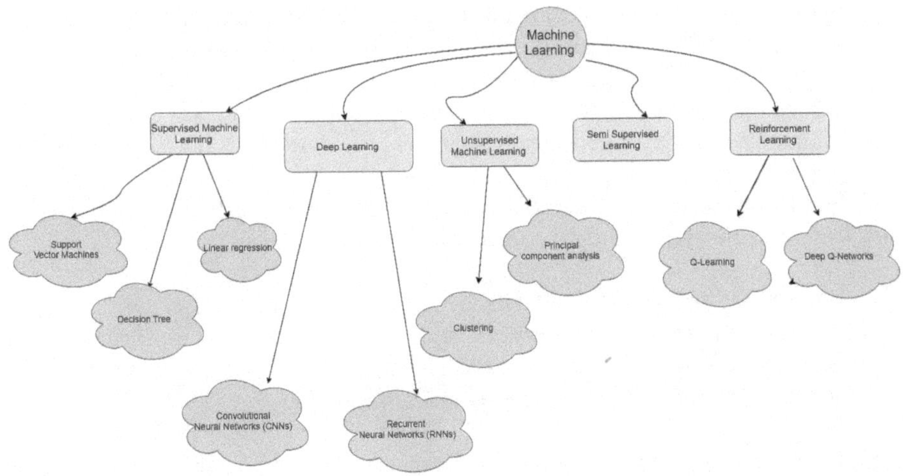

FIGURE 17.2 Schematic classification of machine learning.

value. Linear regression helps to establish a connection between the dependent variable (Y) and one or more independent variables (X) by determining the optimal straight line, also referred to as the regression line, that best fits the data.[27, 28]

- **Support Vector Machines (SVM)**: This strategy works well for classification tasks; SVMs determine the hyperplane that best divides distinct classes in the input space.[29] SVM works by mapping data into a high-dimensional or potentially infinite-dimensional space and attempting to generate a hyperplane or collection of hyperplanes. The goal is to select a hyperplane with the greatest margin from the nearest points of any class in the training dataset, as a larger margin is typically linked with a lower classifier generalization error.[30]
- **Decision Trees and Random Forests**: These have been employed for classification and regression. Decision trees divide data based on certain criteria, whereas random forests mix numerous trees to improve prediction accuracy.[31]

17.3.1.2 Unsupervised Learning

Unsupervised learning algorithms find patterns or structures in data without any labels. These are used for clustering, dimensionality reduction, and association rule learning.

- **K-means Clustering:** A commonly used clustering technique that divides data into k separate clusters based on similarity. It is an efficient, robust, and intuitive approach that produces consistent results for datasets with clearly defined groups. In this method, data points are assigned to clusters in a way that minimizes the total squared distance between the points and the cluster's center, or centroid. Essentially, the K-means method selects a set number of centroids, k, and assigns each data point to the closest cluster, attempting to reduce the size of the centroids as much as feasible. However, because the initial selection of cluster centers is random, the algorithm's output can vary.[32]

Principal Component Analysis (PCA): PCA is a technique for reducing dimensionality in data while maintaining the majority of the variation.[33]

17.3.1.3 Semi-Supervised Learning

Semi-supervised learning is a hybrid of supervised and unsupervised learning that trains on both labeled and unlabeled data. This method is especially beneficial when obtaining a fully labeled dataset is costly or impracticable.

Self-training: This is a simple semi-supervised strategy in which a model is trained with a small quantity of labeled data before using its predictions to label unlabeled data and retrain itself.[34]

17.3.1.4 Reinforcement Learning

Reinforcement learning algorithms learn how to act or make decisions by interacting with an environment to achieve a goal. The learning is driven by rewards and penalties for actions taken.

- **Q-Learning**: This is a prominent reinforcement learning strategy for determining the value of an action in a given state. The "Q" in Q-learning stands for "quality," representing the algorithm's role in estimating the highest expected future rewards for an action taken in a certain state.[35]
- **Deep Q-Networks**: This technique combines Q-learning and deep neural networks, allowing agents to learn directly from high-dimensional sensory inputs. Deep reinforcement learning enables control at the human level. Deep Q-Learning begins by feeding the starting state into a neural network, which then outputs the Q-values for all conceivable actions.[36]

17.3.1.5 Deep Learning

- **CNNs:** Despite their higher computational demands, CNNs eliminate the need for manual feature selection by automatically identifying significant features, making them more potent than traditional ANNs. Numerous advanced DL architectures derived from CNNs, such as AlexNet, Xception, Inception, Visual Geometry Group (VGG), ResNet, and others, are employed in the field to address complex tasks.[37,38]

17.3.2 Role of ML in Medical Image Processing and Recognition

ML, particularly DL, has revolutionized medical image processing and recognition, offering significant advancements in the accuracy, efficiency, and effectiveness of diagnostic procedures. These technologies have been instrumental in detecting, classifying, and predicting diseases from various medical imaging modalities. The role of ML in medical image processing and recognition encompasses several key areas:

- **Automated Disease Detection and Diagnosis**
  ML techniques, particularly DL models such as CNNs, have shown outstanding accuracy in recognizing and diagnosing diseases from medical images, frequently matching or exceeding that of human specialists. A DL method was developed and tested to automatically detect diabetic retinopathy and diabetic macular edema in retinal fundus pictures. In a study, DL was utilized for automated diabetic retinopathy detection, showcasing the capability of ML models to aid in early disease identification.[39]
- **Image Segmentation**
  The U-Net architecture has emerged as a standard in medical image segmentation, providing a robust tool for a variety of segmentation tasks due to its unique design that captures both local and contextual information.[23]
- **Enhanced Image Reconstruction**
  ML methods have enhanced the standard of medical image reconstruction, allowing for the generation of clearer, higher-resolution images from lower-quality data. This advancement is pivotal for precise diagnosis and finds utility in modalities such as MRI, where ML-driven faster image acquisition can enhance patient comfort and mitigate motion artifacts. Research has demonstrated how DL can be utilized to expedite MRI imaging, improving image quality while decreasing scan durations.[40]
- **Predictive Modeling and Prognosis**
  ML models can analyze medical images in conjunction with patient data to predict disease progression, response to treatment, and patient prognosis. This predictive capability supports personalized medicine by facilitating tailored treatment plans based on individual risk profiles and disease characteristics.[41]

  The role of ML in medical image processing and recognition is dynamic and expanding, with ongoing research and development promising to further enhance diagnostic and treatment processes, ultimately improving patient outcomes and healthcare efficiency.

17.4 INTERNET OF THINGS IN SURGICAL ENVIRONMENTS

The Internet of Things (IoT) in surgical environments represents a transformative approach to healthcare, enhancing surgical procedures, patient care, and operational efficiency through interconnected devices and systems. IoT technologies in surgery enable real-time data collection, monitoring, and analysis, facilitating improved decision-making, patient outcomes, and resource management. The several key applications of IoT in surgical environments are:

- **Enhanced Surgical Precision and Navigation**
  IoT devices, including smart surgical instruments and imaging systems, can improve surgical precision and navigation. These systems offer real-time

feedback and guidance during procedures, reducing the risk of errors. In a study, the role of data science and interconnected technologies in enhancing surgical interventions are discussed along with highlighting the potential for IoT to improve precision and outcomes.[5]

- **Remote Monitoring and Telemedicine**
  Wearable devices and sensors in the IoT enable remote monitoring of patient's vital signs and post-surgical recuperation. This capability is crucial for telemedicine applications, allowing healthcare providers to offer continuous care and early detection of complications from a distance. A study explores the early concepts of mobile health (mHealth) and its evolution toward IoT, emphasizing remote monitoring and patient care.[42]
- **Enhanced Training and Simulation**
  IoT, combined with virtual reality and augmented reality (AR), offers immersive training experiences for surgeons and medical staff. These technologies enable the simulation of complex surgical procedures for education and training purposes, improving skills without risking patient safety. A review has found that IoT may also be involved in advancing surgical training and planning through simulations and models.[43]

The integration of IoT in surgical environments promises to revolutionize how surgeries are performed and managed, offering greater efficiency, safety, and outcomes. As technology advances, further innovations in IoT applications are expected to continue shaping the future of surgical care.

17.4.1 Comprehending IoT Technology and Its Significance within the Healthcare Sector

IoT technology has gained increasing significance in healthcare, offering the potential to greatly enhance patient outcomes, streamline healthcare operations, and reduce costs. Here is an overview of the importance of IoT technology in healthcare, substantiated by references. IoT devices enable remote monitoring of patients' health, enabling healthcare providers to monitor vital signs, medication adherence, and other crucial health indicators in real time. This capability is advantageous for managing and controlling chronic health conditions such as diabetes or heart disease and also helps to ensure timely medical interventions. A study has investigated the potential of sensor technologies and IoT in personal health monitoring, along with their broader implications for healthcare.[44] IoT technologies help to empower patients by providing them with more control over their health and treatment plans. Health-related apps encourage active participation in health management, promoting healthier lifestyles for the individuals. Moreover, data collected from these devices can be used to tailor treatments to individual patients, leading to more personalized and effective care. In context, a study highlights the acceleration of digital health technologies, including IoT, in response to the COVID-19 pandemic, underscoring their role in transforming healthcare delivery.[45] IoT devices can also streamline healthcare operations, from inventory management with Radio-frequency identification (RFID) tagging to predictive maintenance of medical equipment. By automating routine tasks and improving resource allocation, healthcare facilities can operate more efficiently and reduce costs. A study has been focused on electronic health record (EHR) portals and touches on the broader theme of digital tools in healthcare, including IoT, improving efficiency and patient engagement.[46] IoT devices also support clinical decision-making by providing healthcare professionals with timely and accurate data. For example, smart beds in hospitals can detect patient movements and alert staff to potential falls, while smart inhalers can monitor asthma patient's adherence to their medication regime, reducing the risk of severe episodes. It has been illustrated in a review that the use of digital health technologies, including IoT, in managing infectious diseases, indicates the potential for improved clinical outcomes.[47]

17.4.2 IoT Devices and Sensors for Surgical Instrumentation

The integration of IoT devices and sensors into surgical instrumentation is revolutionizing the field of surgery, enhancing precision, efficiency, and patient outcomes. These smart surgical tools equipped with IoT capabilities can monitor various parameters during surgery, provide real-time feedback to surgeons, and even assist in remote surgeries. The following are the IoT devices and sensors for surgical instrumentation:

1. **Smart Surgical Instruments**
   Smart surgical instruments, equipped with sensors, can measure pressure, motion, and other variables to ensure procedures are performed with optimal precision. For instance, force-sensing instruments provide feedback on the amount of pressure applied, reducing the risk of tissue damage. It has discussed in a paper that while focused on needle insertion, discusses the principles behind force feedback in surgical instruments, a concept central to smart surgical tools.[48]
2. **Wireless Surgical Tools**
   Wireless sensors embedded in surgical tools can transmit data on tool usage, location, and condition, improving inventory management and operational efficiency in the surgical suite. In a study, real-time imaging was used for guidance in surgery, a concept that extends to the use of wireless tools for enhanced precision and efficiency.[8]
3. **Wearable Sensors for Surgeons**
   Wearable sensors on surgeons can monitor ergonomics and fatigue levels, potentially reducing the risk of errors. These sensors can also track the surgeon's movements for training and skill assessment purposes.[49]
4. **RFID Tagged Surgical Instruments**
   RFID tags on surgical instruments enable real-time tracking of tools, ensuring all instruments are accounted for before and after surgery, thus preventing retained surgical items. Although not directly related to RFID technology, a study underlines the importance of efficiency in the operating room, where RFID can play a critical role in instrument management.[50]
5. **IoT-Enabled Robotic Surgery Systems**
   Robotic surgery systems integrated with IoT can enhance surgical precision through advanced imaging and real-time data analysis, as well as facilitate remote surgeries, expanding access to surgical expertise. A study provides

an overview of robotic technology in surgery, touching on the integration of IoT for improved functionality and outcomes.[51]

17.5 SYNERGISTIC INTEGRATION OF ML AND IoT IN IGS

The synergistic integration of ML and IoT in IGS is driving significant advancements in the field of minimally invasive surgery. This combination enhances the precision, safety, and outcomes of surgical procedures by leveraging real-time data analysis, predictive modeling, and enhanced visualization. The essential facets of the collaborative functioning of ML and IoT in IGS are explored as follows:

(i) **Enhanced Surgical Navigation**
ML algorithms have the capability to analyze data originating from IoT-enabled surgical instruments and imaging devices, thereby furnishing real-time guidance and feedback to surgeons. This integration enhances surgical navigation, aiding surgeons in avoiding critical structures and reducing tissue damage. Such advancements may be elaborated upon in a review delineating technological progressions in image-guided interventions, accentuating the significance of real-time data and image analysis, which form the foundation of ML and IoT integration.[20]

(ii) **Personalized Surgery through Predictive Analytics**
Through the analysis of patient-specific data gathered from IoT devices, ML algorithms have the capability to forecast optimal surgical strategies and potential complications tailored to individual patients. This customized approach enhances surgical preparation and has the potential to enhance patient results.[52]

(iii) **Tracking and Control of Instruments**
The integration of IoT sensors within surgical instruments, alongside ML algorithms, helps to precise monitoring of tool position and movement during surgical procedures. This functionality can automate specific tasks or issue alerts should an instrument deviate from a predefined safe zone, thereby augmenting surgical safety.[53-56] This assertion finds support in a study addressing the burgeoning domain of surgical data science, which underscores the synergy between ML and IoT in advancing surgical interventions.[5]

(iv) **Instantaneous Decision Assistance**
By incorporating ML into IoT devices, surgeons are able to quickly analyze surgical data and receive instant feedback and decision-making assistance. This includes suggestions for selecting instruments, adjusting surgical techniques, and receiving alerts about possible issues based on both current and past data. Furthermore, a research study highlights the use of ML algorithms to evaluate surgical performance and predict outcomes, which can be improved by incorporating IoT data for real-time support.[57]

17.5.1 Conceptual Framework for ML-Enabled IGS

A conceptual framework for ML-enabled IGS involves integrating advanced ML techniques with IGS technologies to enhance surgical planning, execution, and outcomes. This framework capitalizes on the synergy between ML's data processing capabilities and IGS's precision in surgical navigation, aiming to achieve optimal patient outcomes through improved accuracy and efficiency in surgical procedures. It consists of the several components such as:

(i) **Data Acquisition and Preprocessing:**
Image Acquisition
Data Preprocessing

(ii) **ML Model Training and Validation:**
Feature Extraction
Model Training
Validation and Testing[58]

(iii) **Integration with IGS System**
Planning: Surgical planning can be carried out through the ML algorithms which helps by detailed anatomical and pathological insights from preoperative images to the surgeon.[59]
Registration: ML Techniques such as DL-enhanced image registration improve the alignment of preoperative images with the patient's anatomy during surgery.[60]
Instrument Tracking and Navigation: ML algorithms contribute to more accurate and dynamic tracking of surgical instruments, enhancing navigation precision.[5]

(iv) **Intraoperative Decision Support**
Real-time Analysis: Intraoperative data is analyzed in real time by ML models to offer guidance, detect anomalies, and suggest corrective actions.[61]
AR Visualization: ML-integrated AR systems provide surgeons with enhanced visualization tools that overlay crucial information onto the surgical field.[62]

(v) **Postoperative Assessment and Feedback Loop**
Outcome Analysis: Postoperative results are evaluated to assess the efficacy of ML predictions and the success of the surgical intervention.[63]
Feedback Loop: Continuous improvement is facilitated by feeding outcome data back into the ML models, refining their predictive capabilities over time.[5]

17.5.2 Advantages of Combining ML and IoT in Surgical Environments

There are various advantages of combining ML and the IoT in surgical environments leverages the strengths of both technologies to improve surgical outcomes, enhance patient care, and streamline operational efficiency. This amalgamation can pave the way for the creation of intelligent surgical environments that are increasingly responsive, adaptive, and proficient in delivering high-quality care. The benefits of integrating ML and IoT in surgical environments include:

(i) **Augmented Surgical Precision and Safety**
Real-time Monitoring: IoT devices have the capability to continuously monitor patient vitals and surgical conditions in real-time. Concurrently, ML algorithms can analyze this data to anticipate potential adverse events before they manifest, thereby bolstering patient safety.[64]
Predictive Analytics: ML can analyze data from IoT-enabled surgical tools to predict equipment failure or suggest optimal maintenance schedules, reducing the risk of unexpected malfunctions.[65]

(ii) **Improved Surgical Planning and Outcomes**
Preoperative Analysis: ML algorithms can help to process the complex datasets from preoperative IoT devices (e.g., imaging equipment) to assist in planning by identifying risk factors and suggesting the best surgical approaches.[5]
Customized Patient Care: By analyzing patient data collected through IoT devices, ML can help fit surgical strategies to individual patient needs and help to improve the potentially improving outcomes.[66]

(iii) **Operational Efficiency and Cost Reduction**
Resource Optimization: IoT devices can track the usage of surgical equipment and consumables, with ML optimizing inventory management to reduce waste and lower costs.[67]
Enhanced Efficiency in Surgical Procedures: ML algorithms possess the capability to scrutinize data from previous surgeries, thereby optimizing the scheduling and duration of procedures. This optimization contributes to an overall enhancement in the efficiency of surgical operations.[68]

(iv) **Postoperative Monitoring and Care:**
Remote Patient Monitoring: Following surgery, patients can be outfitted with wearable IoT devices designed to monitor their recovery progress. ML algorithms can then analyze the data collected by these devices, detecting complications early and adjusting care plans as necessary.[69]
Personalized Rehabilitation Programs: ML algorithms can utilize data gathered from IoT devices to develop personalized rehabilitation programs for patients. These programs are tailored to individual needs, thereby improving recovery times and diminishing the likelihood of readmission.[70]

17.5.3 Challenges and Considerations Arise When Implementing ML–IoT Solutions for IGS

ML techniques help in providing various benefits; they also pose several hurdles that must be addressed for successful integration into clinical settings. Some delineated key challenges and considerations are discussed here:

(i) **Data Security and Privacy**
The challenge is to ensuring the security and privacy of patient data collected via IoT devices and processed by ML algorithms is crucial, given the significant risk of data breaches and unauthorized access.

The biggest consideration is employing robust encryption techniques, secure data transmission protocols, and adhering to regulations such as GDPR and HIPAA are imperative measures.

(ii) **Data Quality and Integration**
The challenge faced for data quality and integration is that the efficacy of ML models relies on the quality and quantity of data. Obtaining high-quality, comprehensive datasets for training models within the context of IGS can be challenging. While it must be considered to establish standards for data collection, ensuring interoperability among various IoT devices, and employing techniques for data augmentation can help mitigate these challenges.[71]

(iii) **Algorithmic Bias and Equity Challenge:**
Consideration should be given to ensuring fairness requires employing diverse and representative training datasets, along with implementing strategies to detect and mitigate bias.[72]

(iv) **Regulatory Compliance and Certification**
The challenges are for regulatory bodies have stringent requirements for medical devices and software, which can pose barriers to the rapid deployment of ML–IoT solutions in IGS.

Consideration should be given to early engagement with regulatory bodies, adherence to standards like ISO 13485 for medical devices, and conducting rigorous clinical trials are necessary steps.[73]

(v) **Ethical Considerations Challenge:**
Consideration: Establishing ethical guidelines for AI in healthcare, implementing protocols for patient consent, and ensuring a human-centric approach in technology design and implementation is imperative.[74]

17.6 IMAGE PROCESSING AND RECOGNITION

Image recognition techniques can discern and categorize specific objects or patterns within bioimages, providing researchers with insights into molecule behavior and distribution.[75, 76]

17.6.1 Methods for Image Segmentation and Feature Extraction

Image segmentation and feature extraction are vital components of computer vision and image processing applications, spanning medical imaging, object recognition, and surveillance systems. These methods allow for the detection of pertinent patterns, objects, or areas within images, thereby aiding subsequent analysis or decision-making procedures. The different prominent methods for image segmentation and feature extraction include:

Image Segmentation Techniques

- **Thresholding**: This is one of the simplest segmentation techniques, where pixels are The objects are categorized into foreground and background by assessing their intensities relative to a threshold value. Otsu's method is a popular approach for automatically determining the threshold.[77]
- **Region-Based Segmentation**: This approach involves the grouping of neighboring pixels with similar values to form distinct regions. Techniques such as region growing and split-and-merge fall under this category.[78]
- **Edge-Based Segmentation**: Edge detection (e.g., Sobel, Canny) is used to find boundaries between regions based on discontinuities in intensity values. Edge-based segmentation is useful for identifying object outlines.[79]
- **Watershed Segmentation**: Based on topological and morphological concepts, this technique treats an image's intensity values as a topographic surface. Watersheds are used to delineate object boundaries, especially useful in medical imaging.[80]
- **Clustering Methods**: Techniques like K-means clustering and Fuzzy C-means are used to partition image pixels into clusters based on their features. These are unsupervised methods that do not require prior knowledge of the number of segments.[81, 82]
- **DL-Based Segmentation**: CNNs and architectures like U-Net have shown exceptional performance in segmenting complex images, especially in biomedical imaging.[23]

Feature Extraction Techniques

- **Edge Features**: It uses edge detection filters (e.g., Sobel, Prewitt) to identify boundaries and edges in images, which are crucial for object recognition and scene understanding.
- **Texture Features:** Methods like Gray-Level Co-occurrence Matrix and Local Binary Patterns analyze the texture of an image region, useful in classification tasks.[83, 84]
- **Color Features:** It involves extraction of color histograms, color moments, or using color spaces (e.g., RGB, HSV) to capture the color distribution and characteristics of an image.
- **Shape Features:** Descriptors such as Fourier descriptors, Hu moments, and Zernike moments are used to capture the shape information of objects within an image, important for object recognition and classification.
- **DL Features:** Deep CNNs automatically learn hierarchical feature representations from images, leading to state-of-the-art performance in many vision tasks. Features extracted from intermediate layers of pre-trained networks (e.g., VGG, ResNet) can be used for various applications.[85, 86]

17.6.2 ML Algorithms for Image Classification and Object Detection

They consist of two types of fundamental tasks in computer vision that have been significantly advanced with the development of various ML and DL algorithms.

17.6.2.1 Image Classification

Image classification involves assigning a label to an entire image from a fixed set of categories.

17.6.2.2 Fast R-CNN model CNNs

CNN is a form of artificial neural network that predominantly processes data having a grid-like architecture, such as pictures. Artificial Neural Networks (ANN), which are frequently inspired by the functioning of neurons in the human brain, are a popular type of ML models. In an ANN, multiple neurons are joined together to form a large network. These networks frequently comprise numerous layers of neurons sandwiched between the input and output layers, known as hidden layers. The presence of many hidden layers makes the network "deeper," which is why the phrase "deep neural networks" is used, especially when the networks have over a hundred hidden layers. In some cases, each neuron is linked to every neuron in the next layer, resulting in what is known as a fully connected network. The CNN architecture is intended to learn spatial hierarchies of features automatically and adaptively using backpropagation. This is accomplished by utilizing numerous building components, including convolutional layers, pooling layers, and fully connected layers.[87,88]

Convolutional Layers: These layers perform a convolution operation, applying filters to the input data. For images, this means sliding a filter matrix over the image pixels to produce a feature map that emphasizes certain features in the image, like edges or textures. The filters are learned during the training process.

Pooling (Subsampling or Down-sampling) Layers: Pooling layers helps to reduce the spatial size of the representation, making the model more efficient and less sensitive to the exact location of features. Max pooling, which takes the maximum value from each of a cluster of neurons at the prior layer, is a common technique used for this purpose.

Fully Connected Layers: The Fully Connected Layer in a CNN captures complex relationships missed by convolutional layers. It takes a reduced-size input feature vector and often uses softmax activation for classification. This layer contains the majority of parameters that need training in a CNN.

Flattening Layer: The Flattening Layer in a CNN transforms the output from pooling layers into a single column vector, serving as input for the fully connected network. It does not involve learning parameters or tuning hyper-parameters.

Additional Layers: Additional layers in CNNs, such as LRN and dropout, are used to mitigate overfitting by normalizing neuron activity and randomly omitting neurons during training.

Softmax or Classification Layer: The final layer, often a fully connected layer, uses a softmax activation function (for multi-class classification problems) to output probabilities for each class label.[88–90]

17.6.2.3 CNN Architectures

LeNet-5: One of the earliest CNN models designed for digit recognition.[91]

AlexNet: This model significantly outperformed traditional methods in the ImageNet challenge, bringing DL to the forefront of the field.[88]

VGGNet: Known for its simplicity and depth, VGGNet was influential in showing that depth in networks is vital for achieving high accuracy.[85]

ResNet: Introduced residual blocks, making it possible to train up to hundreds or even thousands of layers successfully.[86]

17.6.2.4 Object Detection

Object detection involves identifying instances of objects in an image and typically locating them with bounding boxes.

Region-Based CNNs: In 2013, Girshick and colleagues introduced R-CNN, a complex object detection framework that uses selective search to generate region proposals and then classifies them using CNNs, SVMs, and a region proposal algorithm; however, the training process is computationally intensive and time-consuming, resulting in slow detection speed.[92]

Fast R-CNN (2015): Fast R-CNN improves the efficiency of the original R-CNN by processing the entire image at once using a CNN, eliminating the need for separate feature computation for overlapping regions. It introduces a Region Proposal Network (RPN) to identify regions of interest and a RoI pooling layer to extract uniform-sized feature vectors, resulting in faster detection and streamlined training. It improves efficiency by sharing computation and using RoI pooling.[93]

Faster R-CNN (2015): Faster R-CNN introduces the RPN for generating region proposals directly within the network, significantly speeding up the process. Faster R-CNN uses shared convolutional feature maps and an RPN to speed up object detection, achieving a mean Average Precision (mAP) of 66.9% on the Pascal VOC 2009 dataset and operating at nearly seven frames per second on high-end GPUs.[94]

Single Shot Detectors (SSD): Single Shot Detectors are efficient for real-time detection, SSD predicts bounding boxes and class probabilities in a single pass through the network.[95]

YOLO (You Only Look Once) Series: YOLO is a CNN-based object detection algorithm that adopts a distinct approach for detection, applying a single neural network to the full image and eliminating the need for separate region proposal generation. It is known for its speed and accuracy, YOLO frames object detection as a regression problem.[96]

17.6.3 Case Studies Demonstrating the Effectiveness of ML in Surgical Image Analysis

ML and DL have been increasingly applied to various aspects of surgical image analysis, demonstrating significant effectiveness in improving diagnostic accuracy, automating tedious processes, and enhancing surgical planning and guidance. Here are a few case studies that highlight these advancements, along with references to the original works for more detailed information.

(i) **Preoperative Planning and Prediction**
Case Study: ML for Predicting Liver Disease Severity from CT Images
A study utilized CNNs to analyze CT images for the preoperative prediction of liver disease severity, which is crucial for surgical planning in liver resections and transplantations.[96]

(ii) **Surgical Navigation and Guidance**
Case Study 2: Real-time Polyp Detection During Colonoscopy
The CNNs DL analysis was applied to endoscopic video streams to identify and highlight polyps during colonoscopies in real-time, aiding surgeons in ensuring a thorough examination and reducing the chances of missing lesions. In this study, the researchers created and trained deep CNNs using a heterogeneous sample of 8,641 hand-labeled pictures from screening colonoscopies.[97]

(iii) **Postoperative Monitoring and Complication Detection**
Case Study 3: Detecting Anastomotic Leak from Postoperative Radiographs
The EndoNet approach was created to automatically learn features from cholecystectomy movies and perform phase identification and tool presence detection tasks in a multi-task mode.[98]

(iv) **Tool and Gesture Recognition for Surgical Skills Assessment**
Case Study 4: Automated Assessment of Surgical Skills Using Tool and Gesture Recognition
DL algorithms were applied to laparoscopic video data to recognize surgical tools and gestures, providing a framework for automated surgical skills assessment and feedback, potentially useful in surgical training and credentialing.[99]

Pathology: Diagnosing Prostate Cancer
Case Study: AI for Prostate Cancer Grading on Biopsy Samples
This study looked into the potential of DL to do automated Gleason grading of prostate biopsies. A DL system was developed by the researchers that could grade prostate cancer on biopsy samples with accuracy comparable to expert pathologists. This approach aims to reduce the variability and workload associated with manual grading. A DL system was created utilizing randomly picked biopsies from patients at the Radboud University Medical Center.[100]

Dermatology: Skin Lesion Analysis
Case Study: CNNs for Skin Cancer Classification
In this study, an ML model was trained to categorize skin lesions as malignant or benign based on photographic pictures, demonstrating dermatologist-level accuracy. Such tools can assist in early detection and reduce the need for invasive biopsy procedures. The researchers trained a DL algorithm using a dataset of over 129,000 clinical images of skin lesions, covering more than 2,000 different diseases. The program could classify skin cancer with the same accuracy as dermatologists, highlighting DL's potential for boosting diagnostic accuracy.[22]

Ophthalmology: Diabetic Retinopathy Detection

Case Study: Automated Detection of Diabetic Retinopathy Using DL

An algorithm was developed to screen fundus photographs for diabetic retinopathy, a leading cause of blindness and diabetic macular edema demonstrating the potential to automate the screening process in underserved populations.[39]

Cardiology: ECG Analysis for Arrhythmia Detection

Case Study: DL for Electrocardiogram (ECG) Analysis

In this study, a DL model was used to identify arrhythmias from single-lead ECGs, outperforming the average cardiologist's performance. This technology could enhance remote monitoring and arrhythmia screening efficiency. From the result, it was concluded that DL can classify arrhythmias in ambulatory ECGs with a high potential than the cardiologists.[101, 102]

Gastroenterology: Early Detection of Esophageal Cancer

Case Study: DL for Barrett's Esophagus and Esophageal Cancer Detection

A DL computer-aided detection system was used on endoscopic images was used to detect early signs of Barrett's esophagus and esophageal cancer, achieving high accuracy rates. Engineered for real-time application in clinical settings, the system offers potential as a tool to augment the identification of early neoplasia in patients with Barrett's esophagus.[103]

Pulmonology: Automated Detection of Lung Nodules in CT scans

Case Study: AI for Early Lung Cancer Detection

The study explores the utility of breast multiparametric MRI (BMMR) in anticipating the response to neoadjuvant chemotherapy among breast cancer patients. It assesses the effectiveness of various quantitative imaging characteristics derived from BMMR in predicting chemotherapy outcomes. Additionally, a BMMR2 challenge was undertaken, tasking participants with formulating prediction models based on BMMR data from breast cancer patients. The challenge outcomes underscore the potential of BMMR in furnishing valuable insights for forecasting chemotherapy response in breast cancer patients.[104]

Emergency Medicine: Predicting Hospital Readmission

Case Study: ML for Forecasting Hospital Readmissions among Diabetic Patients

This study employed a ML algorithm to anticipate the likelihood of 30-day hospital readmissions using EHR data, focusing on patients with diabetes.[105] The investigation revealed that diabetic patients at higher risk of readmission include women, Caucasians, outpatients, and individuals undergoing less extensive laboratory or treatment procedures or receiving reduced medication. These patients were discharged without evident improvements or insulin administration despite testing positive for HbA1c. This study highlights the need for effective patient management protocols, especially for non-ICU inpatients, to reduce readmission rates. It suggests that poor management practices, such as inadequate treatments, lab tests, and discharge without significant improvements, contribute to high readmission rates among diabetic patients.[106]

Psychiatry: Identifying Depression from Speech Patterns
Case Study: Detecting Depression Using Vocal and Speech Analysis

An innovative approach used ML algorithms to analyze vocal and speech characteristics from audio recordings, aiming to identify markers of depression. This non-invasive method could supplement traditional diagnostic processes.[107]

These case studies further underscore the versatility and potential of ML to revolutionize healthcare through early detection, diagnosis accuracy improvement, personalized treatment planning, and outcome prediction across a broad spectrum of medical conditions. As data availability and computing power continue to grow, so too will the capabilities and applications of ML in medicine, promising significant advancements in patient care and healthcare efficiency.

17.7 SURGICAL PLANNING OPTIMIZATION

17.7.1 Role of ML in Preoperative Planning

Surgeons undertake difficult, high-risk decisions with enormous consequences for patients' lives, often under time constraints. The team faces difficult problems due to the large volume and variety of diagnostic data, as well as the possible risks of surgical intervention. As a result, preoperative planning, in which surgeons prepare the procedure using medical records, historical methods, and data, is critical to surgical success.

Surgeons make decisions based on their training, experience, and expertise, which can be influenced by their judgment or bias. These restrictions can be solved by AI-based decision-making systems.

AI is utilized as a decision-support technology for two purposes: to compensate for surgeons' varying levels of expertise and experience by objectively and individually evaluating patient data and highlighting clinically relevant correlations that physicians may not detect. Additional benefits of using AI in surgery include objective decision-making, optimal usage of operating theatres, and reduced overtime.[108]

ML tools used for preoperative planning

- **Cognitive Medical Assistant (KoMed):** It helps in projecting risk profile of the individual from laboratory result, image data and diagnosis. It is basically help in predicting the requirement of blood transfusion.
- **Predictive Optimization Trees in Emergency Surgery Risk:** It helps in preoperative planning and preoperative optimization. It is a user-friendly mobile application.[109]
- **American College of Surgeons National Surgical Quality Improvement Program (ACS-NSQIP):** It determines the patient at high risk prior to surgery. This model has been used to optimize perioperative care, facilitate shared decision-making discussions, and determine if surgery is the best

option for the patient. The AVS-NSQIP model has been widely used as a risk assessment tool to predict complications and mortality in surgical patients.[110]

17.7.2 Patient-Specific Modeling

Patient-specific modeling is a crucial aspect of preoperative planning, as it allows for the prediction of individual patients' risks and the optimization of perioperative care. ML models, such as the POTTER calculator, have demonstrated their ability to create patient-specific models based on large datasets like ACS-NSQIP. Patient-specific modeling in preoperative planning serves several important purposes like accurate risk assessment, personalized care, shared decision-making, and optimized resource allocation.[111]

17.7.3 ML-Based Tools for Surgical Simulation and Rehearsal

- Touch surgery app, which provides a user-guided three-dimensional environment to explore the steps of a surgical procedure.
- Simbionix Procedure Rehearsal Studio is a patient-specific simulation software that uses CTA and MRI scan data to produce simulated cases.
- AI-enabled surgical simulators that provide personalized feedback and automate immersive surgical experiences.
- The UNiD Spine Analyzer enables surgeons to view, measure, and simulate the placement of surgical implants.
- D2P device that is used for preoperative image segmentation system for transfer of DICOM visualizations software for surgical planning.[112]

17.8 REAL-TIME INTRAOPERATIVE GUIDANCE

17.8.1 IoT Allows Surgical Instrument and Imaging System

The implementation of IoT in surgery has the potential to revolutionize healthcare by enhancing surgical procedures, improving patient outcomes, and optimizing resource utilization. There are some IoT is being implemented in surgery:

- Smart Surgical Instruments.
- Remote Monitoring and Telemedicine.
- Surgical Workflow Optimization.
- Asset and Inventory Management.
- Surgical Training and Simulation.
- Data Analytics and Decision Support.

It is important to note that the implementation of IoT in surgery requires robust security measures to protect patient privacy and prevent unauthorized access to sensitive data. Additionally, healthcare professionals must be trained to effectively utilize IoT technologies and interpret the data they provide.[113]

Overall, IoT has the ability to improve surgical precision, patient monitoring, and operational efficiency, leading to safer surgeries, faster recoveries, and enhanced healthcare delivery.

17.8.2 Application of ML–IoT Integration in Surgical Navigation and Visualization

- It helps in remote monitoring of post-surgery patients using IoT-enabled smart healthcare system, which can provide reliable and effective solutions for patients care and recovery.
- ML and computer vision can also be used in surgical support systems, such as for preoperative preparation, image registration, anatomical classification detection and segmentation, as well as for real-time contextual awareness, skill assessments and training.
- Mixed reality devices and AI-powered robots can also assist surgeons during surgeries, such as by providing natural 3D imaging, virtual surgery intelligence, remote assistance, surgical guidance, and real-time data access.[114]

17.9 DATA SECURITY

17.9.1 Importance of Data Security in ML-IoT-Enabled Surgical Environments

The importance of data security in ML-IoT-enabled surgical environments cannot be overstated. Medical organizations must implement cutting-edge data encryption algorithms and protection techniques to minimize points of vulnerability in their connected device. This includes securing medical IoT devices, such as insulin pumps, pacemakers, and monitoring sensors, to prevent hacking, malware, and ransomware attacks.[115]

The integration of IoT devices into healthcare brings benefits such as improved patient care and real-time information for healthcare professionals, but it also introduces security risks that can impact healthcare providers. Healthcare IoT devices face greater security and privacy challenges due to the sensitive nature of the data they handle, making them targets for cybercriminals. To address these challenges, organizations should implement strategies to enhance the security of healthcare IoT devices, such as continuous discovery, inventory, and tracking of IoT devices, as well as the implantation of strong encryption protocols for data in transit. Additionally, the use of AI and ML technologies can help in processing and analyzing medical reports, further emphasizing the importance of data security in ML–IoT-enabled surgical environments.[116]

17.10 FUTURE PROSPECTIVE

The future emerging technologies in ML and IoT for IGS can be identified as new imaging modalities (develop novel imaging techniques and nanoparticles for improvement interoperative margin assessment), mathematical models for tracking and registration (enhance the mathematical foundations for IGS which can be integrated with IoT) and tissue deformation compensation model.

17.11 CONCLUSION

The manuscript presents an overview of the integration of ML and IoT in IGS systems. It emphasizes the significance of these technologies in enhancing surgical precision, safety, and outcomes across various surgical disciplines. The integration of ML and IoT technologies into IGS systems represents a notable advancement in surgical technology, offering enhanced precision, safety, and outcomes for patients. ML algorithms play a crucial role in enhancing image analysis, predictive analytics for surgical results, and tailoring patient care plans. Meanwhile, IoT tools enable on-the-spot data gathering and surveillance, as well as intelligent surgical tools and distant patient supervision, resulting in more effective and individualized surgical treatments. Integrating ML and IoT technologies in IGS systems has the potential to establish adaptable and smart surgical settings. Medical environments nowadays can use advanced technology to analyze data in real time, which helps in making well-informed decisions and optimizing surgical plans. However, incorporating these technologies comes with its own set of obstacles, like concerns about data security and privacy, as well as the need to ensure data quality and integration for training ML models. In the future, progress in ML and IoT for IGS could involve the creation of new imaging techniques, mathematical models for tracking and registration, and models to address tissue deformation. These new technologies have the potential to enhance surgical outcomes and shape the future of IGS.

REFERENCES

1. Grimson WE, Kikinis R, Jolesz FA, Black PM. Image-guided surgery. *Scientific American*. 1999 Jun 1;280(6):62–9.
2. Yellu RR, Kukalakunta Y, Thunki P. Medical image analysis-challenges and innovations: Studying challenges and innovations in medical image analysis for applications such as diagnosis, treatment planning, and image-guided surgery. *Journal of Artificial Intelligence Research and Applications*. 2024; 4(1): 93-100.
3. Keereweer S, Kerrebijn JD, Van Driel PB, Xie B, Kaijzel EL, Snoeks TJ, Que I, Hutteman M, Van Der Vorst JR, Mieog JS, Vahrmeijer AL. Optical image-guided surgery—where do we stand? *Molecular Imaging and Biology*. 2011 Apr;13:199–207.
4. Wagner A, Ploder O, Enislidis G, Truppe M, Ewers R. Image-guided surgery. *International Journal of Oral and Maxillofacial Surgery*. 1996 Apr 1;25(2):147–51.
5. Maier-Hein L, Vedula SS, Speidel S, Navab N, Kikinis R, Park A, Eisenmann M, Feussner H, Forestier G, Giannarou S, Hashizume M. Surgical data science for next-generation interventions. *Nature Biomedical Engineering*. 2017 Sep;1(9):691–6.
6. Tangsrivimol JA, Schonfeld E, Zhang M, Veeravagu A, Smith TR, Härtl R, Lawton MT, El-Sherbini AH, Prevedello DM, Glicksberg BS, Krittanawong C. Artificial intelligence in neurosurgery: A state-of-the-art review from past to future. *Diagnostics*. 2023 Jul 20;13(14):2429.
7. Peters T, Cleary K, editors. *Image-guided Interventions: Technology and Applications*. Springer Science & Business Media; 2008 May 21.

8. Kenngott HG, Wagner M, Gondan M, Nickel F, Nolden M, Fetzer A, Weitz J, Fischer L, Speidel S, Meinzer HP, Böckler D. Real-time image guidance in laparoscopic liver surgery: First clinical experience with a guidance system based on intraoperative CT imaging. *Surgical Endoscopy*. 2014 Mar;28:933–40.
9. Azagury DE, Dua MM, Barrese JC, Henderson JM, Buchs NC, Ris F, Cloyd JM, Martinie JB, Razzaque S, Nicolau S, Soler L. Image-guided surgery. *Current Problems in Surgery*. 2015 Dec 1;52(12):476–520.
10. Oldendorf WH. The quest for an image of brain: A brief historical and technical review of brain imaging techniques. *Neurology*. 1978 Jun;28(6):517.
11. Lauterbur PC. Image formation by induced local interactions: Examples employing nuclear magnetic resonance. *Nature*. 1973 Mar 16;242(5394):190–1.
12. Kelly PJ, Kall BA, Goerss S, Earnest F. Computer-assisted stereotaxic laser resection of intra-axial brain neoplasms. *Journal of Neurosurgery*. 1986 Mar 1;64(3):427–39.
13. Gleason PL, Kikinis R, Altobelli D, Wells W, Alexander III E, Black PM, Jolesz F. Video registration virtual reality for nonlinkage stereotactic surgery. *Stereotactic and Functional Neurosurgery*. 1994 Apr 11;63(1–4):139–43.
14. Jolesz FA, Shtern F. The operating room of the future: Report of the national cancer institute workshop, "Imaging-Guided Stereotactic Tumor Diagnosis and Treatment". *Investigative Radiology*. 1992 Apr 1;27(4):326–8.
15. Camara M, Mayer E, Darzi A, Pratt P. Augmented reality and robotic surgery. *Surgical Innovation*. 2010;17(3):256–63.
16. Sutherland JV, Wilson JR, Williams RM. Advances in image-guided urologic surgery. *Journal of Endourology*. 2013;27(4):395–403.
17. Germano IM. Advanced techniques in image-guided brain and spine surgery. (No Title). 2002 May.
18. Nolte LP, Slomczykowski MA, Berlemann U, Strauss MJ, Hofstetter R, Schlenzka D, Laine T, Lund T. A new approach to computer-aided spine surgery: Fluoroscopy-based surgical navigation. *European Spine Journal*. 2000;9(Suppl 1):S78–88.
19. Metson RB, Cosenza MJ, Cunningham MJ, Randolph GW. Physician experience with an optical image guidance system for sinus surgery. *The Laryngoscope*. 2000 Jun;110(6):972–6.
20. Cleary K, Peters TM. Image-guided interventions: Technology review and clinical applications. *Annual Review of Biomedical Engineering*. 2010 Aug 15;12:119–42.
21. Peters TM. Image-guidance for surgical procedures. *Physics in Medicine & Biology*. 2006 Jun 23;51(14):R505.
22. Esteva A, Kuprel B, Novoa RA, Ko J, Swetter SM, Blau HM, Thrun S. Dermatologist-level classification of skin cancer with deep neural networks. *Nature*. 2017;542(7639):115–18.
23. Ronneberger O, Fischer P, Brox T. U-net: Convolutional networks for biomedical image segmentation. In *Medical Image Computing and Computer-Assisted Intervention–MICCAI 2015: 18th International Conference, Munich, Germany, October 5–9, 2015, Proceedings, Part* III (pp. 234–41). Springer International Publishing; 2015.
24. Haskins G, Kruger U, Yan P. Deep learning in medical image registration: A survey. *Machine Vision and Applications*. 2020 Feb;31:1–8.
25. Wang G, Ye JC, Mueller K, Fessler JA. Image reconstruction is a new frontier of machine learning. *IEEE Transactions on Medical Imaging*. 2018 May 15;37(6):1289–96.
26. Obermeyer Z, Emanuel EJ. Predicting the future—big data, machine learning, and clinical medicine. *The New England Journal of Medicine. 2016* Sep 9;375(13):1216.
27. Friedman J, Hastie T, Tibshirani R. *The Elements of Statistical Learning*. Springer series in statistics new. Springer; 2022.
28. Han J, Pei J, Tong H. *Data Mining: Concepts and Techniques*. Morgan Kaufmann; 2022 Jul 2.
29. Cortes C, Vapnik V. Support-vector networks. *Machine Learning*. 1995 Sep;20:273–97.

30. Pedregosa F, Varoquaux G, Gramfort A, Michel V, Thirion B, Grisel O, Blondel M, Prettenhofer P, Weiss R, Dubourg V, Vanderplas J. Scikit-learn: Machine learning in Python. *The Journal of Machine Learning Research*. 2011 Nov 1;12:2825–30.
31. Breiman L. Random forests. *Machine Learning. 2001* Oct;45:5–32.
32. Rokach L. A survey of clustering algorithms. *Data Mining and Knowledge Discovery Handbook*. 2010:269–98.
33. Malegori C, Oliveri P. Principal component analysis. In *Hyperspectral Imaging Analysis and Applications for Food Quality* (pp. 85–107). CRC Press; 2018 Nov 16.
34. Zhu X, Goldberg AB. *Introduction to Semi-supervised Learning*. Springer Nature; 2022 May 31.
35. Watkins CJ, Dayan P. Q-learning. *Machine Learning*. 1992 May;8:279–92.
36. Kaelbling LP, Littman ML, Moore AW. Reinforcement learning: A survey. *Journal of Artificial Intelligence Research*. 1996 May 1;4:237–85.
37. LeCun Y, Bengio Y, Hinton G. Deep learning. *Nature*. 2015 May 28;521(7553):436–44.
38. Hochreiter S, Schmidhuber J. Long short-term memory. *Neural Computation*. 1997 Nov 15;9(8):1735–80.
39. Gulshan V, Peng L, Coram M, Stumpe MC, Wu D, Narayanaswamy A, Venugopalan S, Widner K, Madams T, Cuadros J, Kim R. Development and validation of a deep learning algorithm for detection of diabetic retinopathy in retinal fundus photographs. *JAMA*. 2016 Dec 13;316(22):2402–10.
40. Wang S, Su Z, Ying L, Peng X, Zhu S, Liang F, Feng D, Liang D. Accelerating magnetic resonance imaging via deep learning. In *2016 IEEE 13th international symposium on biomedical imaging (ISBI)* (pp. 514–17). IEEE; 2016 Apr 13.
41. Ardila D, Kiraly AP, Bharadwaj S, Choi B, Reicher JJ, Peng L, Tse D, Etemadi M, Ye W, Corrado G, Naidich DP. End-to-end lung cancer screening with three-dimensional deep learning on low-dose chest computed tomography. *Nature Medicine*. 2019 Jun;25(6):954–61.
42. Istepanian RS, Jovanov E, Zhang YT. Guest editorial introduction to the special section on m-health: Beyond seamless mobility and global wireless health-care connectivity. *IEEE Transactions on Information Technology in Biomedicine. 2004* Nov 30;8(4):405–14.
43. Pietrabissa A, Marconi S, Negrello E, Mauri V, Peri A, Pugliese L, Marone EM, Auricchio F. An overview on 3D printing for abdominal surgery. *Surgical Endoscopy. 2020* Jan;34:1–3.
44. Swan M. Sensor mania! the internet of things, wearable computing, objective metrics, and the quantified self 2.0. *Journal of Sensor and Actuator Networks*. 2012 Nov 8;1(3):217–53.
45. Keesara S, Jonas A, Schulman K. Covid-19 and health care's digital revolution. *New England Journal of Medicine*. 2020 Jun 4;382(23):e82.
46. Tavares J, Oliveira T. Electronic health record patient portal adoption by health care consumers: An acceptance model and survey. *Journal of Medical Internet Research*. 2016 Mar 2;18(3):e5069.
47. Alwashmi MF. The use of digital health in the detection and management of COVID-19. *International Journal of Environmental Research and Public Health*. 2020 Apr;17(8):2906.
48. Okamura AM, Simone C, O'leary MD. Force modeling for needle insertion into soft tissue. *IEEE Transactions on Biomedical Engineering*. 2004 Sep 27;51(10):1707–16.
49. Zulbaran-Rojas A, Najafi B, Arita N, Rahemi H, Razjouyan J, Gilani R. Utilization of flexible-wearable sensors to describe the kinematics of surgical proficiency. *Journal of Surgical Research*. 2021 Jun 1;262:149–58.
50. Macario A. What does one minute of operating room time cost? *Journal of Clinical Anesthesia*. 2010;4(22):233–6.
51. Camarillo DB, Krummel TM, Salisbury Jr JK. Robotic technology in surgery: Past, present, and future. *The American Journal of Surgery*. 2004 Oct 1;188(4):2–15.

52. Senders JT, Staples PC, Karhade AV, Zaki MM, Gormley WB, Broekman ML, Smith TR, Arnaout O. Machine learning and neurosurgical outcome prediction: A systematic review. *World Neurosurgery*. 2018 Jan 1;109:476–86.
53. Majmudar MD, Colucci LA, Landman AB. The quantified patient of the future: Opportunities and challenges. In *Healthcare* (Vol. 3, No. 3, pp. 153–56). Elsevier; 2015 Sep 1.
54. Shen D, Wu G, Suk HI. Deep learning in medical image analysis. *Annual Review of Biomedical Engineering*. 2017 Jun 21;19:221–48.
55. Litjens G, Kooi T, Bejnordi BE, Setio AA, Ciompi F, Ghafoorian M, Van Der Laak JA, Van Ginneken B, Sánchez CI. A survey on deep learning in medical image analysis. *Medical Image Analysis*. 2017 Dec 1;42:60–88.
56. Esteva A, Robicquet A, Ramsundar B, Kuleshov V, DePristo M, Chou K, Cui C, Corrado G, Thrun S, Dean J. A guide to deep learning in healthcare. *Nature Medicine*. 2019 Jan;25(1):24–9.
57. Hung AJ, Chen J, Gill IS. Automated performance metrics and machine learning algorithms to measure surgeon performance and anticipate clinical outcomes in robotic surgery. *JAMA Surgery*. 2018 Aug 1;153(8):770–1.
58. Nagendran M, Chen Y, Lovejoy CA, Gordon AC, Komorowski M, Harvey H, Topol EJ, Ioannidis JP, Collins GS, Maruthappu M. Artificial intelligence versus clinicians: Systematic review of design, reporting standards, and claims of deep learning studies. *BMJ*. 2020 Mar 25;368.
59. Vedula SS, Ishii M, Hager GD. Objective assessment of surgical technical skill and competency in the operating room. *Annual Review of Biomedical Engineering. 2017* Jun 21;19:301–25.
60. Miao S, Wang ZJ, Liao R. A CNN regression approach for real-time 2D/3D registration. *IEEE Transactions on Medical Imaging. 2016* Jan 26;35(5):1352–63.
61. Hashimoto DA, Rosman G, Rus D, Meireles OR. Artificial intelligence in surgery: Promises and perils. *Annals of Surgery. 2018* Jul;268(1):70.
62. Bernhardt S, Nicolau SA, Soler L, Doignon C. The status of augmented reality in laparoscopic surgery as of 2016. *Medical Image Analysis. 2017* Apr 1;37:66–90.
63. Aksamentov I, Twinanda AP, Mutter D, Marescaux J, Padoy N. Deep neural networks predict remaining surgery duration from cholecystectomy videos. In *Medical Image Computing and Computer-Assisted Intervention– MICCAI 2017: 20th International Conference, Quebec City, QC, Canada, September 11–13, 2017, Proceedings, Part II* (pp. 586–93). Springer International Publishing; 2017.
64. Hao Y, Helo P. The role of wearable devices in meeting the needs of cloud manufacturing: A case study. *Robotics and Computer-Integrated Manufacturing*. 2017 Jun 1;45:168–79.
65. Rahman MS, Peeri NC, Shrestha N, Zaki R, Haque U, Ab Hamid SH. Defending against the Novel Coronavirus (COVID-19) outbreak: How can the Internet of Things (IoT) help to save the world? *Health Policy and Technology*. 2020 Jun;9(2):136.
66. Albahri AS, Hamid RA, Alwan JK, Al-Qays ZT, Zaidan AA, Zaidan BB, Albahri AO, AlAmoodi AH, Khlaf JM, Almahdi EM, Thabet E. Role of biological data mining and machine learning techniques in detecting and diagnosing the novel coronavirus (COVID-19): A systematic review. *Journal of Medical Systems*. 2020 Jul;44:200–215.
67. Bharadwaj HK, Agarwal A, Chamola V, Lakkaniga NR, Hassija V, Guizani M, Sikdar B. A review on the role of machine learning in enabling IoT based healthcare applications. *IEEE Access*. 2021 Feb 16;9:38859–90.
68. Romeo L, Petitti A, Marani R, Milella A. Internet of robotic things in smart domains: Applications and challenges. *Sensors*. 2020 Jun 12;20(12):3355.
69. Majumder S, Mondal T, Deen MJ. Wearable sensors for remote health monitoring. *Sensors*. 2017 Jan 12;17(1):130.

70. Giggins OM, Sweeney KT, Caulfield B. Rehabilitation exercise assessment using inertial sensors: A cross-sectional analytical study. *Journal of Neuroengineering and Rehabilitation. 2014* Dec;11(1):1–0.
71. Alsubaei F, Abuhussein A, Shiva S. Security and privacy in the internet of medical things: Taxonomy and risk assessment. In *2017 IEEE 42nd Conference on Local Computer Networks Workshops (LCN Workshops)* (pp. 112–20). IEEE; 2017 Oct 9.
72. Mehrabi N, Morstatter F, Saxena N, Lerman K, Galstyan A. A survey on bias and fairness in machine learning. *ACM Computing Surveys (CSUR)*. 2021 Jul 13;54(6): 1–35.
73. Abomhara M, Køien GM. Security and privacy in the Internet of Things: Current status and open issues. In *2014 International Conference on Privacy and Security in Mobile Systems (PRISMS)* (pp. 1–8). IEEE; 2014 May 11.
74. Luxton DD. Artificial intelligence in psychological practice: Current and future applications and implications. *Professional Psychology: Research and Practice*. 2014 Oct;45(5):332.
75. Uchida S. Image processing and recognition for biological images. *Development, Growth & Differentiation*. 2013 May;55(4):523–49.
76. Lin Z, Lei C, Yang L. Modern image-guided surgery: A narrative review of medical image processing and visualization. *Sensors*. 2023 Dec 16;23(24):9872.
77. Otsu N. A threshold selection method from gray-level histograms. *IEEE Transactions on Systems, Man, and Cybernetics*. 1979 Jan;9(1):62–6.
78. Adams R, Bischof L. Seeded region growing. *IEEE Transactions on Pattern Analysis and Machine Intelligence*. 1994 Jun;16(6):641–7.
79. Canny J. A computational approach to edge detection. *IEEE Transactions on Pattern Analysis and Machine Intelligence*. 1986 Nov(6):679–98.
80. Meyer F. Topographic distance and watershed lines. *Signal Processing*. 1994 Jul 1;38(1):113–25.
81. MacQueen J. Some methods for classification and analysis of multivariate observations. In *Proceedings of the Fifth Berkeley Symposium on Mathematical Statistics and Probability* (Vol. 1, No. 14, pp. 281–97). IEEE; 1967 Jun 21.
82. Bezdek JC, Ehrlich R, Full W. FCM: The fuzzy c-means clustering algorithm. *Computers & Geosciences. 1984* Jan 1;10(2–3):191–203.
83. Haralick RM, Shanmugam K, Dinstein IH. Textural features for image classification. *IEEE Transactions on Systems, Man, and Cybernetics*. 1973 Nov(6):610–21.
84. Ojala T, Pietikainen M, Maenpaa T. Multiresolution gray-scale and rotation invariant texture classification with local binary patterns. *IEEE Transactions on Pattern Analysis and Machine Intelligence*. 2002 Jul;24(7):971–87.
85. Simonyan K, Zisserman A. Very deep convolutional networks for large-scale image recognition. *arXiv preprint* arXiv:1409.1556. 2014 Sep 4.
86. He K, Zhang X, Ren S, Sun J. Deep residual learning for image recognition. In *Proceedings of the IEEE Conference on Computer Vision and Pattern Recognition* (pp. 770–78). IEEE; 2016.
87. Rojas R. *Neural Networks: A Systematic Introduction*. Springer Science & Business Media; 2013 Jun 29.
88. Krizhevsky A, Sutskever I, Hinton GE. Imagenet classification with deep convolutional neural networks. *Advances in Neural Information Processing Systems*. 2012;25.
89. LeCun Y, Bengio Y, Hinton G. Deep learning. *Nature*. 2015 May 28;521(7553):436–44.
90. Goodfellow I, Bengio Y, Courville A, Bengio Y. *Deep Learning* (Vol. 1). Springer; 2022.
91. LeCun Y, Bottou L, Bengio Y, Haffner P. Gradient-based learning applied to document recognition. *Proceedings of the IEEE*. 1998 Nov;86(11):2278–324.
92. Girshick R, Donahue J, Darrell T, Malik J. Rich feature hierarchies for accurate object detection and semantic segmentation. In *Proceedings of the IEEE Conference on Computer Vision and Pattern Recognition* (pp. 580–87). Springer; 2014.

93. Girshick R. Fast R-CNN. In *Proceedings of the IEEE International Conference on Computer Vision* (pp. 1440–48). Springer; 2015.
94. Ren S, He K, Girshick R, Sun J. Faster R-CNN: Towards real-time object detection with region proposal networks. *Advances in Neural Information Processing Systems*. 2015;28.
95. Liu W, Anguelov D, Erhan D, Szegedy C, Reed S, Fu CY, Berg AC. SSD: Single shot multibox detector. In *Computer Vision–ECCV 2016: 14th European Conference, Amsterdam, The Netherlands, October 11–14, 2016, Proceedings, Part I* (pp. 21–37). Springer International Publishing; 2016
96. Redmon J, Divvala S, Girshick R, Farhadi A. You only look once: Unified, real-time object detection. In *Proceedings of the IEEE Conference on Computer Vision and Pattern Recognition* (pp. 779–88). Springer; 2016.
97. Urban G, Tripathi P, Alkayali T, Mittal M, Jalali F, Karnes W, Baldi P. Deep learning localizes and identifies polyps in real time with 96% accuracy in screening colonoscopy. *Gastroenterology*. 2018;155(4):1069–78.e8.
98. Twinanda AP, Shehata S, Mutter D, Marescaux J, De Mathelin M, Padoy N. EndoNet: A deep architecture for recognition tasks on laparoscopic videos. *IEEE Transactions on Medical Imaging*. 2017;36(1):86–97.
99. Zia A, Essa I. Automated analysis of surgical skills using frequency analysis. *International Journal of Computer Assisted Radiology and Surgery*. 2018;13(6):731–9.
100. Bulten W, Pinckaers H, van Boven H, Vink R, de Bel T, van Ginneken B,. . Litjens G. Automated deep-learning system for Gleason grading of prostate cancer using biopsies: A diagnostic study. *The Lancet Oncology*. 2020;21(2):233–41.
101. Rajpurkar P, Hannun AY, Haghpanahi M, Tison GH, Bourn C, Turakhia MP, Ng AY. Cardiologist-level arrhythmia detection and classification in ambulatory electrocardiograms using a deep neural network. *Nature Medicine*. 2017;25(1):65–69.
102. Chen J, Jin W, Zhang XX, Xu W, Liu XN, Ren CC. Prediction of functional outcome in acute ischemic stroke patients using machine learning. *Medical Science Monitor*. 2017;23:5829–38.
103. de Groof AJ, Struyvenberg MR, van der Putten J, van der Sommen F, Fockens KN, Curvers WL, . . . Bergman JJ. Deep-learning system detects neoplasia in patients with Barrett's esophagus with higher accuracy than endoscopists in a multi-step training and validation study with benchmarking. *Gastroenterology*. 2019;158(4):915–29.e4.
104. Setio AAA, Traverso A, de Bel T, Berens MSN, van den Bogaard C, Cerello P,. . .van Ginneken B. Validation, comparison, and combination of algorithms for automatic detection of pulmonary nodules in computed tomography images: The LUNA16 challenge. *Medical Image Analysis*. 2017;42:1–13.
105. Yasaka K, Akai H, Abe O, Kiryu S. Deep learning with convolutional neural network for differentiation of liver masses at dynamic contrast-enhanced CT: A preliminary study. *Radiology*. 2018;286(3):887–96.
106. Desai SN, Shetty A, Nasa P, Chaudhuri S, Srivastava S. Predictive modeling for diabetic patient readmission: Development and implementation of a machine learning approach. *Applied Sciences*. 2019;9(18):3818.
107. Cummins N, Scherer S, Krajewski J, Schnieder S, Epps J, Quatieri TF. A review of depression and suicide risk assessment using speech analysis. *Speech Communication*. 2015;71:10–49.
108. Solanki SL, Pandrowala S, Nayak A, Bhandare M, Ambulkar RP, Shrikhande SV. Artificial intelligence in perioperative management of major gastrointestinal surgeries. *World Journal of Gastroenterology. 2021 Jun 6;27(21):2758.*
109. Marcelo Augusto Fontenelle Ribeiro J, Smaniotto R, Gebran A, Zamudio JP, Mohseni S, da Silva Rodrigues JM, Kaafarani H. The use of POTTER (Predictive Optimal Trees in Emergency Surgery Risk) calculator to predict mortality and complications in patients submitted to Emergency Surgery. *Revista do Colégio Brasileiro de Cirurgiões*. 2023;50.

110. Chiew CJ, Liu N, Wong TH, Sim YE, Abdullah HR. Utilizing machine learning methods for preoperative prediction of postsurgical mortality and intensive care unit admission. *Annals of Surgery. 2020 Dec;272(6):1133.*
111. Neal ML, Kerckhoffs R. Current progress in patient-specific modeling. *Briefings in Bioinformatics*. 2010 Jan 1;11(1):111–26.
112. Park JJ, Tiefenbach J, Demetriades AK. The role of artificial intelligence in surgical simulation. *Frontiers in Medical Technology*. 2022 Dec 14;4:1076755.
113. Huang X, Liu X, Zhu B, Hou X, Hai B, Yu D, Zheng W, Li R, Pan J, Yao Y, Dai Z. Augmented reality surgical navigation in minimally invasive spine surgery: A preclinical study. *Bioengineering*. 2023 Sep 18;10(9):1094.
114. Alsareii SA, Raza M, Alamri AM, AlAsmari MY, Irfan M, Khan U, Awais M. Machine learning and internet of things enabled monitoring of post-surgery patients: A pilot study. *Sensors*. 2022 Feb 12;22(4):1420.
115. Nomikos K, Papadimitriou A, Stergiopoulos G, Koutras D, Psarakis M, Kotzanikolaou P. On a security-oriented design framework for medical IoT devices: The hardware security perspective. In *2020 23rd Euromicro Conference on Digital System Design (DSD)* (pp. 301–8). IEEE; 2020 Aug 26.
116. Pradhan B, Bhattacharyya S, Pal K. IoT-based applications in healthcare devices. *Journal of Healthcare Engineering*. 2021 Mar 18;2021:1–8.

Index

FSC
www.fsc.org
MIX
Papier | Fördert gute Waldnutzung
FSC® C083411

Kolibri 360 GmbH
Ferdinand-Jühlke-Straße 7
99095 Erfurt, Deutschland
produktsicherheit@kolibri360.de